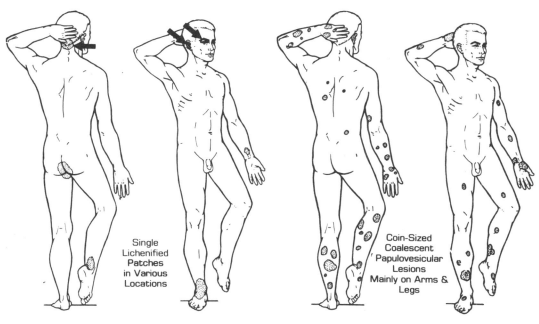

NEURODERMATITIS

Single Lichenified Patches in Various Locations

NUMMULAR ECZEMA

Coin-Sized Coalescent Papulovesicular Lesions Mainly on Arms & Legs

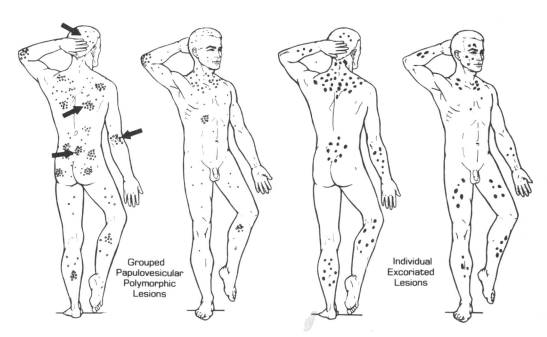

DERMATITIS HERPETIFORMIS

Grouped Papulovesicular Polymorphic Lesions

NEUROTIC EXCORIATIONS

Individual Excoriated Lesions

MANUAL
SKIN D

SAUER, G.C.

6e

90-978

SIXTH EDITION

MANUAL OF SKIN DISEASES

GORDON C. SAUER, M.D.

Clinical Professor of Medicine (Dermatology)
University of Kansas Medical Center
Kansas City, Kansas

Clinical Professor of Medicine
School of Medicine
University of Missouri-Kansas City
Kansas City, Missouri

J.B. LIPPINCOTT COMPANY
Philadelphia

Grand Rapids • New York • St. Louis • San Francisco
London • Sydney • Tokyo

Acquisitions Editor: Darlene Barela Cooke
Developmental Editor: Delois Patterson
Project Editor: Tom Gibbons
Indexer: Mary Rose Muccie
Designer: Doug Smock
Production Manager: Caren Erlichman
Production Coordinator: Kevin P. Johnson
Compositor: Bi-Comp, Inc.
Printer/Binder: R.R. Donnelly & Sons Company

6th Edition

6 5 4 3 2 1

Library of Congress Cataloging-in-Publication Data

Sauer, Gordon C. (Gordon Chenoweth), 1921–
      Manual of skin diseases / Gordon C. Sauer.—6th ed.
            p.   cm.
      Includes bibliographical references.
      ISBN 0-397-51056-X : $49.95
      1. Skin—Diseases—Handbooks, manuals, etc. I. Title.
      [DNLM: 1. Skin Diseases.   WR 140 S255m]
   RL74.S25 1990
   616.5—dc20
   DNLM/DLC
   for Library of Congress   90-5660
                                                          CIP

The authors and publisher have exerted every effort to ensure that drug selection and dosage set forth in this text are in accord with current recommendations and practice at the time of publication. However, in view of ongoing research, changes in government regulations, and the constant flow of information relating to drug therapy and drug reactions, the reader is urged to check the package insert for each drug for any change in indications and dosage and for added warnings and precautions. This is particularly important when the recommended agent is a new or infrequently employed drug.

Dedicated to my grandchildren,
Jennifer, Gordon III, Adam, Michael, Rebecca, and Brian

PREFACE

The way to keep up with the latest in medicine, some say, is to keep up with the current medical journals. Medical books, they say, are out-of-date before they are published. Nonsense. A book on medicine enables you to hold in your hand the condensed compilation of hundreds of journals. You get the author's opinion, as an author and an editor, of the value or nonvalue of the material presented in journals. Diseases don't change, and the management of a patient doesn't change. The color photographs of skin pathology are timeless. These are the advantages of a book. In this dermatology manual you will also be exposed to the author's personal management of patients and skin diseases. Hopefully and humbly I assume my experience has value.

A series of "Sauer Notes" have appeared for several years in the monthly *Schock Letter*, published by the American Academy of Dermatology. The medical editors at J. B. Lippincott thought that the inclusion of similar personal "Sauer Notes" in this sixth edition would enhance the teaching value of this manual.

Dramatic advances in medical therapy are rare. Much "new" therapy is a modification, hopefully an improvement, of existing therapy. Some of the "new" therapy is only beneficial for rarer diseases. The discovery of an agent that can benefit a multitude of patients occurs infrequently, unfortunately. These precious medicines for dermatology, in my lifetime, were sulfonamide, penicillin, undecylenic acid, cortisone, aminopterin, griseofulvin, methoxypsoralen, acyclovir, ketoconazole, isotretinoin, and a few others. The modifications of these drugs have proliferated.

This *Manual of Skin Diseases* has satisfied a need for an intermediate-type book in the field of dermatology. The American, British, and Spanish editions of the book have apparently been purchased by more persons and institutions than any other similar text. This book is not a *brief* outline of dermatology or a *major* compendium. But few dermatoses are left out, even if they are only defined in the Dictionary-Index. Rather uniquely, the first edition in 1959 contained 28 color plates interspersed throughout the text. There are now 102 color plates, which contain 453 individual color photographs. The first edition had dermatologic "silhouettes" to aid in diagnosis, a chapter on geographic skin diseases, and a quite complete Dictionary-Index.

In the past five years since the fifth edition was published, there have been considerable advances in diagnosis, etiology, and therapy of several important groups of diseases, most obviously in the viral and immunologic field. The entire book has been reset to encompass the numerous changes, additions, and deletions in the enlarging field of dermatology.

Many more bibliographical references have been added. Old ones have been updated. A very complete filing system under chapter headings has enabled me, since the last edition was published, to pull out the important article and book references that have delineated the changes and advances in dermatology over this five-year period.

There is a new chapter on cutaneous diseases associated with HIV infection written by Drs. M. Joyce Rico and Neil S. Prose. The chapter on fundamentals of cutaneous surgery has been revised by Dr. Frank Koranda, on cosmetics for the dermatologist by Dr. Earle Brauer, on immunology by Drs. David Norris and Walter Burgdorf, and on photosensitivity by Dr. James Kalivas. Dr. Walter Burgdorf also revised the chapter on genodermatoses, and Dr. Thelda Kestenbaum revised the chapters on diseases affecting the hair and diseases affecting the nails.

The chapters on pediatric and geriatric dermatology really tie together many scattered references in the book, as they relate to both ends of our biologic age spectrum.

The Dictionary-Index has been carefully edited and expanded to keep up with the proliferation of new diseases and new ideas.

Read, learn, and profit.

Gordon C. Sauer, M.D.

PREFACE TO THE FIRST EDITION (ABRIDGED)

Approximately 15 per cent of all patients who walk into the general practitioner's office do so for care of some skin disease or skin lesion. It may be for such a simple treatment as the removal of a wart, for the treatment of athlete's foot or for something as complicated as severe cystic acne. There have been so many recent advances in the various fields of medicine that the medical school instructor can expect his students to learn and retain only a small percentage of the material that is taught them. I believe that the courses in all phases of medicine, and particularly the courses of the various specialties, should be made as simple, basic and concise as possible. If the student retains only a small percentage of what is presented to him, he will be able to handle an amazing number of his walk-in patients. I am presenting in this book only the material that medical students and general practitioners must know for the diagnosis and the treatment of patients with the common skin diseases. In condensing the material many generalities are stated, and the reader must remember that there are exceptions to every rule. The inclusion of these exceptions would defeat the intended purpose of this book. More

complicated diagnostic procedures or treatments for interesting or problem cases are merely frosting on the cake. This information can be obtained by the interested student from any of several more comprehensive dermatologic texts.

This book consists of two distinct but complementary parts.

The first part contains the chapters devoted to the diagnosis and the management of the important common skin diseases. In discussing the common skin diseases, a short introductory sentence is followed by a listing of the salient points of each disease in outline form. All diseases of the skin have primary lesions, secondary lesions, a rather specific distribution, a general course which includes the prognosis and the recurrence rate of the disease, varying subjective complaints and a known or unknown cause. Where indicated, a statement follows concerning seasonal incidence, age groups affected, family and sex incidence, contagiousness or infectiousness, relationship to employment and laboratory findings. The discussion ends with a paragraph on differential diagnosis and treatment. Treatment, to be effective, has to be thought of as a chain of events. The therapy outlined on the first visit is usually different from that given on subsequent visits or for cases that are very severe. The treatment is discussed with these variations in mind. The first part of the book concludes with a chapter on basic equipment necessary for managing dermatologic patients.

The second part consists of a very complete dictionary-index to the entire field of dermatology, defining the majority of rare diseases and the unusual dermatologic terms. The inclusion of this dictionary-index has a twofold purpose. First, it enables me to present a concise first section on *common* skin diseases unencumbered by the inclusion of the rare diseases. Second, the dictionary-index provides a rather complete coverage of all of dermatology for the more interested student. In reality, two books are contained in one.

Dermatologic nomenclature has always been a bugaboo for the new student. I heartily agree with many dermatologists that we should simplify the terminology, and that has been attempted in this text. Some of the changes are mine, but many have been suggested by others. However, after a diligent effort to simplify the names of skin diseases, one is left with the appalling fact that some of the complicated terms defy change. One of the main reasons for this is that all of our field, the skin, is visible to the naked eye. As a result, any minor alteration from normal has been scrutinized by countless physicians through the years and given countless names. The liver or heart counterpart of folliculitis ulerythematosa reticulata (ulerythema acneiforme, atrophoderma reticulatum symmetricum faciei, atrophodermie vermiculée) is yet to be discovered.

What I am presenting in this book is not specialty dermatology but general practice dermatology. Some of my medical educator friends say that only internal medicine, pediatrics and obstetrics should be taught to medical students. They state that the specialized fields of medicine should be taught only at the internship, residency or postgraduate level. That idea misses the very important fact that cases from all of the so-called specialty fields wander in to the general practitioner's office. The general practitioner must have some *basic* knowledge of the varied aspects of all of medicine so that he can properly take care of his general everyday practice. This basic knowledge must be taught in the undergraduate years. The purpose of this book is to complement such teaching.

Gordon C. Sauer, M.D.

ACKNOWLEDGMENTS

For the most realistic presentation of skin diseases, color photography is essential. However, the cost of color reproduction is so great that it is almost impossible to enjoy the advantages of color plates and still keep the price of the book within the range where it will have the broadest appeal. This problem has been solved for the six editions of this book through the generosity of several pharmaceutical companies which contributed the cost of the color plates credited to them.

For this sixth edition the following drug companies contributed money for additional new color plates:

Burroughs Wellcome Company
Glaxo Dermatology (in part)
Hoechst-Roussel Pharmaceuticals Inc.
Neutrogena Skin Care Institute
Ortho Pharmaceutical Corporation
Owen/Galderma
Sandoz Pharmaceuticals, Inc.
Schering Corporation

While the great majority of photographs are from my own private collection, I gratefully acknowledge assistance from the several photographers at the University of Kansas School of Medicine under the direction of Burton Johnson. Several black and white photographs were provided by Larry Brown, Research Medical Center, Kansas City, Mo. The line drawings were done by Jo Ann Clifford, and those for Chapter 7 by Diane Koranda. The physician or institution that furnished illustration material is acknowledged with appreciation under the respective picture.

Drs. M. Joyce Rico and Neil Prose of Duke University have written a chapter on cutaneous diseases associated with HIV infection. They also supplied twelve color photographs for the two color plates in this chapter. Their contribution is greatly appreciated.

Chapters have been rewritten for this sixth edition by Dr. Frank Koranda (Fundamentals of Cutaneous Surgery), Dr. Earle W. Brauer (Cosmetics), Drs. David Norris and Walter Burgdorf (Immunology), and Dr. James Kalivas (Photosensitivity). My profound thanks again to them.

Dr. Thelda Kestenbaum revised the chapters on diseases of the hair and the nails. Dr. Walter Burgdorf revised my chapter on genodermatoses. Their labor and input is appreciated.

Mr. Robert Courtney, R.Ph., answered my questions on pharmaceuticals, and Mr. Gerald Kruse of the Research Medical Center Library assisted with library references. My thanks to them.

Mrs. Barbara Philbrook entered on the word processor the many changes that were necessary for this sixth edition. I am very grateful. The assistance of Mrs. Linda Hammons is also appreciated.

Editorial comments, encouragement and patience have been kindly provided by my wife, Marion.

In the five previous editions further acknowledgements were made, but it would be redundant to repeat them here. Finally, a great deal of credit again goes to the Medical Department of J. B. Lippincott Co., especially to Darlene Cooke, Delois Patterson, and Tom Gibbons. The book and I profited by our association with them.

CONTENTS

LIST OF COLOR PLATES

MANUAL OF
SKIN DISEASES

1

Structure of the Skin

The skin is the largest organ of the human body. It is composed of tissue that grows, differentiates, and renews itself constantly. Since the skin is a barrier between the internal organs and the external environment, it is uniquely subjected to noxious external agents and is also a sensitive reflection of internal disease. An understanding of the cause and the effect of this complex interplay in the skin begins with a thorough understanding of the basic structure of this organ.

LAYERS OF THE SKIN

The skin is divided into three rather distinct layers. From inside out, they are the subcutaneous tissue, the dermis, and the epidermis (Fig. 1–1).

SUBCUTANEOUS TISSUE. The subcutaneous tissue serves as a receptacle for the formation and the storage of fat, is a locus of highly dynamic lipid metabolism, and supports the blood vessels and the nerves that pass from the tissues beneath to the dermis above. The deeper hair follicles and the sweat glands originate in this layer.

DERMIS (CORIUM). The dermis is made up of connective tissue, cellular elements, and ground substance. It has a rich blood and nerve supply. The sebaceous glands and the shorter hair follicles originate in the dermis. Anatomically, the corium can be divided into papillary (upper) and reticular (lower) layers.

The *connective tissue* consists of collagen fibers, elastic fibers, and reticular fibers. All of these, but most importantly the collagen fibers, contribute to the support and elasticity of the skin.

The collagenous fibers are made up of eosinophilic acellular proteins responsible for nearly a fourth of a human's overall protein mass. Under the electron microscope the fibers are seen to be composed of thin, nonbranching fibrils held together by a cementing ground substance. These fibrils are composed of covalently cross-linked and overlapping units called *tropocollagen* molecules. When tannic acid or the salts of heavy metals, such as dichromates, are combined with collagen, the result is leather.

Elastic fibers are thinner than most collagen fibers and are entwined among them. They are composed of the protein elastin. Elastic fibers do not readily take up acid or basic stains such as hematoxylin and eosin, but they can be stained with Verhoeff's stain.

Reticular fibers are believed to be immature collagen fibers, since their physical and chemical properties are similar. They can be stained with silver (Foot's stain). Reticulum fibers are sparse in normal skin but are abundant in certain pathologic conditions of the skin such as the *granulomas* of tuberculosis, syphilis, and sarcoidosis and in the *mesodermal tumors* such as histiocytomas, sarcomas, and lymphomas.

The *cellular elements* of the dermis consist of three groups of mesodermal cells: (1) a reticulohistiocytic group, (2) a myeloid group, and (3) a lymphoid group. Under pathologic conditions, the potentiality of these cells can change.

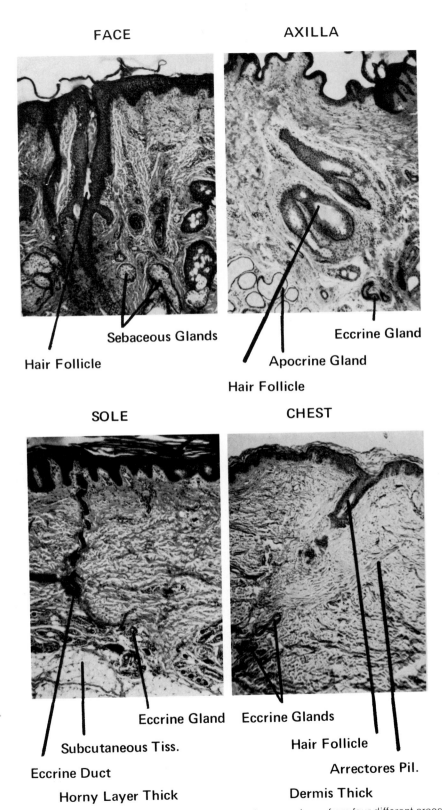

FACE

AXILLA

Sebaceous Glands

Hair Follicle

Eccrine Gland

Apocrine Gland

Hair Follicle

SOLE

CHEST

Eccrine Gland

Subcutaneous Tiss.

Eccrine Duct

Horny Layer Thick

Eccrine Glands

Hair Follicle

Arrectores Pil.

Dermis Thick

Figure 1–1. **Histology of the skin.** Microscopic sections are shown from four different areas of the body. Note the variations in the histologic features, such as the thickness of the horny layer and the presence or absence of the three types of glands and the hair follicles. These photographs were taken at the same magnification. (*Dr. D. Gibson*)

The reticulohistiocytic group consists of fibroblasts, histiocytes, and mast cells. Immature cells of the reticulohistiocytic group are known as reticulum cells.

Fibroblasts form collagen fibers and may be the progenitors of all other connective tissue cells.

Histiocytes normally are present in small numbers around blood vessels, but in pathologic conditions they can migrate in the dermis as *tissue monocytes*. They can also form abundant reticulum fibers. When they phagocytize bacteria and particulate matter, they are known as *macrophages*. Histiocytes, under special pathologic conditions, can also change into epithelioid cells, which in turn can develop into so-called giant cells.

Mast cells are also histiocytic cells. Mast cells have intracytoplasmic basophilic metachromatic granules containing heparin and histamine. The normal skin contains relatively few mast cells, but their number is increased in many different skin conditions, particularly the itching dermatoses, such as *atopic eczema, contact dermatitis*, and *lichen planus*. In *urticaria pigmentosa* the mast cells occur in tumorlike masses.

Plasma cells, rarely seen in normal skin sections, occur in small numbers in most chronic inflammatory diseases of the skin and in larger numbers in granulomas. The origin of plasma cells is unknown, but they are believed to arise from reticulum cells.

In the myeloid group of cells, the polymorphonuclear leukocyte and the eosinophilic leukocyte occur quite commonly with various dermatoses, especially those with an allergic etiology.

In the lymphoid group, the lymphocyte is commonly found in inflammatory lesions of the skin. The myeloid and the lymphoid groups of cells are also found in their specific neoplasms of the skin.

The *ground substance* of the dermis is a gel-like, amorphous matrix not easily seen histologically, but it is of tremendous physiologic importance since it contains proteins, mucopolysaccharides, soluble collagens, enzymes, immune bodies, metabolites, and many other substances.

EPIDERMIS. The epidermis is the most superficial of the three layers of the skin and averages in thickness about the width of the mark of a sharp pencil, or less than 1 mm.

There are two distinct types of cells in the epidermis, the *keratinocytes* and the *dendritic cells*, or clear cells. The keratinocytes, or keratin-forming cells, are found in the basal layer and give rise to all the other cells of the stratified epidermis. The dendritic cells are of three types: (1) melanocytes (melanin-forming cells), (2) Langerhans' cells, and (3) indeterminate dendritic cells.

The epidermis is divided into five layers (Fig. 1–2). From inside out, they include the following:

1. Basal layer
2. Prickle layer
3. Granular layer } Living epidermis
4. Lucid layer
5. Horny layer—Dead end product

The *basal layer* of cells lies next to the corium and contains both keratin-forming and melanin-forming cells. The keratin-forming cells can be thought of as stem cells, which are capable of progressive differentiation into the cell forms higher up in the epidermis. It normally requires 3 or 4 weeks for the epidermis to replicate itself by the process of division and differentiation. This cell turnover is greatly accelerated in such diseases as *psoriasis* and *ichthyosiform erythroderma*.

The *prickle layer*, or stratum malpighii, is made up of several layers of epidermal cells, chiefly of polyhedral shape. This layer get its name from the existence of a network of cytoplasmic threads called prickles, or intercellular bridges, that extends between the cells. These prickles are most readily visible in this layer but, to a lesser extent, are present between all the cells of the epidermis.

The third layer is the *granular layer*. Here the cells are flatter and contain protein granules called keratohyaline granules.

The *lucid layer* is next and appears as a translucent line of flat cells. This layer of the skin is present only on the palms and the soles. The granular and the lucid layers make up the transitional layer of the epidermis and act as a barrier to the inward transfer of noxious substances and outward loss of water.

The outermost layer of the epidermis is the *horny layer*. It is made up of stratified layers of dead keratinized cells that are constantly shedding (Fig. 1–3). The chemical protein in these cells—keratin—is capable of absorbing vast amounts of water. This is readily seen

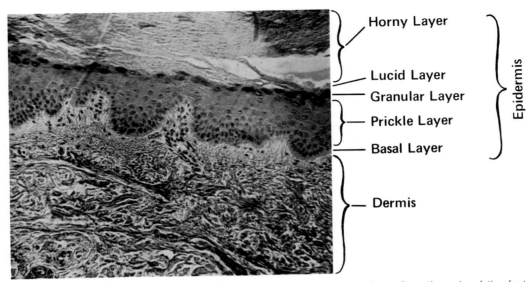

Figure 1–2. **Histology of the epidermis.** A microscopic section is shown from the sole of the foot. (*Dr. D. Gibson*)

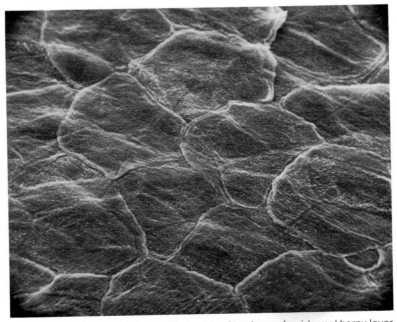

Figure 1–3. **Horny layer cells.** Underside of top layer of epidermal horny layer cells on Scotch tape stripping is seen with Cambridge Mark II Stereoscan at ×1000. (*Drs. J. Arnold, W. Barnes, and G. Sauer*)

during bathing, when the skin of the palms and the soles becomes white and swollen.

The normal oral mucous membrane does not have any granular layer or horny layer.

Of the three types of dendritic cells (melanocytes, Langerhans' cells, and indeterminate cells), only one, the melanocyte, can easily be identified in histologic sections stained with hematoxylin and eosin. The second type, the Langerhans' cell, can only be identified with certainty by histochemical methods or by use of the electron microscope. The third type of dendritic cell, the indeterminate dendritic cell, can be identified only by electron microscopy.

The melanin-forming cells, or melanocytes, are sandwiched between the more numerous keratin-forming cells in the basal layer. These melanocytes are *dopa positive*, because they stain darkly following contact with a solution of levorotatory, 3,4-dihydroxyphenylalanine, or *dopa*. This laboratory reaction closely simulates physiologic melanin formation in which the amino acid tyrosine is oxidized by the enzyme tyrosinase to form dopa. Dopa is then further changed, through a series of complex metabolic processes, to melanin.

Melanin pigmentation of the skin, whether increased or decreased, is influenced by many local and systemic factors (see Chap. 24). The melanocyte-stimulating hormone from the pituitary is the most potent melanizing agent.

VASCULAR SUPPLY

A continuous arteriovenous meshwork perforates the subcutaneous tissues and extends into the dermis. Blood vessels of varying sizes are present in all levels and all planes of the skin tissue and appendages. In fact, the vascularization is so intensive that it has been postulated that its main function is to regulate heat and blood pressure of the body, with the nutrition of the skin as a secondary function.

A special vascular body, the glomus, deserves mention. The glomus body is most commonly seen on the tips of the fingers and the toes and under the nails. Each one of these organs contains a vessel segment that has been called the Sucquet-Hoyer canal. This canal represents a short-circuit device that connects an arteriole with a venule directly, without intervening capillaries. The result is a marked increase in the blood flow through the skin. When this body grows abnormally, the result is a very painful red *glomus tumor*, commonly occurring underneath a nail, which has to be removed by surgical means.

NERVE SUPPLY

The nerve supply of the skin consists of sensory nerves and motor nerves.

SENSORY NERVES. The sensory nerves mediate the sensations of touch, temperature, or pain. The millions of terminal nerve endings, or Merkel cell–neurite complexes, have more to do with the specificity of skin sensation than the better known highly specialized nerve endings, such as the Vater-Pacinian and the Wagner-Meissner tactile corpuscles.

Itching is certainly the most important presenting symptom of an unhappy patient. It may be defined simply as the desire to scratch. Itching apparently is a mild painful sensation that differs from pain in having a lower frequency of impulse stimuli. The release of proteinases (such as follows itch powder application) may be responsible for the itch sensation. The pruritus may be of a pricking type or of a burning type and can vary greatly from one person to another. Sulzberger called those abnormally sensitive persons "itchish," analogous to "ticklish" persons. Itching can occur without any clinical signs of skin disease or from circulating allergens or local superficial contactants.

MOTOR NERVES. The involuntary sympathetic motor nerves control the sweat glands, the arterioles, and the smooth muscles of the skin. Adrenergic fibers carry impulses to the arrectores pilorum muscles, which produce gooseflesh when they are stimulated. This is due to traction of the muscle on the hair follicles to which it is attached.

APPENDAGES

The appendages of the skin include both the cornified appendages (hairs and nails) and the glandular appendages.

HAIRS. Hairs are derived from the hair follicles of the epidermis. Since no new hair follicles are formed after birth, the different types of body hairs are manifestations of the effect of location and of external and internal stimuli. Hormones are the most important internal stimuli influencing the various types of hair growth. This growth is cyclic, with a growing (anagen) phase and a resting (telogen) phase. The catogen cycle is the transition phase between the growing and resting stages and lasts only a few days. Ninety percent of the normal scalp hairs are in the growing (anagen) stage, and 10% are in the resting (falling out) stage, which lasts from 60 to 90 days. The average period of scalp hair growth ranges from 2 to 6 years. However, systemic stresses, such as childbirth, may cause hairs to enter a resting stage prematurely. This *postpartum effect* is noticed most commonly in the scalp when these resting hairs are depilated during combing or washing and the thought of approaching baldness then causes sudden alarm.

SAUER NOTES:

1. Shaving of excess hair, as women do on their legs and thighs, does *not* promote more rapid growth of coarse hair. The shaved stubs *appear* more coarse, but if allowed to grow normally the hairs would appear and feel no different than before shaving.

2. The value of intermittent massage to stimulate scalp hair growth has not been proved.

3. Hair cannot turn gray overnight. The melanin pigmentation, which is distributed throughout the length of the nonvital hair shaft, takes weeks to be shed through the slow process of hair growth.

4. Heredity is the greatest factor predisposing to baldness, and an excess of male hormone may contribute to hair loss in these persons. Male castrates do not become bald.

5. The common male pattern baldness cannot be reversed by over-the-counter "hair restorers." Minoxidil solution (Rogaine), which is physician prescribed, is beneficial for a limited percentage of patients.

Types. The adult has two main types of hairs: (1) the vellus hairs (lanugo hairs of the fetus) and (2) the terminal hairs. The vellus hairs ("peach fuzz") are the fine, short hairs of the body, whereas the terminal hairs are coarse, thick, and pigmented. The terminal hairs are developed most extensively on the scalp, the brows, and the extremities.

Hair Follicles. The hair follicle may be thought of as an invagination of the epidermis, with its different layers of cells. These cells make up the matrix of the hair follicle and produce the keratin of the mature hair. The protein-synthesizing capacity of this tissue is enormous. At the rate of scalp hair growth of 0.35 mm/day, over 100 linear feet of scalp hair is produced daily. The density of hairs in the scalp varies from 175 to 300 hairs per square centimeter.

NAILS. The second cornified appendage, the nail, consists of a nail plate and the tissue that surrounds it. This plate lies in a nail groove, which, like the hair follicle, is an invagination of the epidermis. Unlike hair growth, which is periodic, nail growth is continuous. Nail growth proceeds at about one third of the rate of hair growth, or about 0.1 mm/day. It takes approximately 3 months to restore a removed fingernail and about three times that long for the regrowth of a new toenail. Nail growth can be inhibited during serious illnesses or in old age, increased through nail biting or occupational stress, and altered because of hand dermatitis or systemic disease. Topical treatment of nail disturbances is very unsatisfactory, owing to the inaccessibility of the growth-producing areas.

GLANDULAR APPENDAGES. The two types of glandular appendages of the skin are the sebaceous glands and the sweat glands (Fig. 1–4). The sebaceous glands form their secretion through disintegration of the whole glandular cell, whereas the sweat glands eliminate only a portion of the cell in the formation of secretion.

The *sebaceous glands* are present everywhere on the skin, except the palms and the soles. The secretion from these glands is evacuated through the sebaceous duct to a follicle that may or may not contain a hair. This secretion is not under any neurologic control but is a continuous outflowing of the material of cell

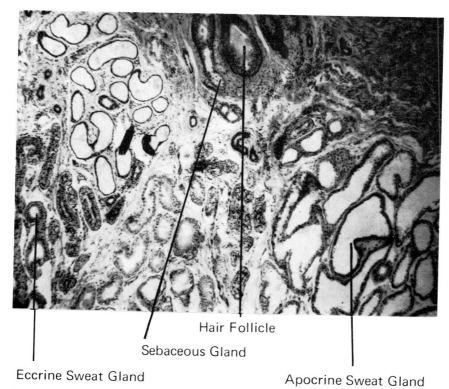

Hair Follicle

Sebaceous Gland

Eccrine Sweat Gland

Apocrine Sweat Gland

Figure 1–4. **Histology of the glands of the skin.** A microscopic section from the axilla is shown. (*Dr. D. Gibson*)

breakdown. These glands produce sebum, which covers the skin with a thin lipoidal film that is mildly bacteriostatic and fungistatic and retards water evaporation. The scalp and the face may contain as many as 1,000 sebaceous glands per square centimeter. The activity of the gland increases markedly at the age of puberty and, in certain persons, becomes plugged with sebum, debris, and bacteria to form the *blackheads* and the *pimples* of acne.

The *sweat glands* are found everywhere in the human skin. They appear in greatest abundance on the palms and the soles and in the axillae. There are two main types of sweat glands: the eccrine, or small sweat glands, open directly onto the skin surface; the apocrine, or large sweat glands, like the sebaceous gland, usually open into a hair follicle.

The *apocrine sweat glands* are found chiefly in the axillae and the genital region and do not develop until the time of puberty. These glands, in humans, have very little im-

portance except for the production of odor (the infamous "B.O."). Any emotional stresses that cause adrenergic sympathetic discharge produce apocrine sweating. This sweat is sterile when excreted but undergoes decomposition when contaminated by bacteria from the skin surface, resulting in a strong and characteristic odor. The purpose of the many cosmetic underarm preparations is to remove these bacteria or block the gland excretion. The main disease of the apocrine glands is *hidradenitis suppurativa*. This uncommon, chronic infection of these glands is caused by blockage of the duct, which usually occurs in patients with the *acne-seborrhea complex*.

The *eccrine sweat glands* and the cutaneous blood vessels are key factors in the maintenance of stable internal body temperatures, despite marked environmental temperature changes. The eccrine glands flood the skin surface with water for cooling, and the blood vessels dilate or constrict to dissipate or to conserve body heat. The eccrine sweat glands

are distributed everywhere on the skin surface, with the greatest concentration on the
palms, the soles, and the forehead. The prime
stimulus for these small sweat glands is heat.
Their activity is under the control of the nervous system, usually through the hypotha-
lamic thermostat. Both adrenergic and cholinergic fibers innervate the glands. Blockage of
the sweat ducts results in the disease entity
known as *prickly heat (miliaria)*. When the
sweat glands are congenitally absent, as in
anhidrotic ectodermal dysplasia, a life-threatening hyperpyrexia may develop.

BIBLIOGRAPHY

Goldsmith L (ed): Biochemistry and Physiology of
the Skin, 2 volumes. New York, Oxford University
Press, 1983

Lever WF, Schaumberg-Lever G: Histopathology
of the Skin, 7th ed. Philadelphia, JB Lippincott,
1989

McKee PH: Pathology of the Skin. Philadelphia, JB
Lippincott, 1989

Sato K, Kang WH, Saga K et al: Biology of sweat
glands and their disorders. J Am Acad Dermatol
20:537, 1989

2

Laboratory Procedures and Tests

In addition to the usual laboratory procedures used in the workup of medical patients, certain special tests are of importance in the field of dermatology. These include *skin tests, fungus examinations, biopsies,* and *cytodiagnosis.* For special problems, additional testing methods are suggested in the sections on the various diseases.

SKIN TESTS

There are three types of skin tests:

1. Intracutaneous
2. Scratch
3. Patch

The *intracutaneous tests* and the *scratch tests* can have two types of reactions: (1) an *immediate wheal reaction* and (2) a *delayed reaction.* The immediate wheal reaction develops to a maximum in 5 to 20 minutes. This type of reaction is elicited in testing for the cause of urticaria, atopic dermatitis, and inhalant allergies. This immediate wheal reaction test is seldom used for determining the cause of skin diseases.

The delayed reaction to intracutaneous skin testing is exemplified best by the tuberculin skin test. Tuberculin is available in two forms: as purified protein derivative (PPD) and as a tuberculin tine test.

The PPD test is performed by using tablets that come in two strengths and by injecting a solution of either one intracutaneously. If there is no reaction following the test with the first strength, then the second strength may be employed.

The tuberculin tine test (Mantoux) is a simple and rapid procedure using OTK. Nine prongs, or tines, covered with OTK are pressed into the skin. If at the end of 48 or 72 hours there is over 2 mm of induration at the site of any prong insertion, the test is positive.

Patch tests are used rather commonly in dermatology and offer a simple and accurate method of determining whether a patient is allergic to any of the testing agents (Figs. 2–1 and 2–2). There are two different reactions to this type of test: (1) *a primary irritant reaction* and (2) an *allergic reaction.* The *primary irritant reaction* occurs in the majority of the population when they are exposed to agents that have skin-destroying properties. Examples of these agents include soaps, cleaning fluids, bleaches, "corn" removers, and counterirritants. The *allergic reaction* indicates that the patient is more sensitive than normal to the agent being tested. It also shows that the patient has had a previous exposure to that agent.

The technique of the patch test is rather simple. However, the interpretation of the test is not that simple. For example, consider that a patient comes in with a dermatitis on the top of his feet. It is possible that shoe leather or some chemical used in the manufacture of the leather is causing the reaction. The procedure for a patch test is to cut out a ½-inch-square piece of the material from the inside of the shoe, moisten the material with distilled water, place it on the skin surface,

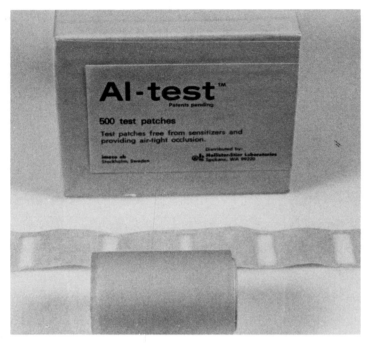

Figure 2–1. **Patch test material.**

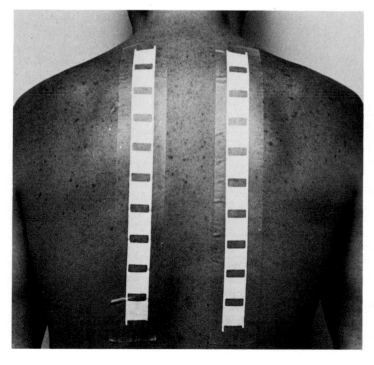

Figure 2–2. **Patch tests.**

and cover it with an adhesive band or some patch-test dressing. The patch test is left on for 48 hours. When the test is removed, the patient is considered to have a positive patch test if there is any redness, papules, or vesiculation under the site of the testing agent. Delayed reactions to allergens can occur and, ideally, a final reading should be made at 96 hours (4 days).

The patch test can be used to make or confirm a diagnosis of poison ivy dermatitis, ragweed dermatitis, or contact dermatitis due to medications, cosmetics, or industrial chemicals. Fisher (1986) and Adams (1982) have compiled lists of chemicals, concentrations, and vehicles to be used for eliciting the allergic type of patch test reaction. However, most tests can be performed very simply, as in the case of the shoe leather dermatitis. One precaution is that the test must not be allowed to become wet in the 48-hour period.

A packaged source of allergy tests is the Allergen Patch Test Kit, which is distributed by the American Academy of Dermatology, Evanson, IL 60201. The kit contains 20 allergen-filled, multiple-dose syringes so that a measured ribbon of petrolatum mixture or a measured amount of solution can be placed on patch test tapes or in the Finn Chamber on Scanpor. This Finn Chamber is available from Allerderm Laboratories, P.O. Box 931, Mill Valley, CA 94942-0931 or from Hermal Pharmaceutical Laboratories, Inc., Route 145, Oak Hill, NY 12460.

A method of testing for allergy when food is suspected is to use the Rowe elimination diet. The procedure is to limit the diet to the following basic foods, which are known to be hypoallergenic: lamb, lemon, grapefruit, pears, lettuce, spinach, carrots, sweet potato, tapioca, rice and rice bread, cane sugar, maple syrup, sesame oil, gelatin, and salt. The patient is to remain on this basic diet for 5 to 7 days. At the end of that time one new food can be added every 2 days. The following foods may be added early: beef, white potatoes, green beens, milk (along with butter and American cheese), and white bread with puffed wheat. If there is a flare-up of the dermatitis, which should occur within 2 to 8 hours after ingestion of an offending food, the new food should be discontinued for the present. More new foods are added until the normal diet, minus the allergenic foods, is regained.

FUNGUS EXAMINATIONS

Fungus examinations are a simple office laboratory procedure. They are accomplished by scraping the diseased skin and examining the material directly under the microscope, culturing the material, and examining the grown culture under the microscope. The skin scrapings are obtained by abrading a scaly diseased area with a knife blade. The material is deposited on a slide and covered with a 20% aqueous potassium hydroxide solution and a coverslip. A diagnostically helpful pale violet stain can be imparted to the fungi if the 20% aqueous potassium hydroxide solution is mixed with an equal amount of Parker Super Quink, Permanent Black Ink. The preparation on the slide can be heated, or allowed to stand for 15 to 60 minutes, to allow the keratin particles to dissolve and reveal the fungi more clearly. The slide is then mounted on a microscope stage and examined for fungus elements with the low-power and high-power lenses (Fig. 2–3).

For a culture preparation, a part of the material from the scraping can be implanted in a test tube containing Sabouraud's media.* In 1 to 2 weeks, a whitish or variously colored growth will be noted (Fig. 2–4). The species of fungus can be determined grossly by the color and the characteristics of the growth in the culture tube and microscopically by study of a small amount of the culture material that has been removed, mixed with a solution of Lacto Phenol Cotton Blue, and placed on a microscope slide. Most species of fungi have a characteristic microscopic appearance.

BIOPSIES

The biopsy of a questionable skin lesion and the microscopic examination of the bi-

---

* *Acuderm Inc., 5370 N.W. 35 Terrace, Ft. Lauderdale, FL 33309; Baker/Cummins, Miami, FL 33269-0670; Dermatologic Lab and Supply, Inc., 201 Ridge #205, Council Bluffs, IA 51503; Derm Medical Company, Inc., 8531 Wellsford Street #3, Santa Fe Springs, CA 90670; Troy Biologicals, 1238 Rankin, Troy, MI, 48084. For cultures that will usually be contaminant free, order the special Sabouraud's media that contains cyclohexamide and chloramphenicol. DTM culture medium has a pH indicator that turns the media red if a dermatophyte is present.*

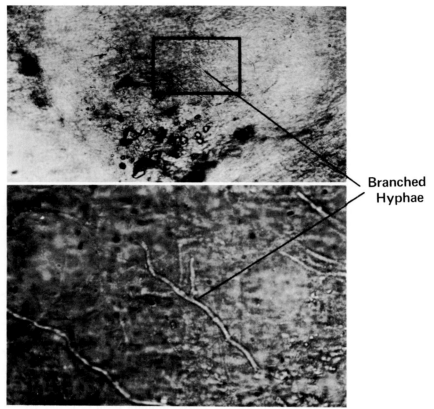

Figure 2–3.   **Fungi from a skin scraping as seen with microscope in a KOH preparation.** (*Top*) Low-power lens (×100) view. (*Bottom*) High-power lens (×450) view of area outlined above. (*Dr. D. Gibson*)

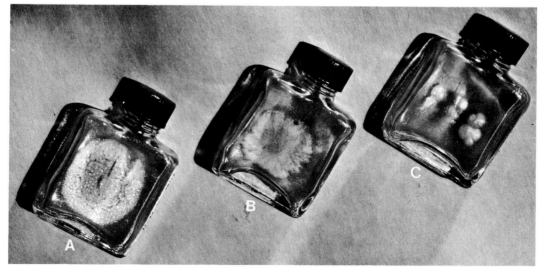

Figure 2–4.   **Fungus cultures.** Cultures grown on disposable bottles of Sabouraud's media (Mycosel, Derm Medical). The three fungi are (*A*) *Trichophyton mentagrophytes,* (*B*) *Microsporum canis,* and (*C*) *Candida albicans.* (*K.U.M.C.*)

opsy section is another important laboratory procedure. The histopathology of many skin conditions is quite diagnostic, particularly when the biopsy specimen is studied by a pathologist who has some knowledge of dermatologic lesions.

The instruments and the materials needed to perform a skin biopsy are listed on page 388 and are shown in Figure 37–2. See also Chapter 7 on Fundamentals of Cutaneous Surgery.

There are three principal techniques for performing skin biopsies: (1) by *surgical excision with suturing*, (2) by *punch*, and (3) by *scissors*. The decision in favor of one method depends on such factors as the site of the biopsy, the cosmetic result desired, the type of tissue to be removed (*e.g.*, flat or elevated), and simplicity of technique.

SAUER NOTE:

The skin biopsy specimen must include adequate tissue for proper interpretation by the pathologist.

SURGICAL EXCISION. The technique of performing surgical excision biopsies with suturing of the skin is well known. In general, this type of biopsy is performed when a good cosmetic result is desired and when the entire lesion is to be removed. The disadvantage is that this procedure is the most time consuming of the three techniques.

PUNCH BIOPSY. Punch biopsies can be done rather rapidly, with or without suturing of the wound. A special punch biopsy instrument of appropriate size is needed. Disposable biopsy punches are available. A local anesthetic is usually injected at the site. The operator rotates the instrument until it penetrates to the subcutaneous level; the circle of tissue is then excised. Bleeding can be stopped with pressure or by the use of one or two sutures. An elliptical wound instead of a circular wound can be produced by stretching the skin perpendicular to the desired suture line before the punch is rotated. The resultant scar, following suturing, is neater.

SCISSORS BIOPSY. The third way to remove skin tissue for a biopsy specimen is to excise the piece with sharp-pointed scissors and stop the bleeding with light electrosurgery. This latter procedure is useful for certain types of elevated lesions and in areas where the cosmetic result is not too important. The greatest advantage of this procedure is the speed and the simplicity with which it can be done.

The biopsy specimen must be placed in appropriate fixative solution, usually 10% formalin. If the specimen is long and tends to curl, it can be stretched out on a piece of paper. Then paper and tissue can be dropped in the fixative solution.

The stain most routinely used is hematoxylin and eosin. With this stain, the nuclei stain blue and collagen, muscles, and nerves stain red. A table of special stains can be found in Lever's book, listed in the bibliography at the end of this chapter.

For immunologic studies, the skin tissue must be processed freshly frozen or from a carrying fixative.

CYTODIAGNOSIS

The cervical Papanicolaou smear is the most common form of cytodiagnosis. In dermatology, cytodiagnosis, known as the Tzanck test, is useful in bullous diseases (pemphigus), vesicular virus eruptions (herpes), and basal cell carcinomas. The technique and choice of lesions is important. For best results select an early lesion. In the case of a blister, remove the top with a scalpel or sharp scissors. Blot the excess fluid with a gauze pad. Then gently scrape the floor of the blister with a scalpel blade. Try not to cause bleeding. Make a thin smear of the cells on a clean glass slide. If you are dealing with a solid lesion, squeeze the material between two slides. The slide may be air dried, but it can also be fixed by dipping it four to five times in 95% ethanol. Stain the slide with Wright's stain, Giemsa's stain, or hematoxylin and eosin. A concise review of this subject is presented by Rook and colleagues (see Bibliography).

In addition to skin testing, fungus examination, biopsies, and cytodiagnosis, there are certain tests for specific skin conditions that will be discussed in connection with the respective diseases.

BIBLIOGRAPHY

Skin Tests

Adams RM: Occupational Skin Disease. Orlando, FL, Grune & Stratton, 1982

Fisher AA: Contact Dermatitis, 3rd ed. Philadelphia, Lea & Febiger, 1986

Fungus Examinations

Koneman EW, Roberts GD: Practical Laboratory Mycology, 3rd ed. Baltimore, Williams & Wilkins, 1985

(See Chapter 19 on Dermatologic Mycology for additional references.)

Biopsies

Epstein E, Epstein E Jr: Skin Surgery, 6th ed. Philadelphia, WB Saunders, 1987

Lever WF, Schaumburg-Lever G: Histopathology of the Skin, 7th ed. Philadelphia, JB Lippincott, 1989

Robinson JK: Fundamentals of Skin Biopsy. Chicago, Year Book Medical Publishers, 1985

Cytodiagnosis

Barr RJ: Cutaneous cytology. J Am Acad Dermatol 10:163, 1984

Rook A, Wilkinson DS, Ebling FJG, Champion RH, Burton JL: Textbook of Dermatology, 4th ed, 3 volumes. Chicago, Year Book–Blackwell, 1986

GENERAL REFERENCE

Beare JM, Bingham EA: The influence of the results of laboratory and ancillary investigations in the management of skin disease. Int J Dermatol 20:653, 1981. The authors conclude that the number of ancillary investigations required by an experienced clinician is quite extraordinarily small. They are (1) biopsy, (2) patch testing, (3) sedimentation rate, and (4) Wood's light. I agree.

3

Dermatologic Diagnosis

To aid in determining the diagnosis of a presenting skin problem, this chapter contains discussions of primary and secondary lesions and also of diagnosis by location. Included are lists of seasonal skin diseases, military dermatoses, and dermatoses of blacks.

PRIMARY AND SECONDARY LESIONS

No two skin diseases look alike, but most of them have some characteristic *primary* lesions, and it is very important to examine the patient closely to find them. Commonly, however, the primary lesions have been obliterated by the *secondary* lesions of overtreat-

ment, excessive scratching, or infection. Even in these cases it is usually possible, by careful examination, to find some primary lesions at the edge of the eruption or on other less irritated areas of the body (Plates 1 through 3).

Combinations of primary and secondary lesions frequently occur as part of the clinical picture.

Primary Lesions

A description of the basic primary lesions follows:

Macules are up to 1 cm and are circumscribed, flat discolorations of the skin. Examples: freckles, flat nevi.

Patches are larger than 1 cm and are circumscribed, flat discolorations of the skin. Examples: vitiligo, senile freckles, measles rash.

Papules are up to 1 cm and are circumscribed, elevated, superficial, solid lesions. Examples: elevated nevi, warts, lichen planus.

A *wheal* is a type of papule that is edematous and transitory. Examples: hives, insect bites.

Plaques are larger than 1 cm and are circumscribed, elevated, superficial, solid lesions. Examples: mycosis fungoides, localized neurodermatitis.

Nodules range to 1 cm and are solid lesions with depth; they may be above, level with, or beneath the skin surface. Examples: nodular secondary or tertiary syphilis, epitheliomas, xanthomas.

SAUER NOTES:

1. One of the dermatologist's tools-of-the-trade is a magnifying lens. *Use it.*

2. A complete examination of the entire body is a necessity when confronted with a diffuse skin eruption or an unusual localized eruption.

3. Touch the skin and skin lesions. You learn a lot by palpating, and the patients appreciate that you are not afraid of "catching" the problem. (For the uncommon contagious problem, use precaution.)

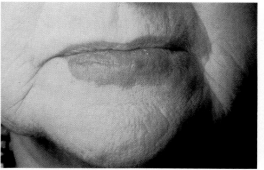

(A) Macule, on lip (port-wine hemangioma)

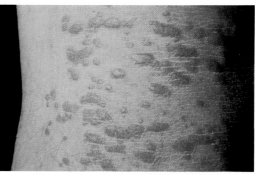

(B) Papules, on knee (lichen planus)

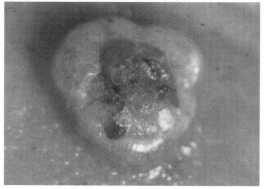

(C) Nodule, on lower eyelid (basal cell carcinoma)

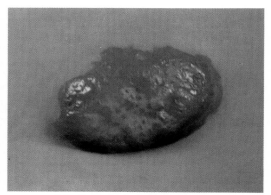

(D) Tumor, of abdomen (mixed hemangioma)

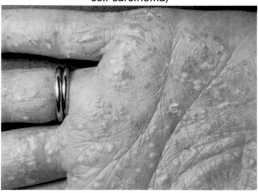

(E) Pustules, on palm (pustular psoriasis)

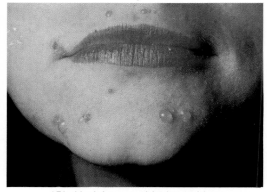

(F) Vesicles, on chin (pemphigus vulgaris)

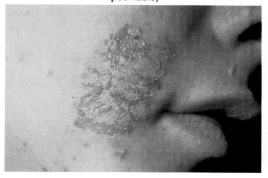

(G) Crust, on cheek (impetigo)

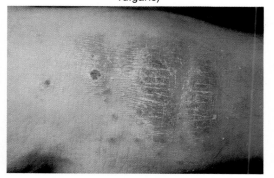

(H) Lichenification, on dorsum of ankle (localized neurodermatitis)

Plate 1. **Primary and secondary lesions.** (*Geigy Pharmaceuticals*)

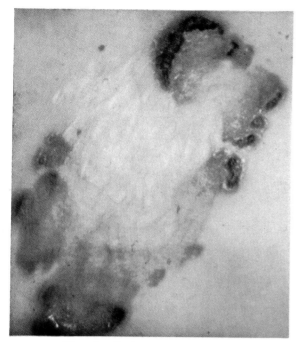
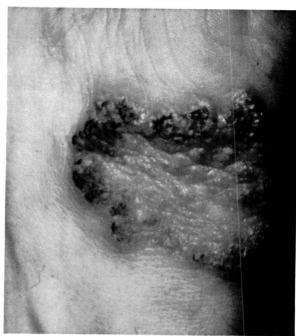

Plate 2. **Nodular lesions.** (*Left*) Grouped nodular lesions with central scarring (tertiary syphilo-derm). (*Right*) Grouped warty, nodular lesions with central scarring (tuberculosis verrucosa cutis). (*Marion B. Sulzberger: Folia Dermatologica, No. 1, Geigy Pharmaceuticals*)

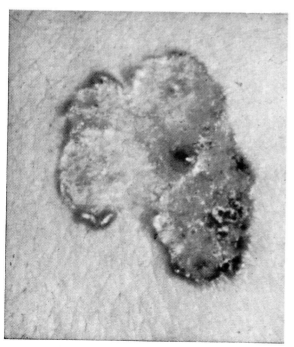
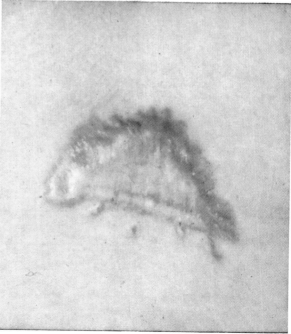

Plate 3. **Nodular lesions.** (*Left*) Polycyclic nodular lesion (superficial basal cell carcinoma). (*Right*) Keloid. (*Marion B. Sulzberger: Folia Dermatologica, No. 1, Geigy Pharmaceuticals*)

Tumors are larger than 1 cm and are solid lesions with depth; they may be above, level with, or beneath the skin surface. Examples: tumor stage of mycosis fungoides, larger epitheliomas.

Vesicles range to 1 cm and are circumscribed elevations of the skin containing serous fluid. Examples: early chickenpox, zoster, contact dermatitis.

Bullae are larger than 1 cm and are circumscribed elevations containing serous fluid. Examples: pemphigus, second-degree burns.

Pustules vary in size and are circumscribed elevations of the skin containing purulent fluid. Examples: acne, impetigo.

Petechiae range to 1 cm and are circumscribed deposits of blood or blood pigments. Examples: certain insect bites and drug eruptions.

Purpura is a larger than 1-cm circumscribed deposit of blood or blood pigment in the skin.

Secondary Lesions

Secondary lesions include the following:

Scales (squamae) are shedding, dead epidermal cells that may be dry or greasy. Examples: dandruff, psoriasis.

Crusts are variously colored masses of skin exudates. Examples: impetigo, infected dermatitis.

Excoriations are abrasions of the skin, usually superficial and traumatic. Examples: scratched insect bites, scabies.

Fissures are linear breaks in the skin, sharply defined with abrupt walls. Examples: congenital syphilis, athlete's foot.

Ulcers are irregularly sized and shaped excavations in the skin extending into the corium. Examples: stasis ulcers of legs, tertiary syphilis.

Scars are formations of connective tissue replacing tissue lost through injury or disease.

Keloids are hypertrophic scars.

Lichenification is a diffuse area of thickening and scaling with resultant increase in the skin lines and markings.

Several combinations of primary and secondary lesions commonly exist on the same patient. Examples: *papulosquamous* lesions of psoriasis, *vesiculopustular* lesions in contact dermatitis, and *crusted excoriations* in scabies.

Special Lesions

There are also some primary lesions, limited to a few skin diseases, that can be called specialized lesions.

Comedones or **blackheads** are plugs of whitish or blackish sebaceous and keratinous material lodged in the pilosebaceous follicle, usually seen on the face, the chest, or the back, rarely on the upper part of the arms. Example: acne.

Milia are whitish nodules, 1 to 2 mm in diameter, that have no visible opening onto the skin surface. Examples: in healed burn or superficial traumatic sites, healed bullous disease sites, or newborns.

Telangiectasias are dilated superficial blood vessels. Examples: spider hemangiomas, chronic radiodermatitis.

Burrows are very small and short (in scabies) or tortuous and long (in creeping eruption) tunnels in the epidermis.

In addition, there are distinct and often diagnostic changes in the nail plates and the hairs that are discussed in the chapters relating to these appendages.

DIAGNOSIS BY LOCATION

A physician is often confronted by a patient with skin trouble localized to one part of the body (Figs. 3–1 through 3–4). The following list of diseases with special localizations is meant to aid in the diagnosis of such conditions, but this list must not be considered as being all inclusive. Generalizations are the rule, and many of the rare diseases are omitted. For further information concerning the particular diseases, consult the Dictionary-Index.

(*text continues on page 23*)

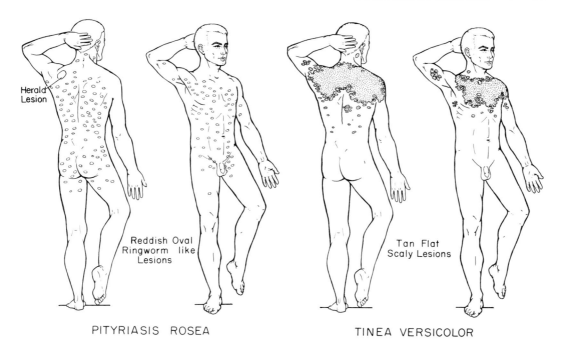

Herald Lesion

Reddish Oval
Ringworm like
Lesions

PITYRIASIS ROSEA

Tan Flat
Scaly Lesions

TINEA VERSICOLOR

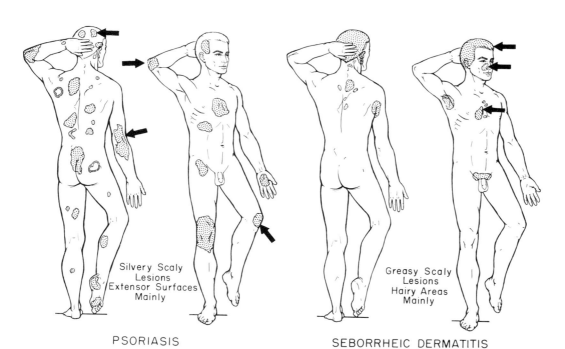

Silvery Scaly
Lesions
Extensor Surfaces
Mainly

PSORIASIS

Greasy Scaly
Lesions
Hairy Areas
Mainly

SEBORRHEIC DERMATITIS

Figure 3–1. **Dermatologic silhouettes.**

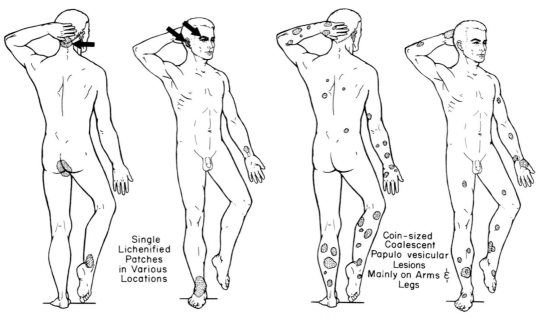

Single
Lichenified
Patches
in Various
Locations

LOCALIZED NEURODERMATITIS

Coin-sized
Coalescent
Papulo vesicular
Lesions
Mainly on Arms &
Legs

NUMMULAR ECZEMA

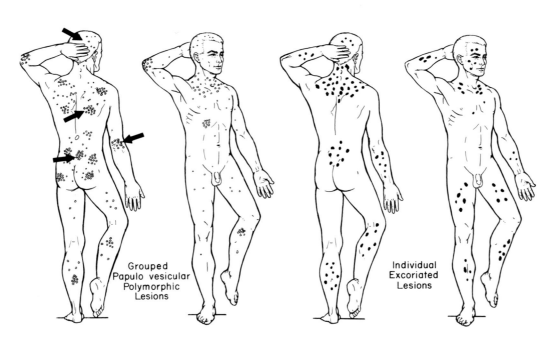

Grouped
Papulo vesicular
Polymorphic
Lesions

DERMATITIS HERPETIFORMIS

Individual
Excoriated
Lesions

NEUROTIC EXCORIATIONS

Figure 3–2. **Dermatologic silhouettes.**

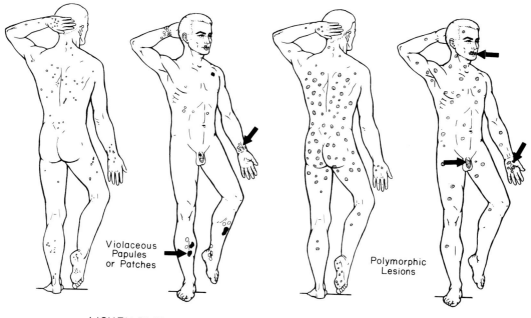

LICHEN PLANUS

SECONDARY SYPHILIS

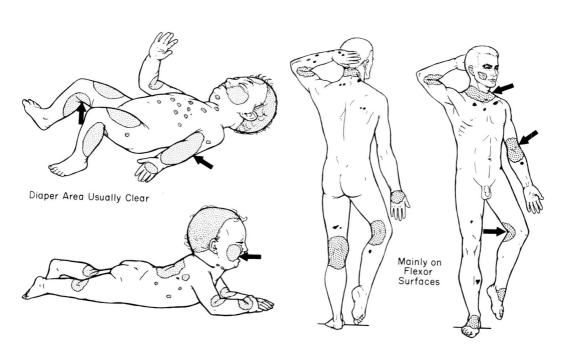

INFANTILE FORM of ATOPIC ECZEMA

ADULT FORM of ATOPIC ECZEMA

Figure 3–3. **Dermatologic silhouettes.**

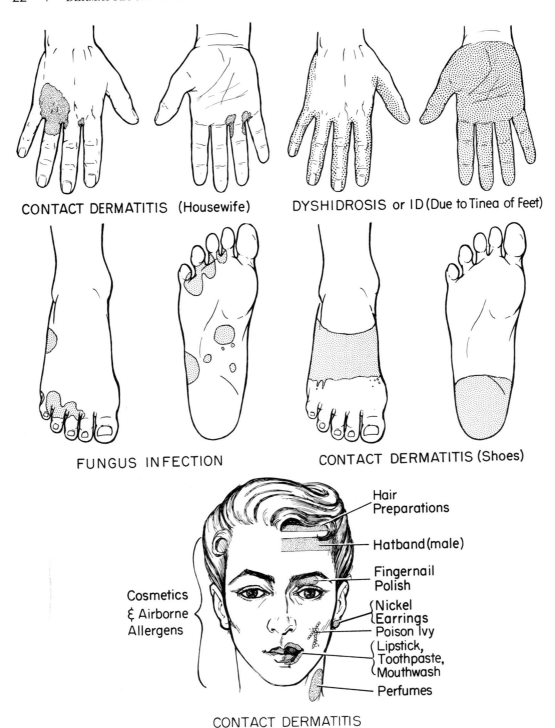

CONTACT DERMATITIS (Housewife)   DYSHIDROSIS or ID (Due to Tinea of Feet)

FUNGUS INFECTION   CONTACT DERMATITIS (Shoes)

Hair
Preparations

Hatband (male)

Fingernail
Polish

Nickel
Earrings

Poison Ivy

Lipstick,
Toothpaste,
Mouthwash

Perfumes

Cosmetics
& Airborne
Allergens

CONTACT DERMATITIS

Figure 3–4.   **Dermatologic silhouettes.**

SAUER NOTES:

In diagnosing a rather generalized skin eruption, the following three mimicking conditions must be considered first, and ruled in or out by appropriate history or examination:

1. Drug eruption
2. Contact dermatitis
3. Infectious diseases, such as secondary syphilis

Scalp: Seborrheic dermatitis, contact dermatitis, psoriasis, folliculitis, pediculosis, and hair loss due to the following: Male or female pattern, alopecia areata, tinea, chronic discoid lupus erythematosus, post pregnancy, or trichotillomania.

Ears: Seborrheic dermatitis, psoriasis, infectious eczematoid dermatitis, actinic keratoses, and, very rarely, fungal infection.

Face: Acne, rosacea, impetigo, contact dermatitis, seborrheic dermatitis, folliculitis, herpes simplex, and, less commonly, lupus erythematosus and actinic dermatitis.

Eyelids: Contact dermatitis due to fingernail polish or hair sprays, seborrheic dermatitis, or atopic eczema.

Posterior Neck: Neurodermatitis, seborrheic dermatitis, psoriasis, or contact dermatitis.

Mouth: Aphthae, herpes simplex, geographic tongue, contact dermatitis, and, less frequently, syphilis, lichen planus, acquired immunodeficiency syndrome, and pemphigus.

Axillae: Contact dermatitis, seborrheic dermatitis, hidradenitis suppurativa, and, less commonly, erythrasma, acanthosis nigricans, and Fox-Fordyce disease.

Chest and Back (Fig. 3–5): Tinea versicolor, pityriasis rosea, acne, seborrheic dermatitis, psoriasis, and secondary syphilis.

Groin and Crural Areas: Tinea infection, candidal infection, bacterial intertrigo, scabies, pediculosis, and granuloma inguinale.

Penis (Fig. 3–6): Contact dermatitis, fusospirochetal and candidal balanitis, chancroid, herpes simplex, primary and secondary syphilis, scabies, and, less frequently, balanitis xerotica obliterans.

Hands (Fig. 3–7): Contact dermatitis, id reaction to fungal infection of the feet, atopic eczema, and, less commonly, pustular psoriasis, nummular eczema, erythema multiforme, secondary syphilis, and fungal infection.

Cubital Fossae and Popliteal Fossae: Atopic eczema, contact dermatitis, and prickly heat.

Elbows and Knees: Psoriasis, xanthomas, and, occasionally, atopic eczema.

Feet (Fig. 3–8): Fungal infection, primary or secondary bacterial infection, contact dermatitis from footwear or foot care, atopic eczema, and, less frequently, psoriasis, erythema multiforme, and secondary syphilis.

(text continues on page 28)

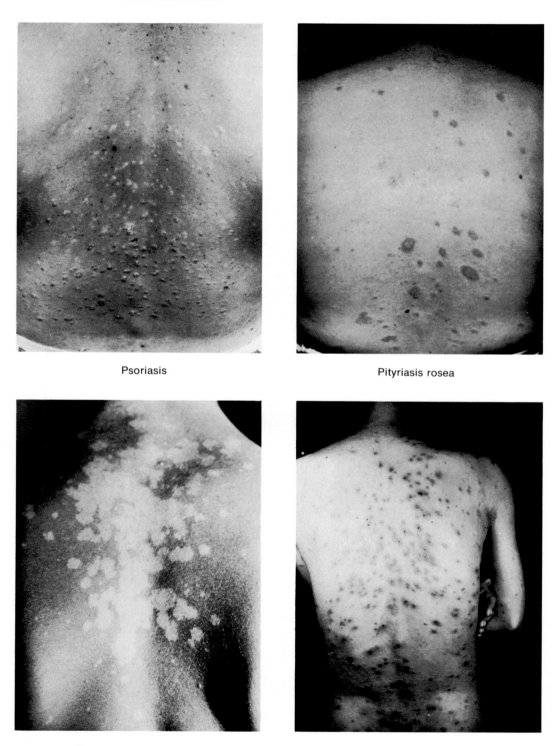

Psoriasis

Pityriasis rosea

Tinea versicolor in a black

Secondary syphilis

Figure 3–5. **Papulosquamous diseases on the back.**

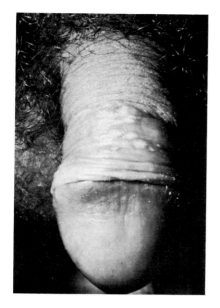

Herpes simplex

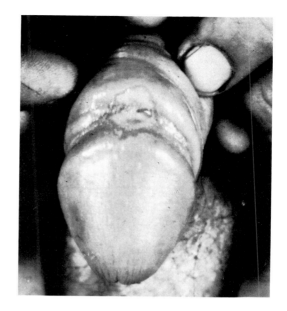

Primary syphilis

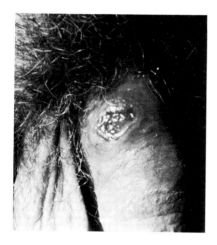

Furuncle

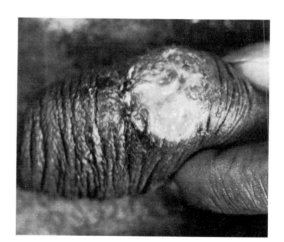

Chancroid

Figure 3–6. **Penile lesions.**

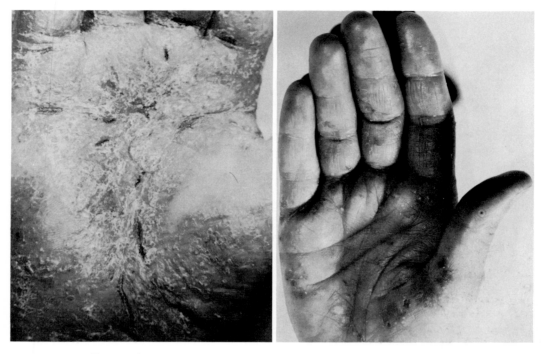

Contact dermatitis   Tinea

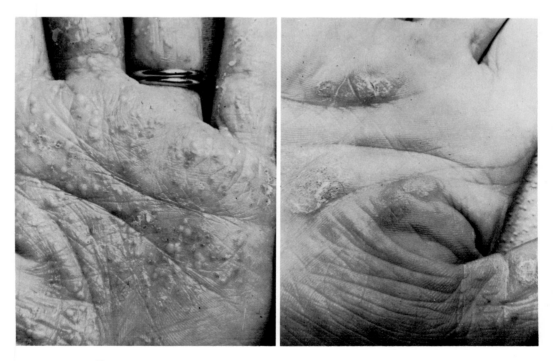

Pustular psoriasis   Psoriasis

Figure 3–7. **Palmar dermatoses.**

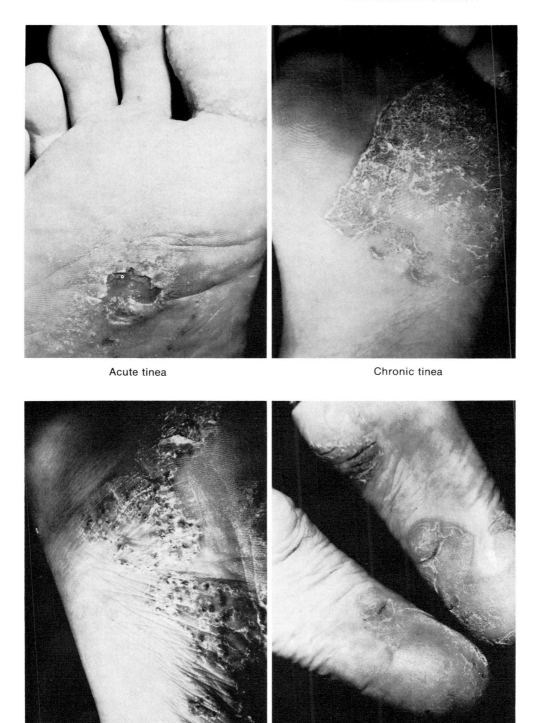

Acute tinea

Chronic tinea

Pustular psoriasis

Psoriasis

Figure 3–8. **Plantar dermatoses.**

SEASONAL SKIN DISEASES

Certain dermatoses have an increased incidence in various seasons of the year. In a busy dermatologist's office one sees literal "epidemics" of atopic eczema, pityriasis rosea, psoriasis, and winter itch, to mention only a few. Knowledge of this seasonal incidence is helpful from a diagnostic standpoint. It will be sufficient simply to list these seasonal diseases, since more specific information concerning them can be found elsewhere in this text. Remember that there are exceptions to every rule.

Winter
Atopic eczema
Contact dermatitis of hands
Psoriasis
Seborrheic dermatitis
Nummular eczema
Winter itch and dry skin (xerosis)
Ichthyosis (rare)

Spring
Pityriasis rosea
Erythema multiforme (Hebra)
Acne (flares)

Summer
Contact dermatitis due to poison ivy
Tinea of the feet and the groin
Candidal intertrigo
Miliaria or prickly heat
Impetigo and other pyodermas
Actinic dermatitis
Insect bites
Tinea versicolor (noticed after suntan)
Darier's disease (uncommon)
Epidermolysis bullosa (uncommon)

Fall
Winter itch
Senile pruritus
Atopic eczema
Pityriasis rosea
Contact dermatitis due to ragweed
Tinea of the scalp (schoolchildren)
Acne (flares)

MILITARY DERMATOSES

Although the major part of the world is now at nominal peace, under the ravages of previous wars the lack of good personal hygiene, lack of adequate food, and the presence of overcrowding, injuries, and pestilence resulted in the aggravation of any existing skin disease and an increased incidence of the following skin diseases:

Scabies
Pediculosis
Syphilis and other sexually transmitted diseases
Bacterial dermatoses
Jungle rot in tropical climates:
    Tinea of the feet and the groin
    Pyoderma
    Miliaria

DERMATOSES OF BLACKS

The following skin diseases are seen with greater frequency in the black race than in the white race (Figs. 3–9 and 3–10):

Keloids
Dermatosis papulosa nigra
Pyodermas of legs in children
Pigmentary disturbances from many causes, both hypopigmented and hyperpigmented
Traumatic marginal alopecia (from braids and from heated irons used in hair straightening)
Seborrheic dermatitis of scalp, aggravated by grease on hair
Ingrown hairs of beard
Acne keloidalis
Annular form of secondary syphilis
Granuloma inguinale
Mongolian spots

On the other hand, certain skin conditions are rarely seen in the black patient:

Squamous cell or basal cell carcinomas
Actinic keratoses
Psoriasis

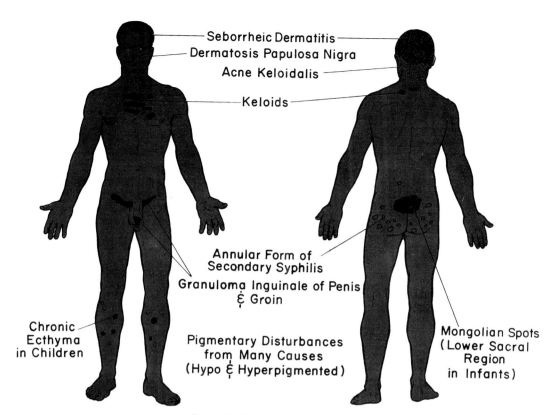

Figure 3–9.   **Black dermogram.**

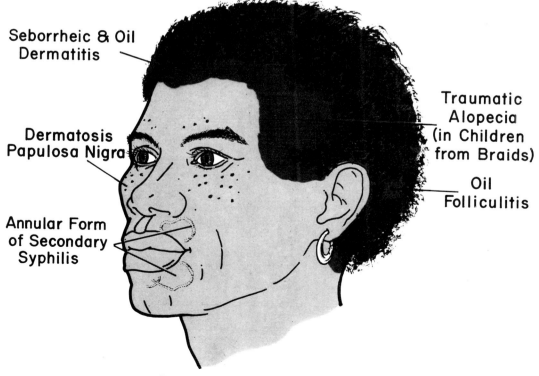

Figure 3–10.   **Black dermogram, head of woman.**

BIBLIOGRAPHY

Ackerman AB, Cockerell CJ: Cutaneous lesions: correlations from microscopic to gross morphologic features. Cutis 37:137–138, 1986

Ackerman AB, Cockerell CJ: Papules. Cutis 37:242–245, 1986

Kenney JA (ed): Black dermatology. Cutis 32:334, 1983

McDonald CJ: Some thoughts on differences in black and white skin. Int J Dermatol 15:427, 1976

Rosen T, Martin S: Atlas of Black Dermatology. Boston, Little, Brown & Co, 1981

4

Your Introduction to the Patient

> SAUER NOTES:
>
> A careful history from the patient taken by the physician is (1) important medically, (2) impresses the patient with your concern, and (3) establishes early-on a necessary favorable rapport between you and the patient.

After the usual conversation introducing yourself to the new patient, the following might transpire:

PHYSICIAN: "What can I do for you, Mrs. Jones?"

MRS. JONES: "I have a bad breaking out on my hands."

PHYSICIAN (*Writes on his chart under present complaint, "hand dermatitis"*): "How long have you had this breaking out?"

MRS. JONES: "Well, I've had this before, but what I have now has been here for only 3 weeks."

PHYSICIAN (*Writes "duration, 3 weeks."*): "When did you have this before, Mrs. Jones?"

MRS. JONES: "Let me see. I believe I had this twice before. The first time I had this breaking out was shortly after our marriage, and I thought that it had to do with the fact that I had my hands in soap and water more than before. It took about a month to heal up. I treated it with salves

that I had at home. It certainly wasn't bad then. The next time I broke out it was a little bit worse. This was after my first child was born. Johnny is 3 years old now. I suppose I should have expected my hands to break out again now because I just had my second baby 3 months ago."

PHYSICIAN: (*Has just finished writing down the following: "The patient states that she has had this eruption on two previous occasions. Home treatment only. Both eruptions lasted approximately 1 month. Present eruption attributed to care of baby born 3 months ago."*): "Mrs. Jones, what have you been putting on your hands for this breaking out?"

MRS. JONES: "Let me take off my bandages, and I'll show you how my hands look."

PHYSICIAN: "Let me help you with those bandages. However, I want to ask you a few more questions before I look at your hands."

MRS. JONES: "Well, first I used a salve that I got over at the corner drugstore that said on the label it was good for athlete's foot. One of my neighbors told me that she used it for her hand trouble, and it had cured her hands. I don't think that her hands looked like mine, though, and I sort of feel that the salve made my hands worse. Then I decided I would burn out the infection, so I soaked my hands in some bleaching solution. This helped some with the itching, but it made the skin too dry. Then I remembered that you had given me some salve for Johnny's 'infantigo,' so I put some of that on. That softened up my hands but didn't seem to help with the itching. So here I am, Doctor."

PHYSICIAN: (*Writing, "Treated with athlete's foot* ℞*, Bleach soaks, Johnny's impetigo* ℞*,"*): "How much itching are you having?"

MRS. JONES: "Well, my hands sting and burn when I get any soap and water on them, but I can sleep without them bothering me."

PHYSICIAN: (*Notes "mild itching."*): "Are you taking any medicine by mouth now for anything? I even want to know about laxatives, vitamins, or aspirin. Have you had any shots recently?"

MRS. JONES: "No, I'm not taking any medicine."

PHYSICIAN: "Now, are you sure?"

MRS. JONES: "Well I do take sleeping medicine at night occasionally, and, oh yes, I'm taking some reducing pills that Dr. Smith gave me about 2 months ago."

PHYSICIAN: (*Writes, "Drugs—takes sleeping medicine h.s. and reducing pills."*): "Mrs. Jones, does anyone in your family have any allergies? Does anyone have any asthma, hay fever, or eczema? Your parents, brothers, sisters, children, other family members?"

MRS. JONES: "No, not that I can recall, Doctor."

PHYSICIAN: "Have you ever had any of those conditions? Any asthma, hay fever, or eczema?"

MRS. JONES: "No, I haven't had any of those. Sometimes I have a little sinus trouble though."

PHYSICIAN: (*Writes, "No atopy in patient or family."*): "Now, let me have a good look at those hands. I also want you to remove your shoes and hose so that I can get a good look at your feet." (*The physician then examines the patient's hands and feet very carefully.*) "Now are you sure that you don't have this anywhere else, Mrs. Jones?"

MRS. JONES: "No I am positive I don't, because I looked all over my skin this morning when I took a bath. However, I do have a mole on my back that I want you to look at, Doctor."

PHYSICIAN: "Has it been bothering you recently?"

MRS. JONES: "Well, no, but my bra strap rubs it occasionally."

PHYSICIAN: (*Examines the mole on her back.*): "That certainly is a small mole, Mrs. Jones. It doesn't have any unusual color, and I see no reason for having it removed. It could be removed if you wish, but I don't think it is necessary."

MRS. JONES: "Well, I don't want it removed if you don't think it is necessary. Now, what do you think about my hands?"

PHYSICIAN: "Let me make a few notes about what I saw and then I'll tell you about your hands and the treatment."

The physician writes, "Physical exam: (1) A crusting, vesicular dermatitis is seen mainly in the webs of the fingers of both hands, worse on the right hand. There is no sharp border to the eruption. The nail of the right ring finger has several transverse furrows. The feet are clear. (2) In the midline of the upper back is a 3 × 3-mm flat, faintly brownish lesion. Diagnosis: (1) Contact dermatitis, probably due to excess soap and water. (2) Pigmented compound nevus."

SAUER NOTES:

As part of a good examination record, one should place in the patient's chart simple diagrams appropriately marked with the site, size, and configuration of growths, scars, rashes, and so on.

1. One need not be an artist to draw a face, a back, a chest, or a hand. One can also use a printed sticker or stamp of the site.

2. Mark in the lesions or configurations and note the size.

3. The value of these simple annotations is multiple. They benefit you, your patient, and, if necessary, your lawyer.

PHYSICIAN: "Mrs. Jones, you have a very common skin condition, commonly called housewives' eczema or housewives' dermatitis. I feel sure that it is aggravated by having your hands in soap and water so many times a day. Most housewives don't even have enough time to dry their hands carefully every time they are wet. Some persons seem to be more sensitive to soaps than others. It isn't a real allergy but just a sensitivity, because the soap and the water have a tendency to remove the normal skin's protective oils and fats. Some of those blisters are infected, and we will have to take care of that infection along with the other irritation. Here is what we will do to treat your hands." (*The physician then gives very careful instructions to* *Mrs. Jones, particularly with regard to the hand soaks, the way the salve is to be applied, advice concerning avoidance of excess soap and water, the use of rubber and cotton gloves, and so on.*)

In the previous play-by-play description, a type of conversation that is repeated many times a month in any busy practitioner's office, I have attempted to show some of the basic points in history-taking.

A careful history is followed by a complete examination of the skin problem, and this, in turn, is followed by therapy, or what I prefer to call *management*. For good management of the patient, I have found it helpful to write out the diagnosis, other information, and instructions on noncarbon forms. (The Drawing Board, Dallas, TX 75221 calls them Mem-O-Grams, Fig. 4-1.) Advantages to the patient and physician are multiple. The patient has an individualized short note about the diagnosis, cause (if known), what the physician can or cannot do (if there is "no cure" as for atopic eczema or psoriasis, say so), and instructions as to diet, bathing, therapy, and so on.

For the physician, the advantage is that a copy can be kept in the patient's chart that could be used later to help refresh the patient's mind about instructions, or it could even be used advantageously in a medicolegal problem regarding information given to the patient.

SAUER NOTES:

1. A careful, thorough medical history from your patient is *very* important.

2. *Local Treatment History.* Find out how much treatment and what kind of local treatment has been administered by the patient or by physicians. Many over-the-counter medications can aggravate a dermatosis.

3. *Systemic Drug History.* Don't just ask "Are you taking any medicines?" Ask "Are you taking any medicine for *any* reason? Are you on birth control pills (if appropriate), are you on vitamins or sleeping pills, do you take aspirin or Tylenol, do you get any shots, etc." This history is important for two reasons. First, something about the patient can be learned from the drugs taken. For example, it is important to know if a person is taking insulin for diabetes or corticosteroids for arthritis. This information can well influence your treatment of the patient. Second, drugs can cause many skin eruptions, and your index of suspicion of a drug eruption will be higher if that information is consistently requested.

4. *Allergy History.* "Do you or did you ever have any asthma, hay fever, eczema, or migraine headaches?" A positive allergy history is important for two reasons. First, a family or a patient history of allergies can aid in making a diagnosis of atopic dermatitis. Second, if there is a positive allergy history, usually it can be predicted that the patient's skin disorder will be slower in responding to treatment than a similar dermatitis in a nonallergic patient. Patients with atopy are more "itchish."

SAUER NOTES:

When a patient is in the hospital, many persons in white coats or with a stethoscope around their neck come and go. The visit of the dermatologic consultant (or others) may be forgotten in the confusion and misery of the hospital confinement.

There is a simple measure that should help the patient remember the dermatologist's visit. You leave your calling card.

This card has your name, address, and phone number. You can even write on the reverse some information you may wish to convey about the skin problem you were asked to see. And when your bill comes, the patient and family will have your calling card as a reminder of your visit.

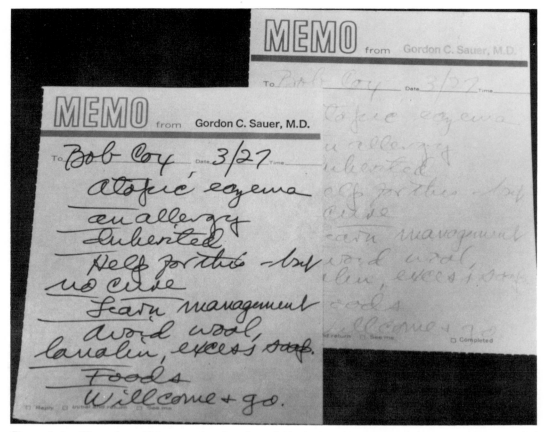

Figure 4–1. **Memo form.** This noncarbon form is useful for both patient and physician to provide a record of information and instructions given in the office.

SAUER NOTES:

The specialty of dermatology, like any medical field, needs good public relations efforts. However, most importantly, we need to promote better public relations in our own sphere of influence.

First, one needs to provide correct diagnoses, correct therapy, and proper management for the patient. This should be our most tangible public relations effort.

Second, it is important to be a visible dermatologist. This can be accomplished by attending medical meetings and assuming offices in medical societies. There are also medical societies in surrounding communities that need speakers. When one begins practice, it helps to go from door to door, at least in your own office building, to meet the possible referring physicians face to face.

Third, after you get a patient referred from another physician, do not fail to thank the physician. Write a note and include the diagnosis with a short description of your treatment.

Fourth, a physician should provide services to the community. One can give medical talks to lay groups and can serve on civic committees.

Five, physicians should have courteous and competent personnel in the office. Pay attention to what goes on at your front desk.

5

Dermatologic Therapy

Many hundreds of medications are available for use in treating skin diseases. However, most physicians have only a few favorite prescriptions that are prescribed day in and day out. These few prescriptions may then be altered slightly to suit an individual patient or disease.

The treatment of the majority of the common skin conditions can be made simpler if the physician is aware of three basic principles:

1. The *type of skin lesion*, more than the cause, influences the kind of local medication used. The old adage, "If it's wet, use a wet dressing, and if it's dry use a salve," is true for a majority of cases. For example, to treat a patient with an acute oozing, crusting dermatitis of the dorsum of the hand, whether due to poison ivy or soap, the physician should prescribe wet soaks. For a chronic-looking, dry, scaly patch of psoriasis on the elbow, an ointment or cream is indicated, since a lotion or a wet dressing would only be more drying. Bear in mind, however, that *the type of skin lesion can change rapidly under treatment*. The patient must be followed closely after beginning therapy. An acute oozing dermatitis treated with soaks can change, in 2 to 3 days, to a dry, scaly lesion that requires a cream or an ointment. Conversely, a chronic dry patch may become irritated with too strong therapy and begin to ooze.

2. The second basic principle in treatment is *never do any harm* and never overtreat. It is important for the physician to know which of the chemicals prescribed for local use on the skin are the greatest irritants and sensitizers. It is no exaggeration to say that the most commonly seen dermatitis is the *overtreatment contact dermatitis*. The overtreatment is often performed by the patient, who has gone to the neighborhood drugstore, or to a friend, and used any, and many, of the medications available for the treatment of skin diseases. It is certainly not unusual to hear the patient tell of using a strong athlete's foot salve for the treatment of the lesions of pityriasis rosea.

3. The third principle is to *instruct the patient adequately regarding the application of the medicine prescribed*. The patient does not have to be told how to swallow a pill but does have to be told how to put on a wet dressing. Most patients with skin disorders are ambulatory, so there is no nurse to help them. They are their own nurse. The success or the failure of therapy rests on adequate instruction of the patient or person responsible for the care. Even in hospitals, particularly when wet dressings or lotions are prescribed, it is wise for the physician to instruct the nurse regarding the procedure.

With these principles of management in mind, let us now turn to the medicine used. It is important to stress that I am endeavoring to present here only the most basic material necessary to treat the majority of skin diseases. For instance, there are many solutions for wet dressings, but Burow's solution is my preference. Other physicians have preferences different from the drugs listed, and their choices

SAUER NOTES ON LOCAL THERAPY: SUMMARY

1. The type of skin lesion (oozing, infected, or dry), more than the cause, should determine the local medication that is prescribed.

2. Do not harm. Begin local therapy for a particular case with mild drugs. The concentration of ingredients can be increased as the acuteness subsides.

3. Do not begin local corticosteroid therapy with the "biggest gun" available, particularly for chronic dermatoses.

4. Carefully instruct the patient or the nurse regarding the local application of salves, lotions, wet dressings, and baths. Many salves should be rubbed in for 5 to 10 seconds.

5. Prescribe the correct amount of medication for the area and the dermatosis to be treated. This knowledge comes with experience. (See p. 43.)

6. Change the therapy as the response indicates. If a new prescription is indicated and the patient has some of the first prescription left, instruct the patient to alternate using the old and the new prescription.

7. If a prescription is going to be relatively expensive, explain this fact to the patient.

8. For many diseases, "therapy plus" is indicated. Here you advise the patient to continue to treat the skin problem for 4 days (5 days, 10 days, *etc.*) after the dermatosis has apparently cleared. This may prevent or slow down recurrences.

9. Instruct the patient to telephone you if there are any questions or if the medicine seems to irritate the dermatosis.

are respected, but to list all of them will not serve the purpose of this book.

Two factors have guided me in the selection of medications presented in this formulary. First, the medication must be readily available in most drugstores; second, it must be a very effective medication for one or several skin conditions. The medications listed in this formulary will also be listed in a complete way in the treatment section concerning the particular disease. However, instructions for the use of the medications will be more nearly complete in this formulary.

FORMULARY

A particular topical medication is prescribed to produce a specific beneficial effect.

Effects of Locally Applied Drugs

1. **Antipruritic agents** relieve itching in various ways. Commonly used chemicals and strengths include menthol (0.25%), phenol (0.5%), camphor (2%), and coal tar solution (liquor carbonis detergens [L.C.D.]) (2% to 10%). These chemicals are added to various bases for the desired effect. Numerous safe and unsafe proprietary preparations for relief of itching are also available. The unsafe preparations are those that contain antihistamines, benzocaine, and related "-caine" derivatives.

2. **Keratoplastic agents** tend to increase the thickness of the horny layer. Salicylic acid (1% to 2%) is an example of a keratoplastic agent. Stronger strengths of salicylic acid are keratolytic.

3. **Keratolytics** remove or soften the horny layer. Commonly used agents of this type include salicylic acid (4% to 10%), resorcinol (2% to 4%), and sulfur (4% to 10%). A *strong* destructive agent is trichloroacetic acid, full strength.

4. **Antieczematous agents** remove oozing and vesicular excretions by various actions. The common antieczematous agents include Burow's solution packs or soaks, coal tar solution (2% to 5%), and hydrocortisone (0.5% to 2%) and derivatives incorporated in lotions or salves.

5. **Antiparasitics** destroy or inhibit living infestations. Examples include Eurax lotion and cream, for scabies, and Kwell cream and lotion, for scabies and pediculosis.

6. **Antiseptics** destroy or inhibit bacteria, fungi, and viruses. *Antibacterial* topical medications include gentamicin (Garamycin), mupirocin (Bactroban) meclocycline sulfosalicylate (Meclan), bacitracin, and neomycin. (Neomycin causes an appreciable incidence of allergic contact sensitivity.) Older antibacterial agents in-

cluded iodochlorhydroxyquin (Vioform) and ammoniated mercury (3% to 10%).

Antifungal and *anticandidal* topical agents include miconazole (Micatin, Monistat-derm), haloprogin (Halotex), clotrimazole (Lotrimin, Mycelex), ciclopirox (Loprox), econazole (Spectazole), oxiconazole (Oxistat), naftifine (Naftin), ketoconazole (Nizoral), and sulconazol (Excelderm). Sulfur (3% to 10%) is an older but effective antifungal.

An *antiviral* topical agent is acyclovir (Zovirax) ointment.

7. **Emollients** soften the skin surface. Nivea oil, mineral oil, and white petrolatum are good examples. Newer emollients are more cosmetically elegant and effective.

SAUER NOTES ON LOCALLY APPLIED GENERIC PRODUCTS:

1. *Advantages:* Less cost—you can prescribe a larger quantity at relatively less expense, and patients appreciate your sharing their concern regarding cost.

2. *Disadvantages:* With a proprietary product you are quite sure of the correct potency of the agent, you know the delivery system, and you know the ingredients in the base.

3. If you prescribe a proprietary medication when a less expensive generic is available, explain to the patient your reason for doing this.

Types of Topical Dermatologic Medications

I. **Baths**
   A. Tar Bath
      Coal tar solution, USP (liquor carbonis detergens [L.C.D.])   120.0
      Sig: 2 tablespoons to the tub of lukewarm water, 6 to 8 inches deep
      Actions: Antipruritic, and antieczematous
   B. Starch Bath
      Linit or Argo Starch, small box
      Sig: ½ box of starch to the tub of cool water, 6 to 8 inches deep

Actions: Soothing, antipruritic
Indications: Generalized itching and dryness of skin, winter itch, urticaria
   C. Aveeno Colloidal Oatmeal Bath
      Sig: 1 cup to the tub of water
      Actions: Soothing and cleansing
      Indications: Generalized itching and dryness of skin and winter and senile itch.
   D. Oil Baths (See Oils and Emulsions, Section VI, below)

II. **Soaps and Shampoos**
   A. Oilatum Soap Unscented, Dove, Neutrogena Soaps, Lowila
      Actions: Mild cleansing agent
      Indications: Dry skin, winter itch
   B. Dial Soap
      Actions: Cleansing, antibacterial
      Indications: Acne, pyodermas
   C. Selsun Suspension or Exsel Shampoo   120.0
      Sig: Shampoo hair with three separate applications and rinses. Can leave the last application on the scalp for 5 minutes before rinsing off. Do not use another shampoo as a final cleanser.
      Actions: Cleansing, antiseborrheic
      Indications: Dandruff or itching scalp (not toxic if used as directed)
   D. Tar Shampoos: Polytar, T/Gel, X Seb T, Sebutone, Ionil-T, Vanseb-T, and so on
      Sig: Shampoo as necessary, even daily
      Actions: Cleansing and antiseborrheic
      Indications: Dandruff, psoriasis, or atopic eczema of scalp

III. **Wet Dressings or Soaks**
   A. Burow's Solution, 1 : 20
      Sig: 1 Domeboro tablet or packet to 1 pint of tap water. Cover affected area with sheeting wet with solution and tie on with gauze bandage or string. Do not allow any wet dressing to dry out. It can also be used as a solution for soaks.
      Actions: Acidifying, antieczematous, antiseptic
      Indications: Oozing or vesicular skin conditions. Do not use over a large area of the body.

B. Vinegar Solution
Sig: ½ cup of white vinegar to 1 quart of water.
For wet dressings or soaks as above.

IV. Powders
A. Purified Talc (USP) or Zeasorb Powder   60.0
Sig: Dust on locally b.i.d. (Supply in a powder can.)
Actions: Absorbent, protective, cooling
Indications: Intertrigo, diaper dermatitis

B. Tinactin Powder, Micatin Powder, Zeasorb-AF Powder, or Desenex Powder
Sig: Dust on feet in morning.
Actions: Absorbent, antifungal.
Indications: Prevention or treatment of tinea pedis, tinea cruris
The above powders are available over the counter.

C. Mycostatin Powder   15.0
Sig: Dust on locally b.i.d.
Actions: Anticandidal
Indications: Candidal intertrigo

V. Shake Lotions
A. Calamine Lotion (USP)   120.0
Sig: Apply locally to affected area t.i.d. with fingers or brush.
Actions: Antipruritic, antieczematous
Indications: Widespread, mildly oozing, inflamed dermatoses

B. Nonalcoholic White Shake Lotion
Zinc oxide   24.0
Talc   24.0
Glycerin   12.0
Distilled water q.s. ad   120.0

C. Alcoholic White Shake Lotion
Zinc oxide   24.0
Talc   24.0
Glycerin   12.0
Distilled water
95% alcohol āā q.s. ad   120.0

D. Colored Alcoholic Shake Lotion
To **V–C** above, add: Sun Chemical pigments (brunette shade)   2.4

E. Proprietary Lotions
Sarna Lotion (with menthol and camphor), Cetaphil Lotion

VI. Oils and Emulsions
A. Zinc Oil
Zinc oxide   40%
Olive oil q.s.   120.0

Sig: Apply locally to affected area by hand or brush t.i.d.
Actions: Soothing, antipruritic, and astringent
Indications: Acute and subacute eczematous eruptions

B. Bath Oils
Nivea Skin Oil or
Alpha-Keri or
Domol or
Geri Bath
Sig: 1 to 2 tablespoonfuls to the tub of water. Be careful to avoid slipping in tub.
Actions: Emollient, lubricating
Indications: Winter itch, dry skin, atopic eczema

C. Hand and Body Emulsions
There are a multitude of products available. Some have phospholipids, some have urea, and some are lanolin free.
Sig: (No prescription required). Apply locally as necessary.
Actions: Emollient, lubricating
Indications: Dry skin, winter itch, atopic eczema

VII. Tinctures and Aqueous Solutions
A. Povidone-iodine (Betadine) Solution (also in skin cleanser, shampoo, and ointment)   15.0
Sig: Apply with swab t.i.d.
Actions: Antibacterial, antifungal, antiviral, and so on.
Indication: General antisepsis

B. Thimerosol Tincture (N.F.)
Merthiolate Tincture, 1 : 1000
Sig: Apply with swab t.i.d.
Actions: Antibacterial, antifungal, and drying

C. Gentian Violet Solution
Gentian Violet   1%

TARS (COAL TAR SOLUTION (L.C.D.), 3–10%;
CRUDE COAL TAR, 1–5%; ANTHRALIN,
0.1–1%)
Consider for use in cases of:

Atopic eczema
Psoriasis
Seborrheic dermatitis
Neurodermatitis, localized

Avoid in intertriginous areas (can cause a
folliculitis).

SULFUR (SULFUR, PRECIPITATED, 3–10%)
Consider for use in cases of:

Tinea of any area of body
Acne vulgaris and rosacea
Seborrheic dermatitis
Pyodermas (combine with antibiotic salves)
Psoriasis

Avoid: Do not mix with mercury (causes
black mercuric sulfide deposit on skin).

MERCURY (AMMONIATED MERCURY, 1–10%)
Consider for use in cases of:

Psoriasis
Pyodermas
Seborrheic dermatitis

Avoid: Do not mix with sulfur (see sulfur,
above).

RESORCINOL
(RESORCINOL MONOACETATE, 1–5%)
Consider for use in cases of:

Acne vulgaris and rosacea (usually with sul-
fur)
Seborrheic dermatitis
Psoriasis

SALICYLIC ACID
(1–5%, HIGHER WITH CAUTION)
Consider for use in cases of:

Psoriasis
Neurodermatitis, localized thick form
Tinea of feet or palms (when peeling is de-
sired)
Seborrheic dermatitis

Avoid in intertriginous areas.

MENTHOL (¼%); PHENOL (½–2%);
CAMPHOR (1–2%)
Consider for use in any pruritic derma-
toses.
Avoid use over large areas of body.

HYDROCORTISONE AND RELATED
CORTICOSTEROIDS (HYDROCORTISONE
POWDER, ½–2%)
Consider for use in cases of:

Contact dermatitis of any area
Seborrheic dermatitis
Intertrigo of axillary, crural, or inframammary
regions
Atopic eczema
Neurodermatitis

Avoid use over large areas of body, because of expense, and possible, but unlikely,
internal absorption.

FLUORINATED CORTICOSTEROIDS LOCALLY
These chemicals are not readily available
as powders for personal compounding, but
triamcinolone, fluocinolone, and others are
available as generic creams and ointments.
Consider for use with or without occlusive
dressings, in cases of:

Psoriasis, localized to small area (see Chap.
14).
Neurodermatitis, localized (see Chap. 11)
Lichen planus, especially hypertrophic type
Also anywhere that hydrocortisone is indi-
cated

Avoid use over large areas of the body (see
Sauer Notes following).

QUANTITY OF CREAM OR OINTMENT
TO PRESCRIBE
Several factors influence any general statements: severity of the dermatosis, acute or
chronic dermatosis, base of the product (a pet-
rolatum-based ointment spreads over the skin
farther than a cream), whether dispensed in a
tube or jar (patients use less from tubes), and
the intelligence of the patient.

15 grams of a cream used b.i.d. will treat a
mild hand dermatosis for 10 to 14 days.
30 grams of a cream used b.i.d. will treat an
arm for 14 days.
60 grams of a cream used b.i.d. will treat a leg
for 14 days.
For the entire body treated b.i.d. for 14 days
one would need 480 to 960 grams or 1 to 2
lbs. This is seldom a practical prescription,
but unmedicated white petrolatum or a
cream base is economical to use over a
large surface area. Other therapeutic
agents should be used to make the derma-

tosis less extensive (*e.g.*, internal corticosteroids).

SAUER NOTES ON LOCAL CORTICOSTEROID THERAPY:

1. Avoid prescribing strong local corticosteroid preparations for generalized body use.

2. Do not prescribe the most potent ("biggest-gun") corticosteroid therapy on the initial visit.

3. The fluorinated corticosteroids should not be used on the face and intertriginous areas where long-term use can result in atrophy and telangiectasia of the skin.

4. The potent corticosteroids have a definite systemic effect.

5. Fluorinated corticosteroid prescriptions only rarely should be written for p.r.n. refills.

6. Continued long-term use of a local corticosteroid can result in a diminished effectiveness (tachyphylaxis).

7. The pros and cons of prescribing *generic* corticosteroids are discussed early in the chapter.

SPECIFIC INTERNAL DRUGS FOR SPECIFIC DISEASES

As in all fields of medicine, there are certain diseases that can be treated best by certain specific systemic drugs. These drugs may not be curative, but they should be considered when beginning to outline a course of management for a particular patient. Many factors will influence the decision to use or not use such a specific drug. Here follows a list of skin diseases and some systemic medicines considered specific (or as specific as "specific" can be) for the disease. *For proper dosage and contraindications, check the appropriate sections in this book or in current books on therapy.*

Acne vulgaris or rosacea in the scarring stage: antibiotics and birth control pills. For severe cases of cystic acne in men, isotretinoin (Accutane) is indicated.

Alopecia areata: rarely corticosteroids in any of three forms—oral, parenteral, and intralesional

Atrophie blanche vasculitis: pentoxifylline (Trental)

Blastomycosis: amphotericin B, administered in hospital

Creeping eruption: thiabendazole

Darier's disease: vitamin A, for controlled periods of time, and possibly isotretinoin

Dermatitis herpetiformis: dapsone and sulfapyridine

Granuloma annulare: intralesional corticosteroids

Herpes simplex: acyclovir (Zovirax)

Inflammation of the skin from many causes: antibiotics are indicated, in some cases, when local therapy is inadequate for control. Nonsteroidal anti-inflammatory drugs are beneficial for some diseases.

Keloids: intralesional corticosteroids

Lupus erythematosus: for systemic lupus erythematosus, use corticosteroids or immunosuppressive agents with care; for discoid form use hydroxychloroquine and related antimalarials (beware of eye damage).

Mycosis fungoides: corticosteroids and antimetabolites

Necrobiosis lipoidica diabeticorum: intralesional corticosteroids

Neurodermatitis, localized: intralesional corticosteroids

Pemphigus: corticosteriods and antimetabolites

Pruritus from many causes: antihistamines and tranquilizer-like drugs. Selected cases can be treated with oral corticosteroids.

Psoriasis, localized: intralesional corticosteroids

Psoriasis, severe: corticosteroids, psoralens and ultraviolet light (PUVA), methotrexate, and, in men or postmenopausal women, etretinate (Tegison)

Pyodermas of skin: systemic antibiotics are valuable, when indicated.

Sarcoidosis: possibly corticosteroids

Sporotrichosis: saturated aqueous solution of potassium iodide and ketoconazole (Nizoral)

Syphilis: penicillin or other antibiotics

Tinea of scalp, body, crural area, fingernails (not feet or toenails): griseofulvin and, for selected cases, ketoconazole

Tuberculosis of the skin: dihydrostreptomycin, isoniazid, *p*-aminosalicyclic acid, and rifampin

Urticaria: antihistamines and corticosteroids

SAUER NOTES:

1. There are potential side-effects from any systemic therapy. Be aware of these possible reactions by being knowledgeable concerning *every* drug you prescribe.
2. The risk–benefit ratio for your patient must always be considered.
3. Be aware of cross-reactions with a patient on multiple medications.

BIBLIOGRAPHY

Arndt KA: Manual of Dermatologic Therapeutics, 4th ed. Boston, Little, Brown & Co, 1989

Council on Scientific Affairs: Vitamin preparations as dietary supplements and as therapeutic agents. JAMA 257:1929, 1987

DiGiovanna JJ, Peck GL: Retinoid toxicity. Prog Dermatol 21(3), 1987

Edwards L: Interferon. Arch Dermatol 123:743, 1987

Goette DK: Salicylic acid. J Assoc Milit Dermatologists 15:24, 1989

Gupta MA, Gupta AK, Ellis CN: Antidepressant drugs in dermatology. Arch Dermatol 123:647, 1987

Hirschmann JV: Topical antibiotics in dermatology. Arch Dermatol 124:1691, 1988

Lin AN, Reimer RJ, Carter DM: Sulfur revisited. J Am Acad Dermatol 18:553, 1988

Lynch PJ: Dermatologic therapy with systemically administered agents. Prog Dermatol 17(3 & 4), 1983

Lynfield YL, Schechter S: Choosing and using a vehicle. J Am Acad Dermatol 10:56, 1984

Physician's Desk Reference (PDR). Oradell, NJ, Medical Economics, published yearly.

Sherertz EF: Pharmacology: I. Topical therapy in dermatology. J Am Acad Dermatol 21:108, 1989

Sherertz EF: Pharmacology: II. Systemic drugs in dermatology. J Am Acad Dermatol 21:298, 1989

Smith MC, Kibbe AH, Brown TR: Dermatologic prescriptions requiring compounding. J Am Acad Dermatol 11:148, 1984

Stoughton RB: Are generic topical glucocorticosteroids equivalent to the brand name? J Am Acad Dermatol 18:138, 1988

6

Physical Dermatologic Therapy

The field of physical medicine embraces therapy with a variety of agents, which include massage, therapeutic exercise, water, air, radiations (heat, light, ultraviolet, x-rays, radium, and lasers), vibrations, refrigeration, and electricity of various forms. Many of these agents are used in the treatment of skin diseases.

HYDROTHERAPY

The physical agent most commonly used for dermatoses is hydrotherapy, in the form of medicated or nonmedicated wet compresses and baths. Distilled water and tap water are the vehicles and may contain any of the following chemicals in varying strengths, sodium chloride, aluminum acetate (Burow's solution), potassium permanganate, silver nitrate, tar, starch, oatmeal (Aveeno), and colloid (Soyaloid). The instructions and the dilutions for Burow's solution compresses, starch baths, and tar baths are listed in the Formulary (see Chap. 5).

Wet Dressings

Wet dressings can be applied as open or closed dressings. The *open* compresses are used most frequently, since excessive maceration of tissue occurs when the dressings are "closed" with plastic wrap or rubber sheeting. The compresses can be *hot, cold,* or *at room temperature.* Instructions to the patient or the nurse concerning correct application of the compresses should be explicit and de-

tailed. For most conditions, the area to be treated should be wrapped with two or three layers of clean gauze sheeting or muslin. Additional gauze 3 inches wide should be wrapped around the sheeting to hold it firmly in place. After that, the dressing can be moistened with the solution by pouring it on or by squirting it under the dressing with a bulb syringe. In most instances the dressing is wet with the solution before it is wrapped on the affected area. The compresses should never be allowed to dry out and should be left on only for the time specified by the physician. The solution used should be made fresh every day. For treating the face, the hands, and the genitalia, special masks, gloves, and slings can be improvised. The indications for wet compresses are any oozing, crusting, or pruritic dermatoses, regardless of cause.

Medicated Baths

Medicated baths should last from 15 to 30 minutes. Cool baths tend to lessen pruritus and are prescribed most frequently. Baths can be used for a multitude of skin diseases except those conditions for which excessive dryness is to be avoided, such as for patients with atopic eczema, senile or winter pruritus, and ichthyosis.

ELECTROSURGERY

Electrosurgery is employed very commonly in treating or removing a multitude of skin lesions. One of several different types of available currents and instruments is employed to achieve a desired result. Five forms of electrosurgery are available. (See also Chapter 7 on Fundamentals of Cutaneous Surgery.)

Electrodesiccation or Fulguration

Electrodesiccation, or fulguration, is produced by an Oudin current of high voltage and low amperage, using a single or monoterminal electrode. The high-frequency current wave is damped. Such a current is produced by the Hyfrecator and by the larger Surgitron, Bovie, or Wappler units, using the spark-gap part of the machine. The effect on the skin is a charring of the tissues.

Electrocoagulation

Electrocoagulation is produced by a d'Arsonval current of relatively low voltage and high amperage, using biterminal electrodes. This current also is damped and can be obtained from the Hyfrecator, Surgitron, Bovie, and the Wappler combination units, using the spark-gap part of the machine. Electrocoagulation is more destructive than electrodesiccation, owing to the intense heat.

Electrosection

Electrosection, or cutting, is produced by a current that is undamped when delivered by a vacuum tube apparatus and moderately damped from a spark-gap apparatus. Biterminal electrodes are used. The large Bovie and Wappler combination units produce a moderately damped current from the spark-gap part of the machine and an undamped current from the vacuum tube part. When the vacuum tube cutting current is used, the cut is clean, with practically no coagulation, whereas the current from a spark-gap machine produces some coagulation of the cut skin edge. Any coagulation can be minimized by making a rapid stroke. Tissue skillfully removed in this manner can be studied histologically, if necessary.

Electrocautery

Electrocautery is simply produced by applying heat to the skin. This can be supplied by many instruments, one of which is the Post Electric Cautery (Andover, NJ). Many operators prefer this form of electrosurgery to electrodesiccation or electrocoagulation.

Electrolysis

Electrolysis uses a direct galvanic current to produce chemical cauterization of tissue due to the formation of sodium hydroxide in the tissues, with liberation of free hydrogen at the negative electrode. Battery machines or rectified direct-current instruments accomplish this. Electrolysis is used mainly to remove superfluous hair. A faster and less painful technique of hair epilation is to use the high-frequency current set at a very low intensity where it will deliver a small electrodesiccation spark.

The dermatoses most commonly treated by electrosurgery are warts of all kinds, actinic and seborrheic keratoses, leukoplakia, pig-

---

SAUER NOTES:

1. Electrosurgery must be used with caution on patients with cardiac pacemakers. If the current is applied in short bursts of only 5 seconds or less, this procedure appears to be safe.

2. If alcohol has been used to prepare the surgery site, make sure it has evaporated and alcohol pledgets are removed from the area before performing electrosurgery.

mented nevi, spider hemangiomas, hypertrichosis, and basal cell and squamous cell carcinomas. The skill and the experience of the therapists will be the factors determining the scope of their use of the surgical diathermy machine. Disposable electrode tips are available.

CRYOSURGERY

Therapeutic refrigeration for the skin can be accomplished by the use of solid carbon dioxide, liquid nitrogen, or freon 114.

Solid carbon dioxide is used quite commonly because it is readily available from a tank of carbon dioxide, or as blocks from ice cream manufacturers, or from the Kidde Dry Ice Apparatus (see p. 389). The temperature of solid carbon dioxide is $-78.5°$ C. The solid carbon dioxide is shaped into an appropriately sized "pencil" for treatment of superficial skin growths, warts, or seborrheic keratoses.

Liquid nitrogen, which provides freezing at $-195.8°$ C, has become more readily available for office use. Many dermatologists now have a 25-liter, refillable container in their office. This amount will last for 3 to 4 weeks, with normal usage. A loosely wound large cotton-tipped applicator is used to hold the smoking liquid (Figs. 6–1 and 6–2). The applicator is applied to the skin for only a few seconds to freeze warts, seborrheic keratoses, actinic keratoses, and other superficial skin growths. The pain varies from moderate to quite marked. A blister forms within 24 hours after the application, and it is hoped that the growth comes off entirely when the dead skin peels away in 10 to 14 days. Additional liquid nitrogen applications may be indicated.

Liquid nitrogen can be sprayed on the skin. There are several spray units available, with varying degrees of sophistication and cost.

Freon 114 is used mainly to freeze and immobilize the skin for the dermabrasion removal of acne scars, tatoos, or senile keratotic skin.

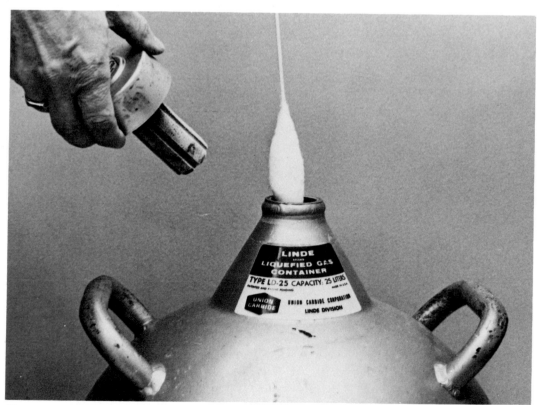

Figure 6–1. **Liquid nitrogen cryosurgery.** A 25-liter container with approximately a 3-week supply of liquid nitrogen. The cotton-tipped applicator is dipped into the liquid for application to the skin.

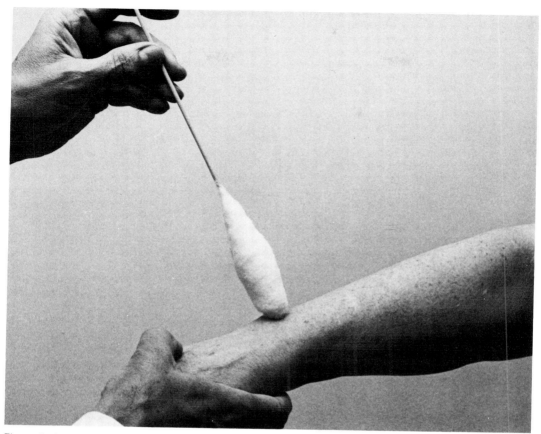

Figure 6–2. **Liquid nitrogen applicator.** One technique of applying liquid nitrogen to skin lesions is with a large or small cotton-tipped applicator.

SAUER NOTES:

1. The length of application of liquid nitrogen cryosurgery should err on the short side rather than on the long side.

2. Seldom does one need to treat a keratosis or wart for longer than 10 to 20 seconds.

3. Overzealous therapy is painful for the patient, is rarely necessary, and will prompt phone calls to the physician at night with concern over a large blood blister and pain.

RADIATION

Radiation agents are important in the field of skin diseases.

Ultraviolet Therapy

Ultraviolet therapy is commonly used and available. There are several sources of artificial ultraviolet radiation.

The *hot quartz mercury vapor lamp* is the most frequently used source for dermatoses. This operates at a high vapor pressure and relatively high temperature, producing middle-wave ultraviolet radiation, in the 290- to 320-nm range, or UVB. These rays cause erythema and tanning of the skin. The dermatoses most commonly treated with the UVB lamp are psoriasis, acne, pityriasis rosea, and seborrheic dermatitis.

The *RS-type bulb* is a commonly used source of ultraviolet radiation for home use. This is a hot quartz, medium pressure, tungsten-filament mercury vapor lamp, with an aluminum reflector. It produces radiation with a peak at 330 nm that tans the skin.

Fluorescent sunlamps are low pressure

mercury vapor lamps in glass tubes internally coated with a white phosphor. They produce waves of moderate intensity, with the main emission in the 280- to 350-nm range. They cause erythema and tanning and are used in specially constructed boothlike units for treatment of psoriasis.

UVA lamps produce high-intensity long-wave ultraviolet radiation, in the 315- to 400-nm range. For decades these wavelengths were believed to be biologically inactive. Newly developed intensified light sources of these wavelengths have been produced. When oral psoralens are given to patients and they are then exposed to this light source, the procedure is known as PUVA therapy. This routine is used to treat psoriasis and vitiligo.

Tanning salons use UVA lamps, but some UVB is emitted. The safety of these units is variable, and regulation, unfortunately, is minimal.

The *cold quartz lamp* operates at a low vapor pressure and low temperature, producing essentially a monochromatic source, at 254 nm, in the UVC range. These rays have insignificant tanning effect and mainly produce desquamation. The use of this lamp in dermatology is limited.

X-ray Therapy

Another of the physical therapeutic agents used for skin diseases is x-ray therapy. A detailed discussion of x-ray therapy is not within the scope of this book, since it is a specialized subject of considerable magnitude. X-ray therapy should be administered only by an adequately trained dermatologist or radiologist. If correct shielding and dosage are observed x-ray therapy is quite safe, as has been proved by many well-controlled studies.

X-ray therapy finds its greatest use in the treatment of skin cancers, various pruritic dermatoses, and cutaneous lymphoblastomas (particularly mycosis fungoides).

For the majority of dermatoses, excluding malignancies, the physical factors of superficial x-ray therapy are 70 to 100 kV-peak, 2 to 5 mA, 20 to 30 cm focal skin distance, and no filter. The half-value layer with these factors varies with the machine from 0.6 to 1.0 mm of aluminum. The average superficial x-ray therapy dose for dermatoses is 75 rad per week. This weekly dose can be given up to a maximum total of 600 to 1,200 rad, if absolutely indicated. The top maximum dose depends on many factors, such as seriousness of the lesion being treated, response of the dermatosis to therapy, complexion and age of the person. *Under no circumstances should such a maximum course of x-ray therapy ever be repeated.* Grenz ray therapy is an even more superficial form of x-ray therapy, and therefore it is potentially less harmful.

Laser

The laser (an acronym for *l*ight *a*mplification by *s*timulated *e*mission of *r*adiation) is an instrument that generates an intensely strong beam of light that is capable of cauterizing, and thus destroying, various skin lesions. The carbon dioxide laser, which produces a beam of intense invisible infrared electromagnetic energy with a wavelength of 10,600 nm, is the laser that at the present is most used for treating dermatologic lesions.

The lesions treated include cutaneous vascular growths, inflammatory masses, tattoos, nevoid lesions, and other growths.

The equipment is very expensive ($25,000 and up) and, to me, for dermatology, is in the category of shooting a mouse with a cannon. Electrosurgical or other surgical procedures appear to accomplish the same task with much less cost. However, the lasers are here to stay in dermatology. (See Chap. 7.)

SAUER NOTES:

My superficial x-ray unit was sold some years ago. The high cost of the malpractice insurance made it impossible to justify my keeping the machine for only occasional usage. But I miss the effectiveness for certain dermatoses, one being palmar psoriasis.

BIBLIOGRAPHY

Anderson TF, Waldinger TP, Voorhees JJ: UV-B phototherapy. Arch Dermatol 120:1502, 1984

Bruyneel-Rapp F, Dorsey SB, Guinn JD: The tanning salon: An area survey of equipment, procedures, and practices. J Am Acad Dermatol 18:1030, 1988

Chue B, Borok M, Lowe NJ: Phototherapy units: Comparison of fluorescent ultraviolet B and ultraviolet A units with a high-pressure mercury system. J Am Acad Dermatol 18:641, 1988

Council on Scientific Affairs: Harmful effects of ultraviolet radiation. JAMA 262:380, 1989

Epstein E, Epstein E Jr: Skin Surgery, 6th ed. Philadelphia, WB Saunders, 1987

Garden JM, O'Banion MK, Shelnitz LS et al: Papillomavirus in the vapor of carbon dioxide laser–treated verrucae. JAMA 259:1199, 1988

Olbricht SM, Arndt KA: Carbon dioxide laser treatment of cutaneous disorders. Mayo Clin Proc 63:297, 1988

Sebben JE: The hazards of electrosurgery. J Am Acad Dermatol 16:869, 1987

Sebben JE: Electrosurgery principles: Cutting current and cutaneous surgery: I. J Dermatol Surg Oncol 14:29, 1988

Sebben JE: Electrosurgery high-frequency modalities. J Dermatol Surg Oncol 14:367, 1988

Sebben JE: Monopolar and bipolar treatment. J Dermatol Surg Oncol 15:364, 1989

Sebben JE: Cutaneous Electrosurgery. Chicago, Year Book Medical Publishers, 1989

Torre D, Lubritz RR, Kuflik EG: Practical Cutaneous Cryosurgery. East Norwalk, CT, Appleton & Lange, 1988

Wheeland RG, Wiley MD: Q-tip cryosurgery for the treatment of senile sebaceous hyperplasia. J Dermatol Surg Oncol 13:729, 1987

7

Fundamentals of Cutaneous Surgery

Frank Custer Koranda, M.D.*

Attention to detail is the essence of surgical perfection. Disregard of or ignorance of any of the fundamentals of surgery is often the difference between the optimal and the merely acceptable scar.

INSTRUMENT SELECTION

If an instrument facilitates one's surgery, it is usually worth its cost. Quality instruments are expensive. For most cutaneous surgery, the Webster needle holder, the neurosurgery needle holder, and the Halsey needle holder are well designed (Fig. 7–1A). Because of the size of the suture and the finer needles that are used, the needle holder should be smooth jawed. For very delicate surgery and for very fine suture, the Castroviejo needle holder is preferred (Fig. 7–1B). The amount of motion necessary to lock and unlock the Castroviejo needle holder is less than for the standard needle holder.

To lessen tissue damage, the skin should be handled in the least traumatic manner. Gentle handling requires the use of skin hooks, such as the single-hook Frazier or the fine double-hook Tyrell. For eyelid tissue it may be advantageous to use the Bishop-Harman ophthalmic forceps (Fig. 7–1C).

The No. 3 scalpel handle is used with the Nos. 10, 11, and 15 blades. It is convenient to obtain scalpels that have a ruler etched into the handle. For scissors dissection, the Metzenbaum, Malis, or Ragnell scissors may be used (Fig. 7–1D). For fine work, a Stevens scissors is well suited (Fig. 7–1E). For cutting sutures precisely and for suture removal, the pointed, delicately curved Gradle scissors are ideal (Fig. 7–1F).

A basic cutaneous surgical pack includes the following:

1. Webster or neurosurgery needle holder
2. Adson forceps with teeth
3. Frazier skin hook (two)
4. Metzenbaum dissecting scissors
5. Stevens curved scissors
6. Gradle scissors
7. Utility scissors
8. Halsted mosquito hemostats (four)
9. Backhaus towel clips, 3½ inch (four)
10. Round toothpicks for marking skin
11. Gauze sponges
12. Cotton-tipped applicators for point control of bleeding

* Associate Clinical Professor of Otolaryngology-Head and Neck Surgery and Dermatology, University of Kansas Medical Center, Kansas City, Kansas

(See also Chapter 37 for an additional listing of basic dermatologic equipment.)

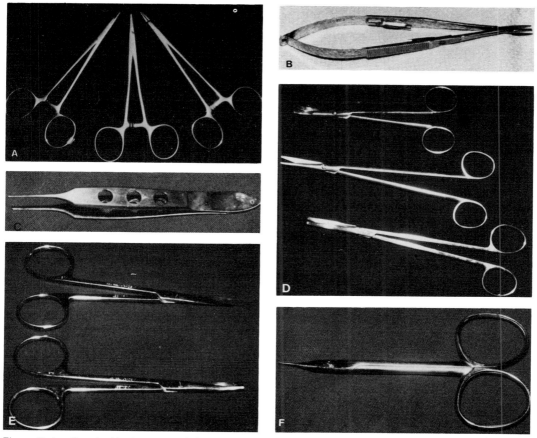

Figure 7–1.   **Surgical instruments.** (*A*) Left to right: Webster needle holder, neurosurgery needle holder, and Halsey needle holder. (*B*) Castroviejo needle holder. (*C*) Bishop-Harmon ophthalmic forceps. (*D*) Metzenbaum, Malis, and Ragnell scissors. (*E*) Stevens scissors. (*F*) Gradle scissors.

SUTURE SELECTION

Sutures may be divided into two general groups: absorbable and nonabsorbable. The absorbable sutures are plain gut, chromic gut, polyglycolic acid (Dexon), polyglactin 910 (Vicryl), and polydioxanone (PDS). Gut sutures undergo degradation by phagocytosis, and the synthetic sutures (Dexon, Vicryl, and PDS) are hydrolytically degraded in the tissues. Plain gut maintains its tensile strength for 14 days; chromic gut, for 21 to 25 days; and Dexon and Vicryl, from 21 to 25 days. The newest absorbable sutures, PDS, maintains tensile strength for 6 to 8 weeks.

The frequently used nonabsorbable sutures are silk and nylon. Sutures of 6-0 silk are preferred for eyelids and lips so that there are no sharp irritating ends. The monofilament nylons such as Ethilon are general purpose sutures. Prolene, a polypropylene type of monofilament suture, has the characteristics of an increased "memory" and high tensile strength. It is a good choice for a running intradermal stitch.

Usually 5-0 and 6-0 size sutures are used on the face. For very fine, delicate work 7-0 nylon may be indicated. With 7-0 nylon, it is easiest to use a Castroviejo needle holder.

For skin and fascia one uses a reverse cutting needle. With the reverse cutting needle, the cutting edge is on the outside. For facial surgery and for fine cutaneous surgery, precision point needles should be used. There is reduced tissue drag and trauma with these super-smooth-finished, highly honed needles. In the Ethicon system, these needles have the code prefix P or PS (plastic or plastic surgery);

and in the Davis and Geck system, PR or PRE. The P 3 or PS 3 size needles have good utility for facial surgery. For general cutaneous surgery, an FS (for skin) reverse cutting needle may be used.

TYPES OF STITCHES

Buried Subcutaneous

The buried subcutaneous stitch (Fig. 7–2A) is used to close the dead space to prevent hematoma and a nidus for infection. It also reduces the tension on the suture line. The knot is buried to decrease superficial tissue reaction, which could disrupt the incision line. This is done by inserting the needle in the deeper tissue and exiting superficially to the entry point and then entering the tissue at the same superficial level on the other side of the incision and exiting at the deeper level. Absorbable suture material is usually used.

Simple Stitch

The simple stitch (Fig. 7–2B) is made through and through the epidermis and dermis from one side to the other. The entry and the exit points of the needle should be about 2 mm from the wound edge. With proper entry of the needle, a greater "bite" of tissue is taken more deeply than superficially. This helps to evert the wound edges.

The simple stitch is not only an approximating and everting stitch, but it may also be used to adjust the height of the wound edges.

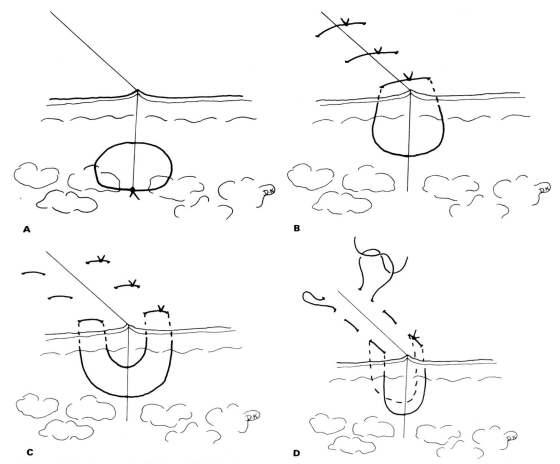

A

B

C

D

Figure 7–2. Types of stitches. (*A*) Buried subcutaneous stitches. (*B*) Simple stitch. (*C*) Vertical mattress stitch. (*D*) Horizontal mattress stitch.

If one side is lower than the other, a slightly deeper bite should be taken on the lower side. The knot may also be placed on the lower side to further finely adjust the height of the wound edges.

Vertical Mattress Stitch

The vertical mattress stitch (Fig. 7–2C) provides for tenting up of the skin edges. This eversion is necessary for good epidermal approximation and to prevent a linear depression in the healed incision line. Alternating this stitch with every two or three simple stitches gives good eversion.

Horizontal Mattress Stitch

The horizontal mattress stitch (Fig. 7–2D) is used for the closure of a wound under tension. It can cause strangulation of the skin. Because of this it is often used with a bolster to reduce the pressure on the skin. It is not a suitable stitch for facial surgery.

Corner Stitch
(Tip Stitch, Half-Buried Mattress)

The corner stitch (Fig. 7–3A) is used for V-shaped corners and T-shaped corners to prevent necrosis of the skin tip. It is inserted

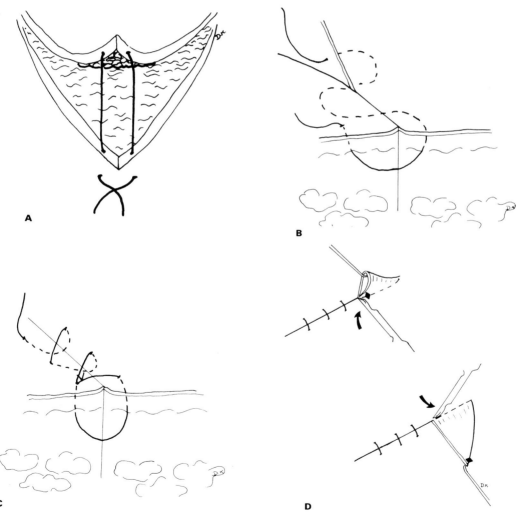

Figure 7–3. **Types of stitches.** (A) Corner stitch (tip stitch, half-buried mattress stitch). (B) Running intradermal stitch. (C) Running simple stitch. (D) Tenting up corner of wound with skin hook to define extent of dog-ear.

vertically down through the main segment of tissue and out through the dermis. It then enters horizontally through the dermal tissue in the tip of the flap and then back up through the main segment of tissue. The suture must enter and leave the flap tip at the same dermal level that it exits and reenters the dermis of the main body of tissue.

Running Intradermal Stitch

The running intradermal stitch (Fig. 7–3*B*) is a dermally placed stitch that may be left in for an extended period without causing crosshatching. On some occasions, this stitch may be left in permanently. This stitch enters the skin at a point 4 to 5 mm beyond the end of the incision. From this point it is brought into the wound and then is placed through the dermis on one side and crosses to the other side. The stitch is continued in a running "S" pattern, staying in the same plane of the dermis on both sides of the wound. In a long running intradermal stitch, it is wise to have it go through and through the skin at midpoint and then proceed intradermally. This will facilitate later removal since this midpoint of the suture may be cut and only half the amount of suture needs to be pulled out from each end.

Although the intradermal stitch will nicely coapt the wound, it is wise to also use a few simple stitches for the first 3 days for additional support and for wound edge eversion.

Running Simple Stitch

The running simple stitch (Fig. 7–3*C*) is a repeated, continuous over-and-over simple stitch that is a rapid method of closure. This stitch lacks great finesse but is useful where the scar is well camouflaged.

SUTURE TYING

Sutures should be tied to coapt the wound edges but not to strangulate. Most physicians err by tying too tightly. The ensuing tissue edema in the wound will also increase the skin tension on the suture. Tying too tightly is a major cause of suture track marks on the skin.

HEMOSTASIS

Meticulous hemostasis is essential to good wound healing. A rule of thumb on controlling bleeding vessels is that named vessels should be clamped and tied and unnamed vessels may be electrocoagulated.

In tying vessels, use the smallest size suture that is practical. The suture should be cut on the knot to leave the least amount of material in the wound that might cause a foreign body reaction.

For electrocoagulation, a biterminal device such as a Bovie is used (see Chap. 6). With the biterminal device, current enters the patient through an active or coagulating electrode. Where tissue contact is made, heat is generated and coagulation occurs. The current passes on through the patient to the dispersing or grounding electrode. The patient usually becomes part of the current circuit.

The grounding pad should be placed as close as possible to the surgical site. The heart should not be in between the active electrode and the grounding pad since it then becomes part of the current pathway.

The area of coagulation should be kept dry with sponging or with suction since copious bleeding into the surrounding area disperses the current and negates the coagulation effect.

Biterminal does not mean bipolar. Bipolar coagulation refers to the system in which a single electrode has both terminals contained in it. Bipolar coagulation is more precise, produces less tissue damage, and does not involve current transmission through the patient.

Electrocautery is essentially a red-hot branding iron that seals blood vessels by the direct application of heat. Electrocautery systems use either low-frequency alternating current or direct current. The current remains in the electrode tip and does not pass into the patient. Electrocautery provides better hemostasis in a very wet field than does electrocoagulation.

PATIENT PREPARATION

Written instructions to the patient before surgery will help to prevent misunderstandings.

1. Do not take aspirin or aspirin-containing products for 2 weeks before surgery since they interfere with blood clotting.
2. Refrain from alcohol for 1 week before surgery.
3. Shampoo hair the night before surgery. Shower or bathe before surgery using pHisoHex or Hibiclens cleanser.
4. Apply no creams or makeup after washing face.
5. Do not wear clothing that pulls over the head.
6. Wear loose and comfortable clothing.
7. Bring a companion to drive you home.

SKIN PREPARATION

It is best to shave as little hair as possible. Do not shave the eyebrows, since they grow at a very slow rate.

Cleanse the skin with a preparation such as Betadine or Hibiclens. Prepare a large enough area so that with sterile draping one may see not only the immediate surgical site but also the relationship to surrounding landmarks, the eye, the ear, the nose, and the mouth.

The incision lines are marked out before any distortion by infiltrative anesthesia. A sterile skin marking pen may be used, or less expensive and just as effective are round toothpicks dipped in gentian violet or Bonney's blue.

ANESTHESIA

Most cutaneous surgery cases require only local infiltrative or regional block anesthesia. The standard agent, 1% lidocaine, is an effective and safe anesthetic in which allergic reactions are virtually unknown. By the addition of epinephrine, systemic absorption of lidocaine is lessened, the duration of action is markedly prolonged, and a local hemostatic effect is achieved. The available commercial preparations usually combine lidocaine with 1:100,000 epinephrine.

Some patients will react to epinephrine with apprehension, body tremors, diaphoresis, palpitations, tachycardia and increased blood pressure. This is usually due to some intravascular injection. These side-effects may be decreased or eliminated by increasing the dilution of epinephrine to 1:200,000 or even to 1:400,000 without significantly changing its efficacy.

The maximum recommended dosage of lidocaine with epinephrine is 500 mg, the equivalent of 50 ml of a 1% solution.

PLACEMENT OF INCISIONS

Incisions should be planned so that they are parallel to or within wrinkle and smile lines. When there is lack of definite wrinkles, place incisions in the direction of relaxed skin tension lines. These lines run at right angles to the contraction vectors of the underlying muscle.

Another guide for camouflaging scars is to place incision lines at the boundaries of aesthetic and anatomical units. Examples are the vermilion junction, the paranasal fold (the junction of the nose and the cheek), the submandibular area (the junction of the cheek and the neck), the submental area (the junction of the chin and the neck), and in the hairline or eyebrow.

INCISIONS

Incisions should be made vertical to the skin surface. Obliquely angled incisions may produce some elevation of the overlying skin. An exception to the rule of vertical incisions is adjacent to the eyebrows where the incision should be angled away from the brow to avoid transecting hair follicles.

Wounds, even small, should be undermined to reduce tension. Undermining may be done with a scissors or scalpel. On the face, the level of undermining is just under the dermal plexus to avoid terminal branches of the facial nerve. On the scalp, the level is between the aponeurosis and the periosteum for a relatively blood-free plane. On the limbs and the trunk, the level above the fascia is less bloody.

EXCISIONS

The standard excision is the fusiform shape; this is often referred to as an ellipse. If the length-to-width ratio of the fusiform excision is less than 4:1 or if one side is longer than the other, redundant tissue will develop at the corner of the closure. These dog-ears or standing cones, if small, will level out and flatten as the wound undergoes contracture. If large, they should be removed by tenting up the corner of the wound with a skin hook to define the extent of the dog-ear. The dog-ear is incised along its base on one side of the incision. This flap of tissue is pulled across the incision line. Where the base of the redundant tissue crosses the incision line, it is transected. The dog-ear is thus eliminated, and the wound is closed (Fig. 7–3*D*).

In the removal of cutaneous malignancies, it is best first to excise the lesion and to have the margins checked histologically. The reconstruction is then planned about the excisional defect rather than planning the excision about the reconstruction. The defect after removal of a carcinoma is usually circular. The wound is closed along the lines of least tension. Excessive tissue at the corners of the closure may be removed by the previously mentioned technique for dog-ears. If the wound is too large for direct linear closure, reconstruction with flaps or grafts may be carried out.

WOUND DRESSINGS

In the first hours, a coagulum forms over the wound. Between 12 and 72 hours, there are two spurts of mitotic activity and epidermal cells begin migrating across the wound. However, the dried crust over the wound is a barrier. Rather than being able to migrate straight and level across the gap between the wound edges, the epidermal cells must form a new plane below the crust. This forms a shallow, linear depression in the healed incision.

To prevent wound crusting and the resultant linear trough in the healed wound, an occlusive dressing is used. For such a dressing, either Dermicel tape or Vigilon is available. For most sized wounds, Dermicel is adequate. Benzoin is applied to the surrounding skin. A 1-inch wide strip of Dermicel is then applied over and along the incision.

A moist environment develops under the dressing that inhibits formation of a crust and accelerates epidermal regeneration. Because of the abundant blood supply of the face, infection has not been a problem. The adhesive on Dermicel tape also has bacteriostatic properties. The tape is left in place for 3 days.

SUTURE REMOVAL

There are no hard and fast rules for suture removal. If there is doubt about whether sutures should be removed, remove every other or every third one and observe for another day or so. Some guidelines for the time of suture removal are as follows:

Face	3 to 5 days
Neck	6 to 8 days
Back	10 to 14 days
Abdomen	7 to 10 days
Extremities	10 to 18 days

It is prudent to examine wounds 4 to 5 days after surgery, since this is when a wound infection is most likely to occur.

In order not to disrupt the wound during suture removal, the sutures may be cut with a fine scissors such as the Gradle or with a No. 11 blade. For correct suture removal, the suture is pulled toward the incision line. Pulling away from the incision line might pull the wound apart.

The time at which sutures are removed from the face is the time when the wound is the weakest since fibroplasia is just beginning and only the epidermal bridging is holding the wound. Therefore, after suture removal, the wound is reinforced with Steri-strips for the next week.

WOUND DYNAMICS

Wound Healing

For understanding, wound healing is divided into four phases. These phases overlap and blend into each other.

During the beginning inflammatory phase, there is initial vasoconstriction with platelet aggregation. After 5 to 10 minutes of vasoconstriction, there is active venule dilatation and increased vascular permeability, lasting about 72 hours. Within a few hours of these vascular responses, a cellular response occurs. Polymorphonuclear leukocytes migrate into the area. There is a diapedesis of monocytes that transform into tissue macrophages. The macrophage is the dominant cell for the first 3 to 4 days. It initiates the fibroblastic phase.

While the inflammatory phase is still proceeding, the proliferative phase commences. Epidermal cells undergo changes and begin migrating into the wound. By the third day, migration of epidermal cells across an apposed incision is completed. Fibroblasts within the dermis begin to proliferate at 24 to 36 hours after the tissue injury.

By the fourth day, the fibroblastic phase is heralded by the synthesis of collagen and proteoglycans by the proliferating fibroblasts. Collagen fibers are laid down in a random pattern without orientation.

Overlapping and toward the latter part of the fibroblastic phase the remodeling phase begins. This is a phase of differentiation, resorption, and maturation. Fibroblasts disappear from the wound, and collagen fibers are modeled into organized bundles and patterns.

Wound Contraction

In an open wound healing by second intention there is an active drawing of the full thickness of the surrounding skin toward the center of the wound. Wound contraction begins during the proliferative phase of wound healing. There is a differentiation of fibroblasts into contractile fibroblasts or myofibroblasts, which are responsible for this dynamic process. Wound contraction usually proceeds until the wound is closed or until surrounding forces on the skin are greater than the contractile forces of the myofibroblasts.

Contracture

All scars undergo contracture, with a resultant shortening along their longitudinal axis. This process of contracture is due to collagen cross-linking, which occurs during the remodeling phase. Contracture is distinct and different from wound contraction.

Wound Strength

By 2 weeks, the wound has gained 7% of its final strength; by 3 weeks, 20%; by 4 weeks, 50%. At full maturation, the healed wound regains only 80% of the strength of the original intact skin.

DOCUMENTATION AND ASSESSMENT

Although success or failure in cutaneous surgery may be readily apparent, it is important to document results with objective photography. Only by consistent, standardized photographs may one judge progress and analyze techniques and methods. Preoperative and postoperative photographs are essential, as are intraoperative photographs. Uniform clinical photography is a form of self-assessment and serves as a stimulus and a direction for improvement.

CUTANEOUS LASER SURGERY

Lasers have been used for more than 2 decades for cutaneous surgery. The carbon dioxide and argon lasers have been most widely applied, but greater and greater roles are being identified for the pulsed tunable dye laser and for the neodymium:yttrium–aluminum garnet (Nd:YAG) laser.

Laser is the acronym for *l*ight *a*mplification by *s*timulated *e*mission of *r*adiation. The electromagnetic radiations of lasers have three key characteristics. They are monochromatic, in phase, and highly collimated (nondivergent). Because they are monochromatic, specific tissue damage may be inflicted. Because they are in phase, a sufficient energy intensity can be generated for surgical demands. Because they are collimated, nearly all the energy can be focused and reflected onto the target.

The precision of the carbon dioxide laser makes it an ideal instrument for cutaneous surgery. It generates electromagnetic energy with a wavelength of 10,600 nm, which is in the invisible mid-infrared portion of the electromagnetic spectrum. The carbon dioxide laser has several surgical advantages. The thermal energy generated by the laser beam is sterilizing. When the beam vaporizes tissue, there is limited heat diffusion beyond the point of impact. Therefore, histologic detail is preserved up to the incision line. The laser seals lymphatics, nerve endings, and blood vessels up to 0.5 mm in diameter. There is less postoperative discomfort and less operative oozing. A laser with a maximum output of 35 watts is usually sufficient for cutaneous surgery.

With the hand-held adapter on the articulated arm, the carbon dioxide laser may be used as an incisional device. The incision is 0.2 mm wide, compared with a 0.25-mm wide incision with a No. 15 scalpel blade. The carbon dioxide laser may be coupled to the operating microscope to enhance visualization and to provide a sensitive yet stable firing platform. With a 200-mm microscope lens the laser can be focused to an impact point of 0.4 mm, and with a 400-mm lens it can be focused to an impact point of 0.8 mm.

At times the carbon dioxide laser may be preferred over the traditional steel scalpel for patients with certain medical problems. Patients with angina, arrhythmias, or hypertension may be jeopardized if local infiltrative anesthesia with epinephrine is used. The bleeding in patients with thrombocytopenia or on anticoagulation therapy may complicate the simplest incision or skin flap. By using the carbon dioxide laser as an incisional instrument, one may be able to operate in a less bloody field.

The carbon dioxide laser may be used for the excision of skin cancers, including melanomas. Since there is less tissue manipulation with the laser and since the lymphatics are sealed, there may be less chance of milking neoplastic cells into the perioperative field and into the circulation.

The carbon dioxide laser is not only used for incisions and excisions but also for undermining and mobilizing skin flaps for reconstruction. Skin grafts may be rapidly affixed by using the laser to "spot weld" the graft to the recipient site rather than suturing or stapling it.

There is usually less postoperative pain with laser surgery. With the scalpel, frayed nerve endings are left in the cut tissue. This leads to an increased release of prostaglandins producing pain. With the laser, the cuts are sharp and the nerve endings are sealed.

Actinic cheilitis is a premalignant condition usually of the lower lip. The standard method of treatment is a vermilionectomy or lip shave. However, the atypical epidermis of the vermilion surface may also be vaporized away with the carbon dioxide laser. The advantages of the laser vermilionectomy are that it is rapid, heals quickly, maintains the lip contour, and avoids most sensory alterations.

Numerous cutaneous conditions are amenable to treatment with the carbon dioxide laser: syringoma, trichoepithelioma, adenoma sebaceum, lymphangioma circumscriptum, and Hailey-Hailey disease.

Intranasal verrucae and squamous papillomas can be destroyed accurately without damaging septal cartilage. The laser is practical for verrucae vulgaris on other areas of the body. If destructive methods are used for warts on the palms and soles, persistent, painful postoperative scars may occur that are more troublesome than the warts were. With the laser, tissue destruction can be limited to the area of the wart. Since the wart is intraepidermal, the destructive process should not extend into the dermis. By using the operative microscope one may better distinguish between normal and wart tissue. By not using local anesthesia one may also use pain sensation as a guide to the depth of laser vaporization. For warts on other areas of the body (except periungual warts), the laser is usually reserved for those that have been recalcitrant. Condylomata accuminata may also respond to laser treatment.

Both professional and homemade tattoos may be removed with the carbon dioxide laser. As with other methods, the laser still leaves a scar. However, there may be less of a scar since there is greater control of the depth of ablation. Homemade tattoos are more difficult to remove than professional ones since the pigment is instilled into the dermis at varying levels. With the laser, particularly when coupled with a microscope, the degree of vaporization may be adjusted according to the depth of pigment. Not only may the carbon dioxide laser be used for removing tattoos, but with allergic reactions to tattoo pigments, it can also selectively vaporize away the sensitizing pigment without destroying the integrity of the rest of the tattoo.

Hypertrophic scars and keloidal scars from acne and trauma may be leveled with the carbon dioxide laser. There is usually rapid reepithelialization without renewed hypertrophy. Keloids of the earlobe are amenable to laser resection and seem to have a lesser incidence of recurrence with this approach.

With the development of contact tips, the Nd:YAG laser is having increased applications in cutaneous surgery. Its output is in the near-infrared portion of the spectrum at 1060 nm. The Nd:YAG laser has been reported to suppress collagen formation both in tissue cultures and in normal skin. However, its role in the treatment of scar tissues requires further study.

Capillary hemangiomas (port-wine stain hemangiomas) have been effectively treated in many cases with the argon laser. The argon laser is a spectrum absorption laser. Its blue-green light (480 to 521 nm) should be selectively absorbed by the red blood cell hemoglobin within blood vessels. However, there is also some coagulation of the adjacent tissues and the overlying epidermis. This is due to both reflection into adjoining tissues and absorption by interposing tissues, particularly those with melanin.

The pulsed tunable dye laser may have the greatest application for vascular lesions. The dye laser's wavelength output may be adjusted by using different dyes for the lasing medium. A selective increase in blood vessel thermal damage is achieved by using a rhodamine dye that achieves a wavelength output of 577 nm.

Although lasers are widely used in cutaneous surgery, modifications of current lasers and new innovations should increase their applications.

BIBLIOGRAPHY

Davidson TM, Webster RC, Gordon BR: The Principles and Dynamics of Local Skin Flaps. Washington, DC, American Academy of Otolaryngology—Head and Neck Surgery Foundation, 1983

Fuller TA: Surgical Lasers. New York, Macmillan, 1987

Peacock EE: Wound Repair. Philadelphia, WB Saunders, 1984

Rudolph R: Problems in Aesthetic Surgery. St. Louis, CV Mosby, 1986

Thomas JR, Holt GR: Facial Scars—Incision, Revision, and Camouflage. St. Louis, CV Mosby, 1989

8

Cosmetics for
the Dermatologist

Earle W. Brauer, M.D.*

Archeological, historical, and anthropological studies confirm that body adornment has been practiced by men and women of all cultures and societies. A walk through the portrait galleries of our nation's capital provides vivid evidence of the evolution in our own personal grooming habits over the past 200 years. Modern observations of remote cultures dramatically demonstrate the importance skin painting, scarification, and hair coloring play in societal behavior. In our present culture, by comparison, this trait is not diminished, just more subtle and less vividly portrayed.

The need for skin adornment is so basic that if all commercial cosmetic products were removed from the marketplace, the consumer would contrive and fabricate his or her own: animal, vegetable, and mineral substances would be mixed, kneaded, boiled, and baked in secret family recipes for grooming, coloring hair, and ironing face wrinkles; schoolgirls would hoard the red jelly beans that, after being moistened and stroked on the skin, brighten cheeks and lips; eyebrows, hair lines, and "beauty marks" would come and go

to meet the current social perception of attractiveness.

Skin health deserves a broader interpretation than merely the absence of disease. Because the appearance of skin, hair, and nails is used to project status and influence and to create impressions on others, thus promoting self-confidence and personal satisfaction, the person who believes that his or her otherwise normal external body structures are not meeting current standards of beauty is also suffering from a "dis-ease." It behooves the dermatologist, therefore, to take an active interest in basic skin care and adornment. This responsibility should not be abdicated to barbers, beauticians, and salespersons at toiletry and cosmetic counters. The patient is eager to accept counseling from the physician and is easily stimulated to initiate a self-improvement effort.

To function easily and efficiently with cosmetics, the physician should understand a few basic principles concerning the ingredients of cosmetics, rather than depending on brand names. The cosmetic industry, like many others (such as food, clothing, and automobile industries) in our modern society, is fashion oriented and moves rapidly; brand designations and package graphics are short lived. However, ingredient disclosure on the product label is now a legal requirement. If the list of ingredients is not found on the bottle, tube, or jar, then it appears on the outer

* Associate Professor of Clinical Dermatology, New York University School of Medicine; Vice President for Medical Affairs, Revlon Research Center, Inc.

box. (Fragrance, although a complex mixture, is listed as a single ingredient.) Standard terminology is used, and complete technical information about an ingredient, such as the chemical designation, trade name, source of supply, and other details, can be obtained from the third edition of the *CTFA Cosmetic Ingredient Dictionary* (published by the Cosmetic, Toiletry and Fragrance Association, Inc., 1110 Vermont Avenue, NW, Washington, DC 20005).

CLASSIFICATION AND GENERAL DESCRIPTION

Cosmetics may be defined, broadly, as topical agents used to effect personal grooming, influence appearance, and improve self-image. Ordinarily, they do not act physiologically on the skin or mucous membranes. A few products that do act physiologically, such as antiperspirants (not deodorants), sunscreens, skin lighteners, and hair products with genuine active antidandruff agents, are loosely called *cosmetic drugs*. The Food and Drug Administration (FDA) considers them to be both drugs and cosmetics and subjects them to all regulations for over-the-counter (OTC) drugs as well as for cosmetics.

A convenient classification of cosmetics in general is presented below:

1. *Toiletries:* Soaps, shampoos, hair rinses and conditioners, hair dressings, sprays and setting lotions, hair color preparations, waving preparations, straightening (relaxer) agents, deodorants, antiperspirants, sun-protective agents
2. *Skin Care Products*:* Shaving agents, cosmetic cleansers, astringents, toners, moisturizers, masks, night creams, baths
3. *Makeup (Color) Products:* Foundations, eye makeup (shadows, liners, mascaras), lipsticks, rouges, blushers, nail enamel

4. *Fragrance Products:* Perfumes, colognes, toilet waters, bath water additives, bath powders, aftershave agents

The vast majority of these products are manufactured by reputable companies whose research, developmental, and manufacturing practices and quality assurance programs match those of the pharmaceutical industry. The consumer is offered a safe, stable product that will perform as designed. Product presentation using extravagant imagery and word-puffery is common in a competitive industry serving the mercurial fluctuations in mood and fashion of a fast-moving society. The physician familiar with cosmetic product types can easily guide the patient to product selection, use, and satisfaction. A discussion of each of the major types of cosmetics follows.

TOILETRIES

Skin cleansing is efficiently achieved with the use of the classic soap that results from the chemical reaction between fats and alkalis. The common milled and white floating bars are serviceable soaps; french-milled bars receive added production details that create a steadfast bar of fine texture and bouquet, lasting through the life of the product. Transparent soaps permit better control of alkaline residue. Special soaps may incorporate medicaments, germicides, abrasive granules, or encapsulated emollients to perform particular functions. Detergent bars consist of synthetic, non-soap cleansing agents in which pH control may even be accomplished on the acid side of neutral pH. Since cleansing is a daily ritual, the user often seeks variety; therefore, bar color, fragrance, and lather richness are factors in selection.

Hair cleansing, or shampooing, may be a daily event for a large segment of the population. Short, casual hair styles and quick, efficient appliances for drying foster this practice. Shampoos presently cleanse with synthetic detergents. Soap shampoos are obsolete and deserve to be. The cosmetic chemist can finely tune a synthetic shampoo product to perform at a designated pH within strict parameters, so that the product will work with equal efficiency in hard or soft water, without

---

* *Within the cosmetic industry, such products are referred to as "treatment products." This is not meant to imply treatment in a medical sense. Originally, the description was a convenient means of separating skin care products from the more familiar color cosmetics that create camouflage and illusion.*

the deposition of dulling salt precipitates that occurs with soap products.

The integrity of the hair cuticle is the critical factor in the selection of a shampoo. Hair care services (such as waving, relaxing, and coloring), the degree of manipulation (combing and brushing, styling, shampoo and drying cycles), and exposure to sun, swimming, and the environment will lift hair cuticular cells or dislodge them. The porosity of such hair is increased; when wet, it imbibes excess water and acts like a soggy sponge; when dry, it takes on a frizzy and fragile quality. These damaged hair strands easily tangle with their neighbors. Alkaline shampoos will exaggerate these problems by further disruption in the cuticular layer. Slightly alkaline, neutral or slightly acid shampoos will temporarily "shrink down" the irregular cuticular layer to make the shampooing process and immediate postshampoo care easier and more successful. Thoroughness of cleansing may be sacrificed, but this is hardly a factor unless long intervals, or excessive buildup of hair spray or setting preparations, occurs between shampoos. For the more normal and intact hair cuticle, the alkaline shampoo will perform well, and a product should be selected that conforms to the degree of seborrhea of the scalp, environmental soil, and grooming preferences of the individual.

The *postshampoo hair rinses* and *conditioners* perform a significant function. Through the application of chemically substantive ingredients such as resins, quaternary salts, coating agents, and antistatics the hair acquires sheen and gloss, gains body, and loses undesirable static charges of electricity. The hair is then easier to comb and retains fiber flexibility. The more hair care services and manipulation to which the hair is subjected, the greater is the satisfaction resulting from the regular use of these conditioners.

Hair waving is achieved by the application of thioglycolates. The glyceryl monothioglycolate (GMTG) salts, known as the "cold" or "acid" perm, which is less damaging to the hair strand structure and imparts a more natural feel to the hair, have gained in popularity over the standard ammonium thioglycolate product. However, atopic persons, in particular, whether salon operator or client, tend to easily develop an allergic sensitivity to the GMTG salts. Switching such persons to the

ammonium product has been known to afford hair styling satisfaction while avoiding the allergic reaction. Hair relaxing (curl straightening) is achieved by hydroxyl ions obtained through the use of sodium, lithium, or calcium hydroxide. These chemicals are primary irritants, which produce permanent effects on the hair shaft. Such products demand careful conformity to package directions. Injudicious use of these products may cause temporary physical injury, such as hair-shaft breakage and primary skin irritation. Rare instances have been reported of allergic dermatitis in the non-atopic to GMTG.

The face-framing effect of scalp hair, as well as its color (see the discussion below), plays a vital role in a person's social, economic, and political life. The physician must help patients to achieve the hair styles that they desire, while also showing them how to avoid damage to either hair or skin. Unskilled application of hair-waving or hair-relaxing preparations by the patient or operator should be evaluated and discussed with the patient, who needs the physician's understanding and help.

The physician should do more than admonish the patient to stop using the product. He or she should explain the effect of the agent, suggest alternate methods for the hair waving or curling, and especially insist on proper adherence to the directions for use. Frustration of the patient due to the physician's lack of interest in giving proper advice has usually resulted in the patient's seeking hair "knowledge" and education from the beauty salon operator.

Hair coloring is important to both sexes and to all age-groups; it is estimated that at least 50 million persons color their hair. A convenient survey of the types of hair-coloring preparations that are available, along with their attributes and limitations, is presented in Table 8–1. For the most part, adverse reactions are of the allergic, contact dermatitis type. For such allergic patients to whom the interdiction of oxidation dye procedures poses serious compromise with personal need, the physician can offer a practical alternative. For the 3 days immediately preceding and following the next exposure to the coloring procedure, the patient can be protected with 10 mg of oral prednisone, three times daily. This has offered adequate protection

Table 8–1
Coloring Products and Their Key Characteristics

TYPE OF COLORING PRODUCT	RECOGNITION	SKILL INVOLVED	TYPE OF DYES	COLOR CHANGE RANGE	SITE OF ACTION	LASTING QUALITY	OVERALL PERFORMANCE	DEGREE OF ABUSE OF HAIR STRUCTURE	POTENTIAL FOR DERMATOLOGIC COMPLAINTS
Temporary "color rinses"	Multiple-use package	Minimal Apply and dry	High molecular weight acid dyes as used in textiles, and certified food colors in a hydro-alcoholic suspension	Covers gray	Surface of shaft	Poor Removed by shampooing	Poor	Negligible	Negligible
Semi-permanent	Single- or multiple-use package More viscous than No. 1 to prevent dripping off hair	Moderate Applied to freshly shampooed hair and left in place for 15–40 minutes Skin patch test required	Low molecular weight dyes: nitro-phenylenediamines, nitroaminophenols, aminoanthroquinones in shampoo vehicle or a solvent system	Covers gray One to three shades on dark side of normal hair color	Penetrates to cortex	Gradually lost through three to five shampoos	Fair	Negligible	Negligible
Permanent oxidation type Single process	Two-unit system for mixing just prior to use	Moderate Skin patch test required	Several classes of dyes including PPD* intermediates in an alkaline peroxide "shampoo"	Covers gray and two to three shades on each side of normal	Cortex	Permanent New growth touch-up every 4–8 weeks	Excellent	Moderate	Modest
Double process	Same as above	Professional attention necessary	As above, but hair must be previously decolorized (stripped)	Unlimited	Cortex	As above	Excellent	Significant	Moderate Hair breakage; local and systemic peroxide reactions
Progressive	Multiple-use package	None	Metallic salts, particularly lead in solution, cream, or pomade form	Discolors hair only	Surface and some beneath cuticle	As long as product is used regularly	Poor	Minimal	Negligible A public health problem; incompatible with other chemical hair services
Vegetable Henna	For all practical purposes, this does not exist and is not available. Although true henna is a vegetable dye, its color properties and lasting abilities make it unacceptable. Products are being marketed currently with this name but are actually henna coloring in the second and third categories above.								

* p-phenylenediamine.

in *p*-phenylenediamine-class sensitive patients, permitting them to maintain their usual hair coloring routine without suffering any disability. Of course, cooperation and coordination among patient, salon operator, and physician are essential.

SKIN CARE PRODUCTS

The *cosmetic cleansers* are emulsions of oil and water, occasionally with small amounts of detergents. They are not a total substitute for soap or detergent-bar cleansing, but they have a useful place in skin care. The makeup user will find it easier, more efficient, and infinitely less messy to wash basin, clothes, and surroundings if a cotton ball or facial tissue saturated with a cosmetic cleanser is used to float off and remove colored eye makeup, face foundations, and blushers. The younger person may then prefer following with conventional soap; the mature woman, with "dry," sebum-deficient skin, will not.

Astringents, fresheners, and *toners* are dilute, aqueous alcoholic solutions applied with a cotton ball that permit efficient removal of excess sebum, soil, and cellular debris from isolated areas of the face, such as mid forehead, nose, nasolabial folds, and chin.

Moisturizers constitute a broad group of products. Their purpose is to increase the water content of the stratum corneum. Water may be added extraneously to the skin surface, while a lipid-type film retards evaporation of endogenous water from the epidermis. The hydrophilic keratin layer will then become softer and smoother by "filling out" any accentuated normal skin-surface markings.

Most moisturizers are water-in-oil (w/o) or oil-in-water (o/w) emulsions. In general, the w/o products are "heavier" and deposit a thicker and longer-lasting oily film on the skin surface. They are preferred by the mature person with "dry" skin. The o/w emulsion is "lighter," since its film is thinner and less obvious. It is preferred by the person with less sebum deficit. Both types of persons will benefit from use of these products at bedtime (night creams) or as "prime coats" for use under makeup. The under-makeup moisturizer eases application of makeup and affords better wear characteristics. The young, sebum-rich skin does not need moisturizers.

Moisturizer products are offered in abundance by all manufacturers. By finely balancing the w/o and o/w ratios, a variety of products can be achieved that fit the needs of particular skin types while satisfying aesthetic tastes. It is not possible to determine this from reading package labels. A good, generally reliable "rule of thumb" that the physician may use to distinguish w/o from o/w products brought to the office is to apply a few drops to a palm and rub the palms together for a moment or two. If the product feels warm and the skin surface appears glossy, then the product is probably a w/o preparation. If the product feels cool (due to evaporation of its higher water content) and the skin surface feels smooth but exhibits no gloss or apparent film, then the product probably is the "lighter" o/w type. Of course, the heaviest products are anhydrous (without water) preparations, such as petroleum jelly. These are good moisturizers, with the worst aesthetics: they are difficult to remove, mat the hair, and soil bedclothes.

MAKEUP (COLOR) PRODUCTS

Makeup products are used to camouflage, adorn, highlight, or deemphasize surface contours through the artistic use of color—manipulating the reflection and absorption of light. Elevations and depressions on the skin, or any surface, are appreciated by the shadows that they cast and by the manner in which light is reflected from them to the eye of the observer. Similarly, pigmentation becomes visible because it absorbs light, which cannot be reflected to the observer's eye. Foundation makeup creates a remarkably uniform surface by simultaneously applying transparent and opaque color qualities. Eye makeup, lipstick, and rouges (blushers) add highlights and contouring, which create enhanced interest and attractiveness in the features. The basics of applying makeup can be easily learned by any interested person, but it takes practice and experimentation, trial and error, to achieve any degree of success. It also requires well-manufactured materials and the right combination of color products. Complimentary shades of eye shadow blended about the lid surfaces, eyeliner to marginate the shape of the eye, and mascara to emphasize the cilia create an attractive and flattering appearance that captures the observer's attention. Cosmetic defects elsewhere on the face are minimized.

The use of customized high-coverage makeup for camouflaging major cosmetic deficits, such as port-wine stains, as well as the successful use of standard cosmetics to minimize significant cosmetic deficits (*e.g.*, facial hemiatrophy, telangiectasia, pigmentary alterations), are special situations not considered in this chapter. The reader is referred to a chapter by the author in *Clinical Dermatology* (see Bibliography).

It is important, however, in this discussion of makeup products that some clarification is given to the increasingly important *product comedogenicity index* and the commonly used term *hypoallergenic*.

A person whose skin has active sebaceous gland activity, or an acne-prone person, should probably avoid the use of "heavier" moisturizers and makeup products. Although the total oil content is a factor, comedogenic potential is equally dependent on the qualitative and quantitative relationship among particular components. Unlike the classic dermatologic shake-lotion of powders placed in momentary suspension with water, a makeup that achieves adequate coverage and spreadability requires nonaqueous fluids. This gives the user time to work with the product, known in the industry as "play time." Ideal nonaqueous fluid makeup products are available, which, on bioassay, score extremely low on an index for comedogenicity. In identifying these complex components the reading of ingredient disclosure statements on labels is of little help and relying on medical publications for product comedogenicity scores is haphazard at best. Major cosmetic companies perform comedogenic bioassays, making this information available on request. These indices of comedogenicity are not the valuable tools the physician anticipated in the management of acne-prone persons who insist on using cosmetics. These assays apparently do not reflect or predict what happens in the human in actual use conditions. Those who have pioneered these assays have discredited them in public. Further information on treatment for acne can be found in Chapter 13.

Stripped to its roots, the meaning of the term *hypoallergenic* seems simple: a lessened tendency to evoke an allergenic response in a person with the acquired ability to react.

However, applying the name to a cosmetic product is meaningless without knowing to what substance(s) the person is allergic. For example, most cosmetics, including those labeled "hypoallergenic" or "allergy tested," commonly contain paraben as well as mercurial preservatives. How can such a product be hypoallergenic to a paraben- or mercurial-sensitive consumer? Since all cosmetic manufacturers eliminate substances known to possess undesirably high-sensitivity indices, comparable products, regardless of manufacturer, are broadly hypoallergenic, whether so labeled or not. Perhaps this word has promotional value in marketing; however, the practicing physician should not be influenced by it.

FRAGRANCE PRODUCTS

Fragrance products come in a variety of forms. In earlier times, when bathing was not commonly practiced, perfumes and incense masked undesirable odors. In our culture we use fragrance to evoke nonvisual, romantic imagery of the present, as well as memories of the past. *Perfumes* are very complex compounds. As few as 20 and as many as 300 individual essential oils and fragrance components may be blended to achieve a particular odor. One group of chemical agents will react with another: for example, alcohols react with aldehydes to form hemiacetals; aldehydes react with amines to form Schiff's base; esters interchange; and the multitude of chemicals combinate and permutate until equilibrium is finally reached. This is why perfumes must age before the final, true fragrance is developed. Consequently, a fragrance is more precisely a complex compound unto itself rather than a simple sum of its initial parts. Perhaps broad classes of chemicals used in perfumes are identifiable, but not specific chemical substances. To try to identify the chemical ingredient in a fragrance to which a patient has an allergic sensitivity is a heroic and frustrating task. A practical solution is to educate the patient in self-testing. Most cosmetic counters have "tester" samples available. Application of the product to a confined area of an antecubital fossa for a 24-hour period of limited exposure will usually reveal the potential for allergy.

BIBLIOGRAPHY

Adams RM, Maibach HI: A five year study of cosmetic reactions. J Am Acad Dermatol 13:1062, 1985

Balsam MS, Sagarin E (eds): Cosmetics: Science and Technology, 2nd ed. 3 volumes. New York, Wiley-Interscience, 1972–1974

Brauer EW: Cosmetics. In Baran R, Dawber RPR (eds): Diseases of the Nails and Their Management. Oxford, Blackwell Scientific Publications, 1984

Brauer EW: Cosmetics for the dermatologist. In Demis DJ, Dobson RL, McGuire J (eds): Clinical Dermatology. Philadelphia, JB Lippincott, 1984

Brauer EW: Coloring and corrective makeup preparations. In Abramovits W (ed): Clinics in Dermatology, chap 10. Philadelphia, JB Lippincott, 1988

Brauer EW: Cosmetics. In Newcomer VD, Young EM Jr (eds): Geriatric Dermatology: Clinical Diagnosis and Practical Therapy. New York, Igaku-Shoin, 1989

de Groot AC, Bruynzeel DP, Bos JD et al: The allergens in cosmetics. Arch Dermatol 124:1525, 1988

Elder RL: The cosmetic ingredient review—a safety evaluation program. J Am Acad Dermatol 11:1168, 1984

Larsen WG: Perfume dermatitis. J Am Acad Dermatol 12:1, 1985

Nelson FP, Rumsfield J: Cosmetics: content and function. Int J Dermatol 27:665, 1988

Wehr RF, Krochmal L: Considerations in selecting a moisturizer. Cutis 39:512, 1987

Wickett RR: Permanent waving and straightening of hair. Cutis 39:496, 1987

Journal

Cosmetic Dermatology is a journal published by Knolls Publishing Group, Inc (Cedar Knolls, NJ).

9

Dermatologic Allergy

Contact dermatitis, industrial dermatoses, atopic eczema, and *drug eruptions* are included in this chapter because of their obvious allergenic factors. (However, some cases of contact dermatitis and industrial dermatitis are due to irritants.) *Nummular eczema* is also included because it resembles some forms of atopic eczema and may even be a variant of atopic eczema.

CONTACT DERMATITIS
(Plates 4 through 7)

Contact dermatitis, or dermatitis venenata, is a very common inflammation of the skin caused by the exposure of the skin either to *primary irritant substances,* such as soaps, or to *allergenic substances,* such as poison ivy resin. Industrial dermatoses will be considered at the end of this section.

PRIMARY LESIONS. Any of the stages, from mild redness, edema, or vesicles to large bullae with a marked amount of oozing, are seen.

SECONDARY LESIONS. Crusting from secondary bacterial infection, excoriations, and lichenification occur.

DISTRIBUTION AND ETIOLOGY. Any agent can affect any area of the body. However, certain agents commonly affect certain skin areas.

Face and Neck (Fig. 9–1): Cosmetics, soaps, insect sprays, ragweed, perfumes or hair sprays (sides of neck), fingernail polish (eyelids), hatband (forehead), mouthwashes, toothpaste or lipstick (perioral), nickel metal (earlobes), industrial oil (facial chloracne)

Hands and Forearms: Soaps, hand lotions, wrist bands, industrial chemicals, poison ivy, and a multitude of other agents. Irritation from soap often begins under rings.

Axillae: Deodorants, dress shields, or dry cleaning solutions

Trunk: Clothing (new, not previously cleaned), rubber or metal attached to, or in, clothing

Anogenital Region: Douches, dusting powder, contraceptives, colored toilet paper, poison ivy, or too strong salves for treatment of pruritus ani and fungal infections

Feet: Shoes, foot powders, too strong salves for "athlete's feet" infection

Generalized Eruption: Volatile airborne chemicals (paint, spray, ragweed), medicaments locally applied to large areas, bath powder, or clothing

---

SAUER NOTES:

1. In obtaining a history, question the patient carefully concerning home, over-the-counter, other physicians' and well-meaning friend's remedies. A contact dermatitis on top of a contact dermatitis is quite common.

2. When you are unable to find the cause of a generalized contact dermatitis, determine the site of the *initial* eruption and think of the agents that touch the area.

(text continues on page 74)

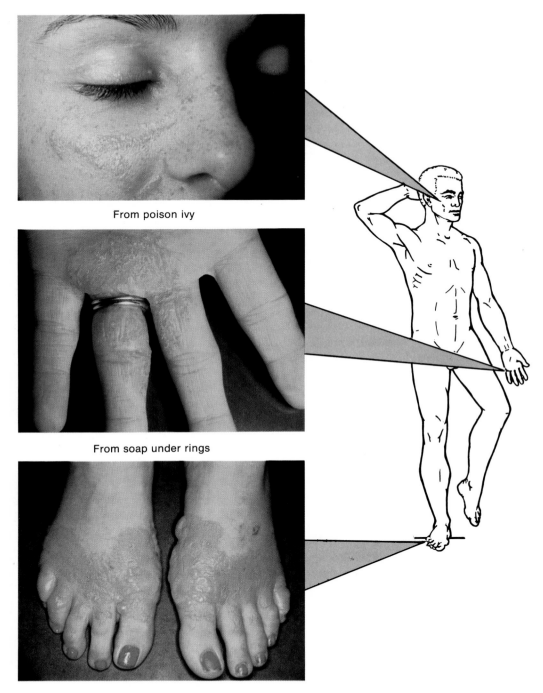

From poison ivy

From soap under rings

From shoe material

Plate 4. **Contact dermatitis.** (*Burroughs Wellcome Co.*)

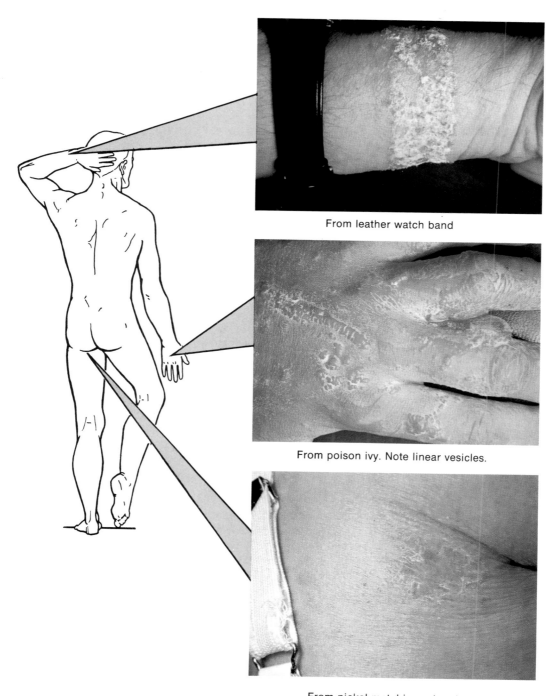

From leather watch band

From poison ivy. Note linear vesicles.

From nickel metal in garter strap

Plate 5. **Contact dermatitis.** (*Burroughs Wellcome Co.*)

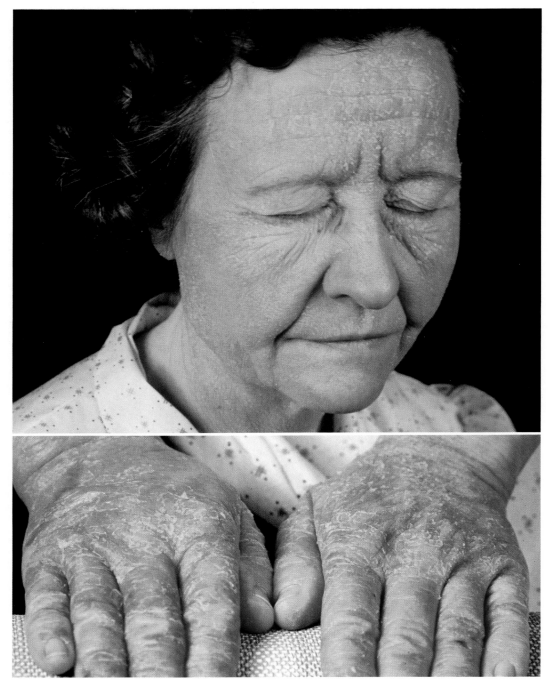

Plate 6. **Contact dermatitis in a nurse due to chlorpromazine.** The hands and the face were involved most severely. This eruption was aggravated following exposure to sunlight. (*K.U.M.C.*) (*Burroughs Wellcome Co.*)

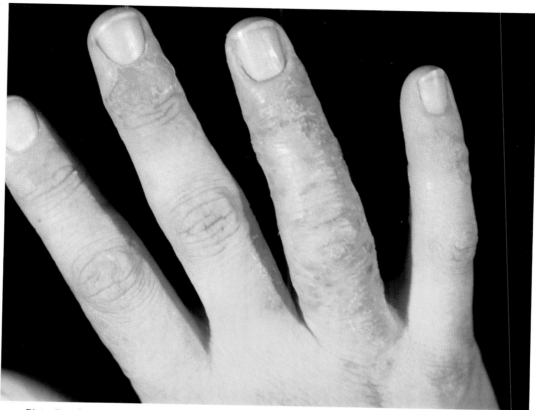

Plate 7. **Contact dermatitis of the hand.** This common dermatitis is usually due to continued exposure to soap and water. (*K.U.M.C.*) (*Burroughs Wellcome Co.*)

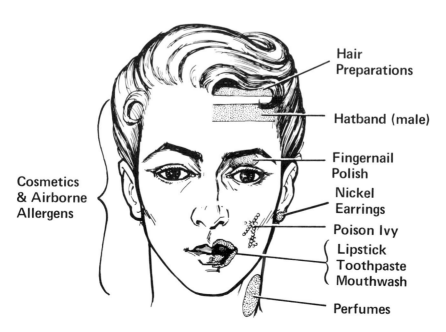

Hair Preparations

Hatband (male)

Fingernail Polish

Nickel Earrings

Poison Ivy

Lipstick Toothpaste Mouthwash

Perfumes

Cosmetics & Airborne Allergens

FIGURE 9-1. **Contact dermatitis of the face.**

COURSE. Duration can be very short to very chronic. As a general rule, successive recurrences become more chronic (*e.g.*, seasonal ragweed dermatitis can become a year-round dermatitis). An established hypersensitivity reaction is never lost. Also, certain persons have greater susceptibility for allergic and irritant contact dermatitis than others.

SEASON. A very careful seasonal history of the onset, in chronic cases, may lead to discovery of an unsuspected causative agent, such as ragweed.

FAMILY INCIDENCE. This is not evident.

CONTAGIOUSNESS. The eczematous reaction (*e.g.*, the blister fluid of poison ivy) contains no allergen that can cause the dermatitis in another person. However, if the poison ivy oil or other allergen remains on the skin of the affected person, contact of the allergen with a susceptible individual could cause a dermatitis.

LABORATORY FINDINGS. Patch tests (see Chap. 2) are of value in eliciting the cause in a problem case. Careful interpretation is required.

Differential Diagnosis

A contactant reaction must be considered and ruled in or out in any case of eczematous dermatitis on any body area.

Treatment

Two of the most common contact dermatoses seen in the physician's office are *poison ivy* (or *poison oak*) *dermatitis* and *hand dermatitis*. The treatment of these two conditions will be discussed.

Treatment of Contact Dermatitis due to Poison Ivy

A patient comes to the office with a linear, vesicular dermatitis of the feet, the hands, and the face. He states that he spent the weekend fishing and that the rash broke out the next day. The itching is rather severe but not enough to keep him awake at night. He had "poison ivy" 5 years ago (Fig. 9–2).

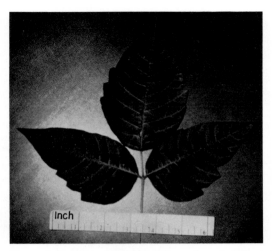

Figure 9–2.　**Large leaves of the poison ivy plant.**

TREATMENT ON FIRST VISIT

1. There are several mistaken notions about poison ivy dermatitis. Assure the patient that he cannot give the dermatitis to his family, or spread it on himself, from the blister fluid.
2. Suggest that the clothes warn while fishing be washed or cleaned to remove the allergenic resin.
3. Perform debridement. The blisters should be opened with manicure scissors, not by sticking with a needle. Cutting the top open with the scissors will prevent that blister from re-forming.
4. Prescribe Burow's solution wet packs.
   Sig: One packet of powder (Domeboro or Bluboro) to 1 quart of cool water.
   Apply sheeting or toweling, wet with the solution, to the blistered areas for 20 minutes twice a day. The wet packs need not be removed during the 20-minute period.
   (For a more widespread case of poison ivy dermatitis, cool baths, with ½ box of Aveeno (Colloidal Oatmeal) or soluble starch to the tub, give considerable relief from the itching.)
5. 1% hydrocortisone lotion q.s.　　　60.0
   (Acticort 100 lotion; 1% Hytone lotion, *etc.*)
   Sig: Apply t.i.d. to the affected areas.
6. Prescribe　chlorpheniramine　tablets, 8 mg　　　　　　　　　　　　　#60
   Sig: 1 tablet t.i.d. (for relief of itching).
   Warn patient about side effect of drowsiness. This drug is available over the

counter but is less expensive if a generic prescription is written.

7. Use cortisone-type injection. Short- but rapid-acting corticosteroids are moderately beneficial, such as Celestone Phosphate (3 mg/ml) in a dose of 1 to 2 ml subcutaneously.

SUBSEQUENT VISITS

1. Continue the wet packs only as long as there are blisters and oozing. Extended use is too drying for the skin.
2. After 3 to 4 days of use, the lotion may be too drying. Substitute:

Fluorinated corticosteroid emollient cream q.s. 60.0

Sig: Apply small amount locally t.i.d., or more often if itching is present.

SEVERE CASES OF POISON IVY DERMATITIS

An oral corticosteroid is indicated in severe poison ivy dermatitis:

Prednisone, 10 mg #40

Sig: 2 tablets b.i.d. for 6 days, then 2 tablets every morning for 8 days.

SAUER NOTES:

1. Most failures in the therapy for severe poison ivy or oak dermatitis result from the failure to continue the oral corticosteroid for 10 to 14 days or longer.

2. Medrol Dos-pak therapy does not provide enough days of treatment for most cases of poison ivy dermatitis.

3. Explain to the patient that it is common for new lesions, even blisters, to continue to pop out during the entire duration of the eruption.

The use of poison ivy vaccine orally or intramuscularly is contraindicated during an acute episode. Desensitization may occur following a long course of oral ingestion of graduated doses of the allergen. Desensitization does not occur following a short course of intramuscular injections of the vaccine, and this form of prophylactic therapy is worthless.

Treatment of Contact Dermatitis of the Hand Due to Soap

A young housewife states that she has had a breaking-out on her hands for 5 weeks. The dermatitis developed about 4 weeks after the birth of her last child. She states that she had a similar eruption after her previous two pregnancies. She has used a lot of local medication of her own, and the rash is getting worse instead of better. The patient and her immediate family never have had any asthma, hay fever, or eczema.

Examination of her hands reveals small vesicles on the sides of all of her fingers, with a 5-cm sized area of oozing and crusting around her left ring finger.

TREATMENT ON THE FIRST VISIT

1. General instructions must always be given to these patients.
   A. Assure the patient that the hand eczema is not contagious to her family.
   B. Inform the patient that soap irritates the dermatitis and that it must be avoided as much as possible. A housewife will find this avoidance very difficult. One of the best remedies is to wear protective gloves when extended soap-and-water contact is unavoidable. Rubber gloves alone produce a considerable amount or irritating perspiration, but this is absorbed when thin white cotton gloves are worn under the rubber gloves. Lined rubber gloves are not as satisfactory because the lining eventually becomes dirty and soggy and cannot be cleaned easily.
   C. For body cleanliness a mild soap, such as Dove, can be used, or any of the following:

   Oilatum Soap
   Basis Soap
   Neutragena Soaps

   D. Tell the patient that the above prophylactic measures will have to be adhered to for several weeks *after* the eruption has apparently cleared, or there will be a recurrence. Injured skin is sensitive and needs to be babied for an extended time.

2. Burow's Solution Soaks
   Sig: 1 packet of powder (Domeboro or Bluboro) to 1 quart of cool water.
   Soak hands for 15 minutes twice a day.
3. Fluorinated corticosteroid cream (See Formulary in Chapter 5).   15.0
   Sig: Apply sparingly, locally, q.i.d.

SAUER NOTES:

1. *Housewives' "eczema"* cannot usually be cured with a corticosteroid salve alone without observing the other protective measures.

2. After the dermatitis is clear, it is very important to advise the patient to treat the area for at least another week to prevent a recurrence. I call this "therapy-plus."

RESISTANT, CHRONIC CASES
1. To the corticosteroid cream add, as indicated, sulfur (3% to 5%), coal tar solution (3% to 10%), or an antipruritic agent such as menthol (0.25%) or camphor (2%).
2. Oral corticosteroid therapy. A short course of such therapy will rapidly improve or cure a chronic dermatitis.

INDUSTRIAL DERMATOSES

Sixty-five percent of all the industrial diseases are dermatoses. The patient with an average case of occupational dermatitis is compensated for 10 weeks, resulting in a total cost of over $100 million a year in the United States. The most common cause of these skin problems is contact irritants, of which cutting oils are the worst offenders. Lack of adequate cleansing is a big contributing factor.

It is not possible to list the thousands of different chemicals used in the hundreds of varied industrial operations that have the potential of causing a primary irritant reaction or an allergic reaction on the skin surface. Excellent books on the subject of occupational dermatitis are listed in the bibliography at the end of this chapter.

Management of Industrial Dermatitis

A cutting-tool laborer presents with a pruritic, red, vesicular dermatitis on his hands, forearms, and face of 2 months' duration.

1. Obtain a careful, detailed history of his type of work, and any recent change, such as use of new chemicals, new cleansing agents, exposure at home with hobbies, painting, and so on. Question him concerning remission of the dermatitis on weekends or while on vacation.
2. Question the patient concerning the first-aid care given at the plant. Too often this care aggravates the dermatitis. Bland protective remedies should be substituted for potential sensitizers, such as sulfonamide and penicillin salves, antihistamine creams, benzocaine ointments, nitrofuran preparations, and strong antipruritic lotions and salves.
3. Treatment of the dermatitis with wet compresses, bland lotions, or salves is the same as for any contact dermatitis (see previous discussion). Unfortunately, many of the occupational dermatoses respond slowly to therapy. This is due, in part, to the fact that most patients continue to work and are reexposed, repeatedly, to small amounts of the irritating chemicals, even though precautions are taken. Also, certain industrial chemicals, such as chromates, beryllium salts, and cutting oils, injure the skin in such a way as to prevent healing for months and years.
4. The legal complications with compensation boards, insurance companies, the industry, and the injured patient can be discouraging, frustrating, and time consuming. However, most patients are not malingerers, but they do expect and deserve proper care and compensation for their injury.

My comprehensive paper on the percentages of skin impairment is entitled "A Guide to the Evaluation of Permanent Impairment of the Skin" (Arch Dermatol 97:566, 1968). A rather similar guide published by the American Medical Association is listed in the bibliography at the conclusion of this chapter.

ATOPIC ECZEMA
(Plates 8 through 12)

Atopic eczema, or atopic dermatitis, is a rather common, markedly pruritic, chronic skin condition that occurs in two clinical forms: *infantile* and *adult.*

CLINICAL LESIONS. *Infantile form:* blisters, oozing, and crusting, with excoriation. *Adolescent and adult forms:* marked dryness, thickening (lichenification), excoriation, and even scarring.

DISTRIBUTION. *Infantile form:* on face, scalp, arms, and legs, or generalized. The diaper area is usually clear. *Adolescent and adult forms:* on cubital and popliteal fossae and, less commonly, on dorsa of hands and feet, ears, or generalized. Atopic eczema of the soles of the feet is quite common in adolescents.

COURSE. The course varies from a mild single episode to severe chronic, recurrent episodes resulting in the "psychoitchical" person. The infantile form usually becomes milder or even disappears after the age 3 or 4. At the age of puberty and the late teens, flare-ups or new outbreaks can occur. Young housewives may have their first recurrence of atopic eczema since childhood due to their new job of dishwashing and child care. Thirty percent of patients with atopic dermatitis eventually develop allergic asthma or hay fever.

ETIOLOGY. The following factors are important:

1. *Heredity* is the most important single factor. The family history is usually positive for one or more of the triad of allergic diseases: asthma, hay fever, or atopic eczema. Determination of this history in cases of hand dermatitis is important because often it will enable the physician, on the patient's first visit, to prognosticate a more drawn out recovery than if the patient had a simple contact dermatitis.
2. *Dryness of the skin* is important. Most often atopic eczema is worse in the winter. The factor here is the decrease in home or office humidity that causes a drying of the skin. For this reason, bathing and the use of soap and water should be reduced.
3. *Wool and lanolin* (wool fat) commonly irritate the skin of these patients. The wearing of wool clothes may be another reason for an increased incidence of atopic eczema in the winter.
4. *Allergy to foods* is a factor often overstressed, particularly with the infantile form. The mother's history of certain foods causing trouble should be your guide for eliminating foods. The correctness of her belief can be tested by adding these incriminated foods to the diet, one new food every 48 hours, when the dermatitis is stable. Scratch tests and intracutaneous tests uncover very few dermatologic allergens.
5. *Emotional stress and nervousness* aggravate any existing condition such as itching, duodenal ulcers, or migraine headaches. Therefore, this "nervous" factor is important but not causative enough to label this disease *disseminated neurodermatitis.*

Differential Diagnosis

Dermatitis venenata: positive history, usually, of contactants; no family allergic history; distribution rather characteristic (see Chap. 9).

Psoriasis: patches localized to extensor surfaces, mainly knees and elbows (see Chap. 14).

Seborrheic dermatitis in infants: absence of family allergy history; lesions scaling and greasy (see Chap. 13).

Localized neurodermatitis: single patches, mainly; no family allergy history (see Chap. 11).

General Management for Atopic Eczema

Inform the patient or family that this is usually a chronic problem; that this is an inherited allergy; that skin tests usually are not helpful; and that relief can occur from the dermatitis and the itch but there is no "cure" except time. The forms shown in Figure 4–1 are very useful to convey this type of information to the patient.

Treatment of Infantile Form

FIRST VISIT

A child, aged 6 months, presents with mild oozing, red, excoriated dermatitis on face, arms, and legs.

(text continues on page 83)

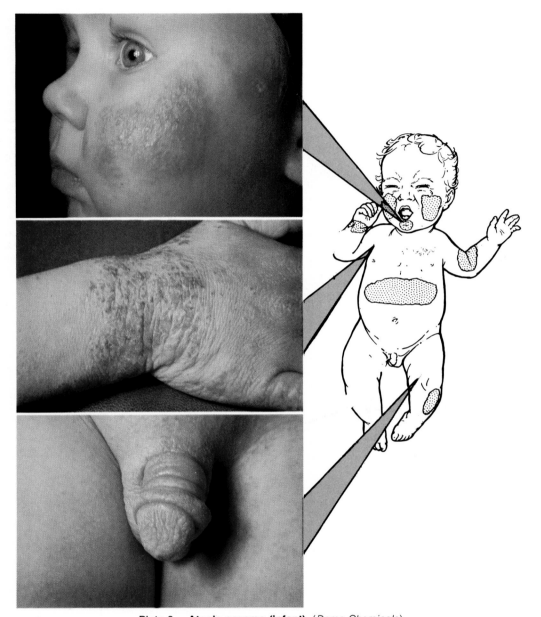

Plate 8. **Atopic eczema (infant).** (*Dome Chemicals*)

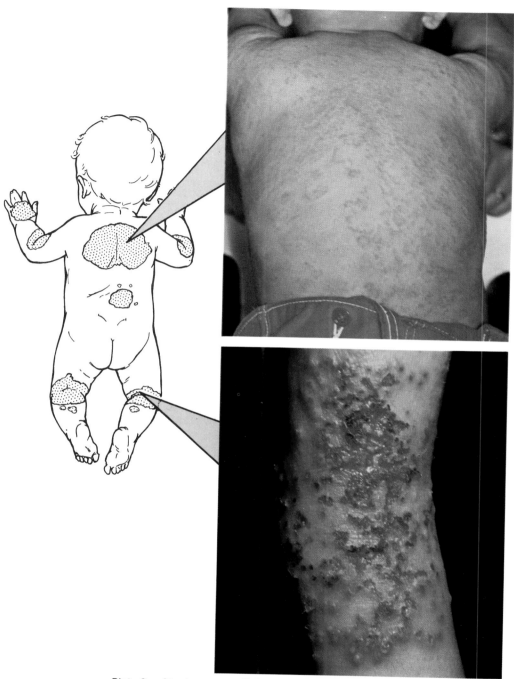

Plate 9. **Atopic eczema (infant).** (*Roche Laboratories*)

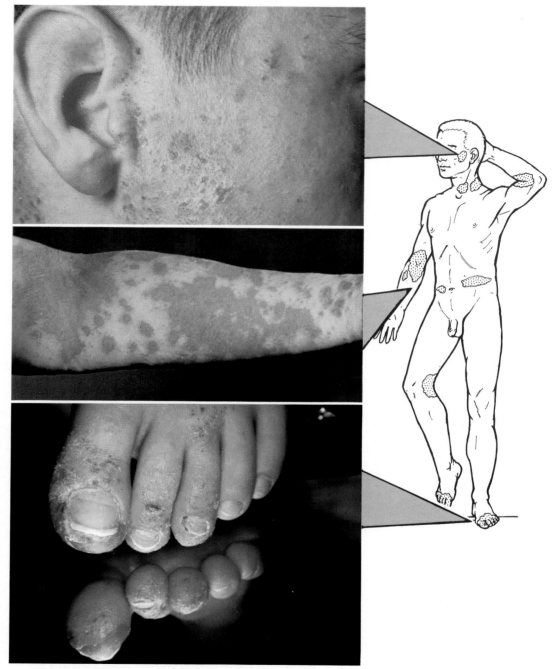

Plate 10. **Atopic eczema.** The bottom photograph, by the use of a mirror, demonstrates the under-surface of the toes. (*Sandoz Pharmaceuticals*)

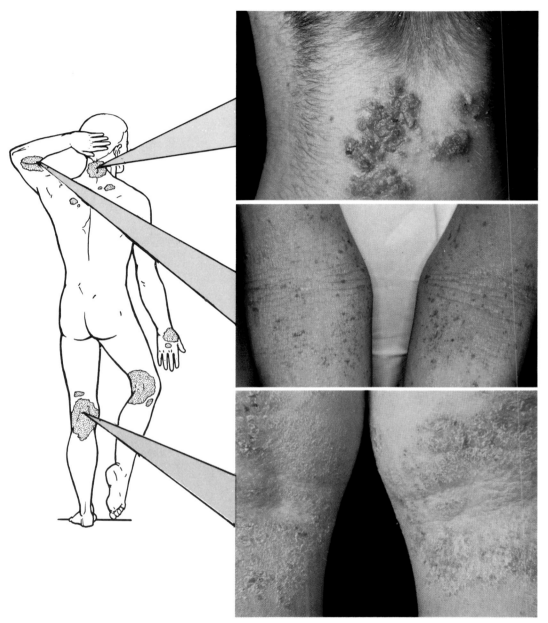

Plate 11. **Atopic eczema.** (*Geigy Pharmaceuticals*)

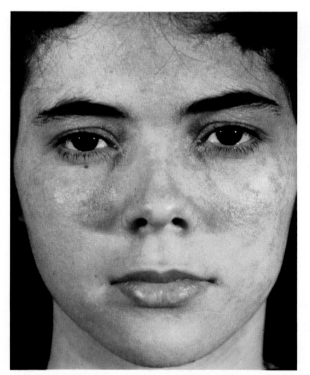

Plate 12. **Atopic eczema.** This case of facial atopic eczema resembled acute lupus erythematosus. The arm eruption is on another patient and exemplifies the chronic lichenified form of atopic eczema. (*K.U.M.C.*) (*Dome Chemicals*)

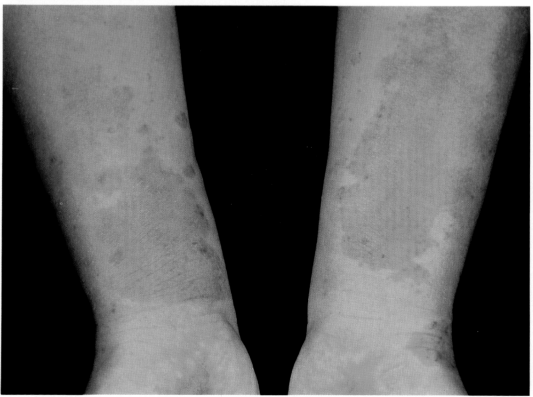

1. Follow regular diet except for the avoidance of any foods that the mother believes aggravate the eruption.
2. Avoid exposure of infant to excessive bathing with soaps and to contact with wool and products containing lanolin.
3. Coal tar solution (L.C.D.)   120.0
   Sig: ½ tablespoon to the lukewarm bath water. Bathe only once or twice a week.
4. Hydrocortisone ointment, 1%   30.0
   (1% Hytone ointment is in a petrolatum base without lanolin; I use it frequently.)
   Sig: Apply sparingly b.i.d. to affected areas. (Other proprietary corticosteroid preparations are listed in the Formulary; see Chap. 5.)
5. Benadryl elixer   90.0
   Sig: 1 teaspoonful b.i.d. Warn parent that this drug may stimulate the child.

SUBSEQUENT VISITS
1. Add coal tar solution (3% to 10%) to the above ointment.

SEVERE OR RESISTANT CASES
1. Restrict diet to milk only, and after 3 days add one different food every 24 hours. An offending food will cause a flare-up of the eczema in several hours.
2. Hydrocortisone liquid
   (Fluid Cortef)   90.0
   Sig: 1 teaspoonful (10 mg) q.i.d. for 3 days, then 1 teaspoonful t.i.d. for 1 week. (Decrease the dose or discontinue as improvement warrants. Vary the dosage according to the weight of the child.)
3. Hospitalization with change of environment may be necessary for a severe case.

Treatment of Adult Form

FIRST VISIT
A young adult presents with dry, scaly, lichenified patches in cubital and popliteal fossae:

1. Stress avoidance of excess soap and water for bathing, of lanolin preparations locally, and of contact with wool.
2. Coal tar solution (L.C.D.)   5%
   Fluorinated corticosteroid ointment or emollient cream (see Chap. 5) q.s. 30.0
3. Chlor-trimeton 8 mg or 12 mg   #60
   Sig: 1 tablet b.i.d.
   Warn patient about side-effect of drowsiness. (Available generically and over-the-counter.)

> **SAUER NOTE:**
>
> Do not *initiate* local corticosteroid therapy with the strongest "big guns." Save these for later use, if necessary.

Terfenadine (Seldane), 60 mg, b.i.d.; astemizole (Hismanal), 10 mg, once a day (2 hours after a meal); or clemastine (Tavist-1), 1 tablet b.i.d., relieves itching.

SUBSEQUENT VISITS
1. Gradually increase the concentration of the coal tar solution in the previously mentioned salve up to 10%.
2. Increase the potency of the corticosteroid ointment or emollient cream.
3. For patients with infected crusted lesions (all patients have an element of infection), an antibiotic such as erythromycin, 250 mg, could be prescribed b.i.d., or t.i.d., for several weeks.
4. Systemic corticosteroid therapy may be indicated for severe and resistant cases.

> **SAUER NOTES:**
>
> 1. With every visit, reemphasize the fact of the chronicity of this disease and the ups and downs that occur, particularly with seasons and stress.
> 2. Nonspecific protein injections. These are of some value. An example is Bacterial Vaccine (Hollister-Stier), beginning with 0.05 ml and increasing very gradually weekly or biweekly, as tolerated, up to 1.0 ml. A mildly sore arm reaction for 24 hours is normal.
>   I know that my suggestion of the use of such nonspecific injection therapy is open to skepticism and criticism, but I strongly believe in the value of this therapy.

NUMMULAR ECZEMA
(Plate 13)

Nummular eczema is a moderately common, distinctive eczematous eruption characterized by coin-shaped (nummular), papulo-

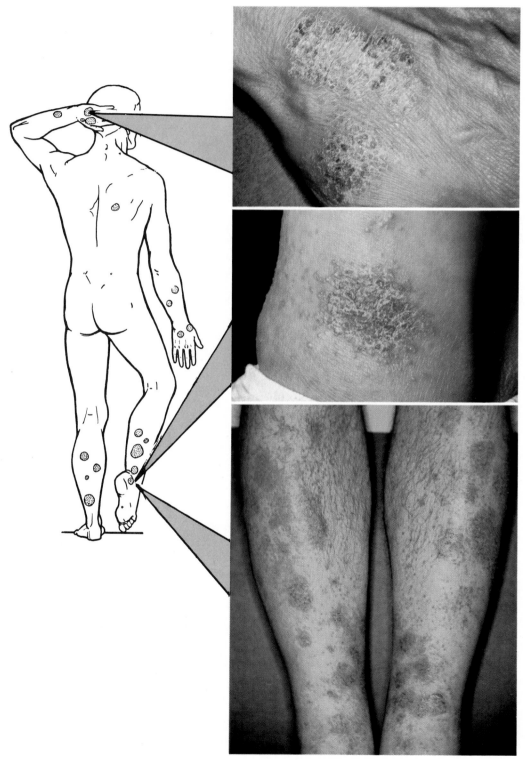

Plate 13. **Nummular eczema.** (*Schering Corp.*)

vesicular patches, mainly on the arms and the legs of young adults and elderly patients.

PRIMARY LESIONS. Coin-shaped patches of vesicles and papules are usually seen on the extremities, occasionally on the trunk.

SECONDARY LESIONS. Lichenification and bacterial infection occur.

COURSE. This is very chronic, particularly in the older age-group. Recurrences are common.

SUBJECTIVE COMPLAINTS. Itching is usually quite severe.

ETIOLOGY. Nothing is definite, but these factors are important:

1. History is usually positive for asthma, hay fever, or atopic eczema, particularly in the young adult.
2. Ingestion of iodides and bromides aggravates the disease.
3. Bacterial infection of the lesions is common.
4. In the older age-group a history of a low-protein diet is common.
5. The low indoor humidity of winter causes dry skin, which intensifies the itching, particularly in the elderly patients.

Differential Diagnosis

Atopic eczema: mainly in cubital and popliteal fossae, not coin-sized lesions (see preceding section).
Psoriasis: not vesicular; see scalp and fingernail lesions (Chap. 14).
Contact dermatitis: will not see coin-sized lesions on both arms and legs (see beginning of this chapter).
"Id" reaction, from stasis dermatitis of legs or a localized contact dermatitis: impossible to differentiate this clinically from nummular eczema but have history of previous primary dermatitis that suddenly became aggravated.

Treatment

FIRST VISIT
An elderly man presents in the winter with five to eight distinct, coin-shaped, excoriated, vesicular, crusted lesions on the arms and the legs.

1. Instruct the patient to avoid excess bathing with soap and water.
2. Tell the patient to avoid these foods, which are rich in iodides and bromides: chocolate, salted nuts, cheeses (except cottage cheese), seafoods, iodized salt (can use plain salt), tomatoes, melons, and dark greens.

SAUER NOTES:

1. The value of a low iodine and bromide diet is important for nummular eczema and dermatitis herpetiformis.
2. My teacher at the New York Skin and Cancer Clinic, Dr. Max Jessner, patch tested these patients to fresh iodine and bromide preparations and found them positive.

---

3. Increase the intake of protein-rich foods, such as beef products, liver, and gelatin.
4. Corticosteroid ointment   60.0
   Sig: Apply t.i.d. locally.
   The use of the *ointment* base is particularly important in the therapy for nummular eczema.
5. Benadryl, 50 mg   #15
   Sig: 1 capsule h.s. for antipruritic and sedative effect. (Available generically and over-the-counter.)

RESISTANT CASES
1. Add coal tar solution, 3% to 10%, to the previously mentioned salve.
2. Oral antibiotic therapy is beneficial because all cases have an element of infection. Prescribe erythromycin, 250 mg, t.i.d. for several weeks.
3. A short course of oral corticosteroid therapy is effective, but relapses are common.

DRUG ERUPTIONS
(Plate 14)

It can be stated almost without exception that any drug systemically administered is capable of causing a skin eruption.

To jog the memory of patients I often ask, "Do you take any medicine for any condition? What about medicated toothpaste, laxatives,

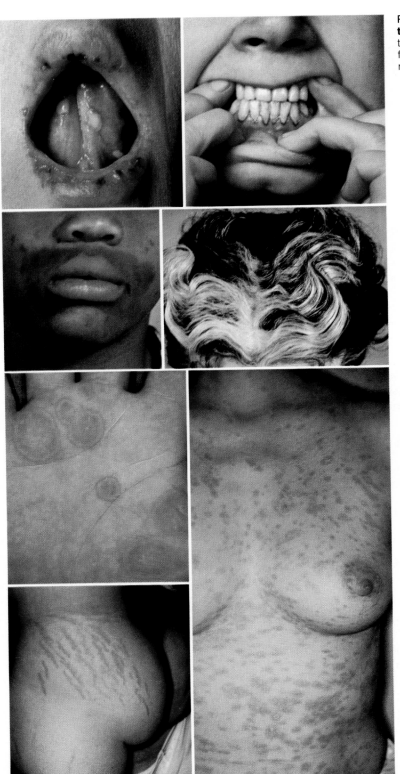

Plate 14. Drug eruptions. (*Left*) Erosions of tongue and lips from sulfonamides. (*Right*) Bismuth line of gums.

(*Left*) Phenolphthalein fixed eruption of lips of a black boy. (*Right*) Whitening of scalp hair from chloroquine therapy for lupus erythematosus.

(*Left, upper*) Erythema multiforme–like eruption of palm from oral antibiotic therapy. (*Left, lower*) Striae of buttocks of 30-year-old man following 9 months of corticosteroid therapy. (*Right*) Papulosquamous eruption of chest from phenolphthalein. (*E. R. Squibb*)

vitamins, aspirin, and tonics? Have you received any shots in the past month?" As stated in Chapter 4, this questioning also gives the physician some general information regarding other ills of the patient that might influence the skin problem. (An eruption due to allergy or primary irritation from *locally* applied drugs is a contact dermatitis.)

SAUER NOTE:

Any patient with a generalized skin eruption should be carefully questioned concerning the use of oral or parenteral medicinal drugs.

Any of the larger dermatologic texts have extensive lists of common and uncommon drugs, with their common and uncommon skin reactions. These books must be consulted for the rare reactions, but the following paragraphs will cover 95% of these idiosyncrasies.

Photosensitivity reactions from drugs are also covered in Chapter 31.

Drugs and the Dermatoses They Cause

Drug eruptions are usually not characteristic for any certain drug or group of drugs. However, the following drugs most commonly cause the associated listed skin lesions. Systemic drug reactions will not be stressed in this chapter.

ACCUTANE. (See Isotretinoin.)

ACETAMINOPHEN (TYLENOL). This drug is an infrequent cause of drug eruption.

ACETOPHENETIDIN (PHENACETIN). This drug is found in Empirin Compound, Phenaphen, A.S.A. Compound, A.P.C., BC, Nembudeine, Bromo Quinine, Super-Anahist and many other remedies. Urticaria and erythematous eruptions are noted.

ACTH. Cushing's syndrome, hyperpigmentation, acneiform eruptions, seborrheic dermatitis–like eruptions, and hirsutism have been seen.

ALLOPURINOL (ZYLOPRIM). Erythema, maculopapular rash, and severe bullae are noted.

AMANTADINE. Livedo reticularis is seen.

AMINOSALICYLIC ACID. Scarlatiniform or morbilliform rash, fixed drug eruption, and nummular eczema–like rash are seen.

AMPHETAMINE (BENZEDRINE). Coldness of extremities and redness of neck and shoulders occur; it increases itching in neurodermatitis.

AMPICILLIN. (See Antibiotics.)

ANTABUSE. Redness of face and acne may be noted.

ANTIBIOTICS. Various agents have different reactions, but in general, candidal overgrowth in oral, genital, and anal orifices results in pruritus ani, pruritus vulvae, and generalized pruritus. Candidal skin lesions may spread out from these foci. Also common are urticaria and erythema multiforme–like eruptions, particularly from penicillin. Ampicillin not infrequently causes a generalized maculopapular rash. (See Streptomycin and also Photosensitivity Reactions at end of chapter.)

ANTICOAGULANTS. Bishydroxycoumarin (Dicumarol), sodium warfarin (Coumadin), and heparin can cause severe hemorrhagic skin infarction and necrosis.

ANTIHISTAMINES. These drugs are found in Coricidin, Super-Anahist, and many other preparations. They cause urticaria, eczematous dermatitis, and pityriasis rosea–like rash.

ANTINEOPLASTIC AGENTS. These can cause many skin and mucocutaneous reactions, including alopecia, stomatitis, radiation recall reaction, and erythemas.

ANTITOXIN. Immediate reaction occurs with skin manifestations of pruritus, urticaria, and sweating; delayed serum sickness reaction is evidenced by urticaria, redness, and purpura.

APRESOLINE. Systemic lupus erythematosus–like reaction occurs.

ARSENIC. Inorganic arsenic (Fowler's solution, Asiatic pills) causes erythematous, scarlatiniform, vesicular, or urticarial rashes. Delayed reactions include palmar and plantar keratoses and eventual carcinomatous changes. Organic arsenic (Mapharsen, Neoarsphenamine, Tryparsamide) causes similar skin changes plus a severe form of exfoliative dermatitis. A mild erythema on the ninth day of therapy is not unusual. British Antilewisite (BAL) is effective therapy if given early for the skin reactions due to organic arsenicals.

ASPIRIN AND SALICYLATES. Aspirin is found as an ingredient in a multitude of cold and anti-pain remedies. Pepto-Bismol contains salicylates. Urticaria, purpura, and bullous lesions result.

ATABRINE. Universal yellow pigmentation, blue macules on face and mucosa, and lichen planus—like eruption are found.

ATROPINE. Scarlet fever—like rash occurs.

BARBITURATES. This class of drugs causes urticarial, erythematous, bullous, or purpuric eruptions and fixed drug eruptions.

BISMUTH. Bluish pigmentation of gums and erythematous, papulosquamous, and urticarial skin eruptions have been reported.

BORIC ACID. Accidental oral ingestion can cause exfoliative dermatitis and severe systemic reaction.

BROMIDES. (See Iodides.) Bromides are found in Neurosine, Bromo Quinine, Bromo-Seltzer, Shut-eye, and other drugs. Acnelike pustular lesions that can spread to form deep granulomatous pyodermas that heal with marked scarring are mainly seen. These must be differentiated from other granulomas.

BUTAZOLIDIN. (See Phenylbutazone.)

CAPTOPRIL. Pemphigus-like eruption may occur.

CHEMOTHERAPY AGENTS. (See Antineoplastic Agents.)

CHLORAL HYDRATE. Urticarial, papular, erythematous, and purpuric eruptions occur.

CHLOROQUINE. Erythematous or lichenoid eruptions with pruritus and urticaria have been noted. (Ocular retinal damage from long-term use of chloroquine and other antimalarials can be irreversible.)

CHLOROTHIAZIDE DIURETICS. (See Photosensitivity Reactions at end of chapter.)

CHLORPROMAZINE (THORAZINE). Maculopapular rash, increased sun sensitivity, purpura with agranulocytosis, and icterus from hepatitis may occur. With long-term therapy a slate gray to violet discoloration of the skin can develop.

CIMETIDINE. Dry, scaly skin may result.

CLOFIBRATE. Alopecia may occur.

CODEINE AND MORPHINE. Erythematous, urticarial, or vesicular eruption has been noted.

COLLAGEN, BOVINE, INJECTED. Skin edema, erythema, induration, and urticaria may be seen at implantation sites.

CONTRACEPTIVE DRUGS. Chloasma-like eruption, erythema nodosum, and hives occur, and some cases of acne are aggravated.

CORTISONE AND DERIVATIVES. Cutaneous allergy is rare.

COUMADIN. (See Anticoagulants.)

DAPSONE. Red, maculopapular, vesicular eruption with agranulocytosis occurs, occasionally resembling erythema nodosum.

DICUMAROL. (See Anticoagulants.)

DIETHYLPROPION HYDROCHLORIDE (TENUATE, TEPANIL). Measles-like eruption has been reported.

DIGITALIS. An erythematous, papular eruption is seen rarely.

DIGITOXIN. Thrombocytopenic purpura has been noted.

DILANTIN. (See Phenytoin.)

DORIDEN. (See Glutethimide.)

ESTROGENIC SUBSTANCES AND STILBESTROL. Edema of legs with cutaneous redness progressing to exfoliative dermatitis is seen.

FELDENE. (See Piroxicam under Photosensitivity Reactions at end of chapter.)

FLAGYL. (See Metronidazole).

FUROSEMIDE. Bullous hemorrhagic eruption occurs.

GLUTETHIMIDE (DORIDEN). Erythema, urticaria, purpura, or (rarely) exfoliative dermatitis has been reported.

GOLD. There is eczematous dermatitis of hands, arms, and legs or a pityriasis rosea—like eruption. Seborrheic-like eruption, urticaria, or purpura has also been found.

10

Dermatologic Immunology

David A. Norris, M.D.,* and Walter H. C. Burgdorf, M.D.†

THE IMMUNE RESPONSE AND DERMATOLOGY

A large proportion of dermatologic patients present with diseases characterized by cutaneous inflammation. Although the skin has long been thought of as an effective barrier between humans and their environment, it is now clear that it is not an inert shield but instead a major participant in the complex immunologic reactions that protect humans against foreign antigens. The skin is the most exposed of all epithelial surfaces, separated from irritants, toxins, and microorganisms by a thin barrier of dried epithelial cells. Because it is so accessible, minor degrees of inflammation are readily observed. Whether the triggering agent is a bacterial infection such as impetigo, bacterial and lipid products as in acne, or a contact allergen as in poison ivy, the common denominator is the tissue change induced by the humoral and/or cellular mediators of the immune response. In this brief section, the basic features of this response will be

reviewed and correlated with many of the skin diseases discussed elsewhere in the text. The reader is referred to the bibliography for more thorough introductory works on basic immunology.

THE IMMUNE RESPONSE: DESIGN AND ORGANIZATION

The main purpose of the immune response is to recognize foreign substances (antigens) and implement their removal from the host. This role response is complex because antigens differ: some are large, some are small; some are polysaccharides, some are proteins; some are soluble, some are tightly bound to cells; some are presented in the circulation, some in tissue, some on mucosal surfaces, and some to the stratum corneum. The immune response can be divided in a number of different ways. First, there is both an afferent and efferent limb. The afferent limb refers to the events between initial exposure to an antigen and developing hypersensitivity to it, while the efferent limb refers to the events producing inflammation as the specific immune response is amplified in response to the antigen.

There are both nonspecific and specific responses. The former occur in many situations without evoking immunologic memory, such as when the body reacts to a splinter. The latter require earlier exposure to an antigen and

* Professor, Department of Dermatology, University of Colorado School of Medicine, Denver, Colorado

† Professor and Chairman, Department of Dermatology, University of New Mexico School of Medicine, Albuquerque, New Mexico

then an antigen-specific response involving memory cells. Many factors are responsible for nonspecific immune response. The main one is phagocytosis, in which polymorphonuclear white blood cells and monocytes and macrophages from the circulation and a variety of tissues engulf foreign objects. This process can be enhanced by cells and soluble products of the specific immune response. The complement cascade can also be nonspecifically initiated to produce inflammation. Finally, some specialized lymphocytes (natural killer, or NK, cells) and eosinophils can attack foreign cells, such as tumor cells, or parasites without specific recognition or sensitization.

The most widespread separation of the immune response is into humoral and cellular immunity. Lymphocyte stem cells develop into B and T lymphocytes, responsible for humoral or antibody-mediated and cellular immune responses, respectively (Fig. 10–1). Fortunately for the body, there is a series of complex interactions between these two branches, mediated both by direct cellular interactions and by a variety of soluble factors. First we will briefly review the traditional B and T cell functions and then even more briefly consider these interactions. The major "actors" in this process are summarized in Table 10–1.

The humoral immune response develops when a B cell coated with an immunoglobulin (monomeric IgM) recognizes an antigen of a given shape that binds with its surface IgM.

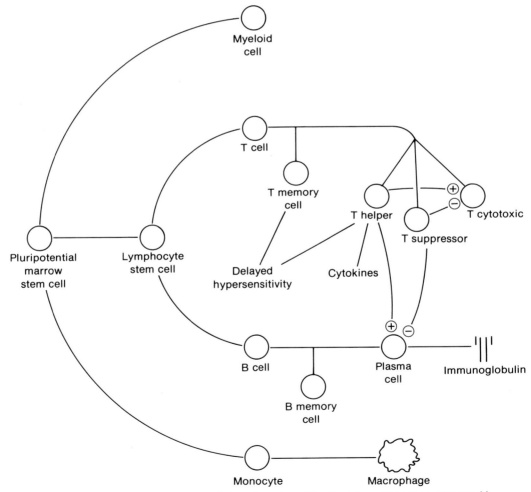

Figure 10–1. Development of T and B lymphocytes. (*Modified from Chapel H, Haeney M: Essentials of Clinical Immunology. Oxford, Blackwell, 1984; courtesy of Dr. C. Littler*)

Table 10–1
Components of the Immune Response

TYPE	DIFFERENTIATION	LOCATION	FUNCTION
Cellular Components			
T lymphocyte	1. Derived from lymphoid cells in bone marrow 2. Induced to differentiate by direct and humoral influence of thymus	1. Peripheral blood 2. Tissue fluids (recirculating small lymphocyte) 3. Lymph nodes 4. Spleen 5. Marrow	1. Specific antigen recognition to trigger cell–mediated response 2. Mobilizes other cells to participate in cell-mediated response (lymphokine production) 3. Regulate B-cell function 4. "Memory cell"
B lymphocyte	1. Derived from marrow lymphoid cells 2. Induced to differentiate in "gut-associated lymphoid tissue" (GALT)	1. Lymph nodes 2. Spleen 3. Peripheral blood	1. Sensitization with specific antigen causes differentiation into plasma cell 2. "Memory cell"
Plasma cell	Derived from sensitized B lymphocyte	1. Lymph nodes 2. Spleen 3. GALT 4. Bone marrow	Antibody production
Monocyte/ macrophage	1. Myeloid origin in bone marrow 2. Monocytes released from marrow populate peripheral tissue and differentiate into macrophages	1. Peripheral blood 2. All tissues, specialized functions in different tissues—long-lived	1. "Present" antigens to B and T lymphocytes 2. "Garbage collectors" 3. Cytotoxic cells—nonspecific 4. Engulf opsonized bacteria 5. Production of regulating proteins
Neutrophil	1. Myeloid origin in marrow 2. Short-lived end-stage cell	1. Peripheral blood 2. "Marginal pool" 3. Tissue sites of inflammation—short-lived	1. Engulf and kill opsonized microorganisms 2. Engulf tissue deposits of immune complexes
Mast cell	? Mesenchymal origin	Around blood vessels in most organs	1. Modulate vascular permeability by release of vasoactive amines 2. Mobilize eosinophils
Basophil	Myeloid origin in bone marrow	Peripheral blood	Similar to mast cell
Platelet	Derived from bone marrow	Peripheral blood	1. Modulate vascular permeability 2. Participate in clot formation
Eosinophil	Myeloid origin in bone marrow	1. Peripheral blood 2. Tissue sites of inflammation	1. Kill parasites 2. Counteract mast cell–initiated changes in vascular permeability
Soluble Factors (Antibodies)			
IgG (1200 mg/dl)	Produced by plasma cells	Blood, tissue fluid	1. Long-lasting immunity 2. Placental transfer
IgM (100 mg/dl)		Blood > tissue	1. Early antibody response 2. Antigen recognition
IgA (200 mg/dl)		Secretions > blood	Protective barrier in secretions
IgE (0.05 mg/dl)		Cell-bound in tissue blood	Anaphylaxis, bound to mast cells
IgD (3 mg/dl)		B-cell surface during differentiation	Surface receptor (?)

There then occurs a clonal expansion of this particular B cell into plasma cells that produce immunoglobulin identical in configuration to that which initially recognized the foreign antigen. Imprinted B memory cells are retained in the body so that on subsequent exposure there is a rapid and greater production of protective immunoglobulin.

The five major groups of immunoglobulin are constructed from a widely distributed molecule of two heavy chains and two light chains, which on one end (the variable region) has the capacity to assume many shapes and interact with many specific antigens. Similar structures are involved in many other aspects of the immune response; the major histocompatibility complex antigens and the T-cell receptor are similar to immunoglobulin. Antibodies work in many ways to produce destruction of antigen. By coating a microorganism, they can facilitate phagocytosis. They also serve to activate complement, producing cell membrane destruction.

Complement is a complex system of proteins that has bedeviled students for many years. As Figure 10–2 shows, there is a cascade effect with a variety of biologic roles. These include (1) opsonization (making it easier for phagocytes to take up material coated with complement fragments), (2) production of biologically active fragments that can stimulate leukocyte chemotaxis and mast cell release (to mention two examples), and (3) membrane destruction to kill cells.

The cellular or T-cell response is primarily directed against intracellular antigens. T cells are introduced to antigens via antigen-presenting cells, such as phagocytes or, in the skin, Langerhans' cells. The T cells interact with a variety of presenting cell surface antigens along with the foreign antigen expressed on the cell surface. In this way T cells with memory for an antigen develop and then are capable of producing classic cell-mediated immunity on reexposure and complement (clean-up phagocytes). The specific T cells recognize the antigen and call in nonspecific cells such as phagocytes to complete the task of destroying the antigen.

The T-cell subsets and mediators have become at least peripherally familiar to most physicians and many patients because of the acquired immunodeficiency syndrome (AIDS) epidemic. T cells are recognized by a variety of antigens on their surfaces. In simplest terms, there are at least two major types of T cells in peripheral blood: the T-helper/inducer (T_H) cells (identified by the T4 or CD4 antigen on its surface) and the T-suppressor/cytotoxic cell (T_S) (with T8, CD8). The T_H interacts with antigen-presenting cells to produce a variety of soluble lymphokines, which then control the nonspecific arm of the immune response. Included in this group are interleukins, which further drive the cell-mediated response; interferons, which provide protection against viral infections; and macrophage activating and controlling factors. This subset of T_H cells is the one that is selectively reduced in patients with human immunodeficiency virus (HIV) infection and is thus responsible for at least some of the panoply of immune defects in patients with AIDS. Some T_H cells help B lymphocytes proliferate, while others activate T_S cells. These T_S cells interact with B cells to suppress immunoglobulin production, while one subset (T_C) is cytotoxic, binding to cells via surface antigen to provide direct cell killing. This brief overview shows how these

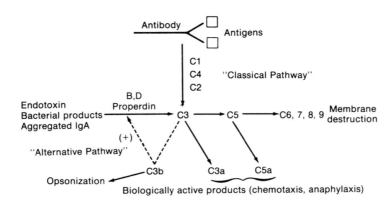

Figure 10–2. **Complement activation.**

complex interactions modulate the immune response.

THE GELL AND COOMBS' CLASSIFICATION OF IMMUNE RESPONSE

The Gell and Coombs' classification of immunologic injury is presented in Table 10–2. This is a convenient format for discussing the different mechanisms of tissue damage induced by the immune response. Types I through III are antibody mediated. Type IV encompasses all of the classic cell-mediated immune responses. However, all of the antibody-mediated processes require nonspecific effector cells to complete antigen destruction.

Type I reactions involve specific IgE, bound either to mast cells or to basophils. Interaction of IgE with specific antigen triggers the release of histamine and other vasoactive amines, creating increased vascular permeability, smooth muscle contraction, and either anaphylactic or allergic symptoms, depending on the principal target organs involved, the route of antigen administration, and the location of specific IgE-containing mast cells.

Type II reactions involve antibody binding specifically to cell walls, basement membranes, or bacteria in tissue. Destruction of antigens bound to antibody is accomplished either by direct lysis, complement-mediated lysis, phagocytosis by neutrophils, or antibody-dependent cellular cytotoxicity (ADCC) involving nonspecific effector cell recognition of antibody bound to cell surface antigen.

In *Type III reactions*, immune complexes composed of antigens and antibody in varying proportions form in tissue or localize from the circulation, fix complement, and attract neutrophils, which induce nonspecific cellular damage. The role of mast cells, basophils, or platelets in altering vascular permeability and promoting tissue deposition of circulating complexes is believed to be important in this type of reaction.

Type IV reactions are classic cell-mediated immune responses, as seen in delayed-type hypersensitivity reactions, contact dermatitis, skin graft rejection, and destruction of obligate intracellular organisms such as *Mycobacterium leprae*.

DISEASES AFFECTING THE SKIN

Diseases Characterized by Type I Injury

Anaphylaxis

Generalized immediate hypersensitivity reactions, known historically as anaphylaxis, cause airway obstruction secondary to bron-

Table 10–2
Gell and Coombs' Classification of Immunologic Injury

TYPE	DESCRIPTION	EFFECTORS INVOLVED	DISEASES
I	IgE-mediated	IgE—mast cell IgE—basophil Histamine	Anaphylaxis Acute urticaria Allergic rhinitis, asthma
II	Antimembrane antibody	1. Direct cell lysis 2. Phagocytosis Neutrophils Macrophages 3. Complement-mediated lysis 4. Antibody-dependent cellular cytotoxicity (ADCC)—macrophage/monocyte, neutrophil, lymphocyte	Pemphigus vulgaris Bullous pemphigoid Herpes gestationis
III	Immune-complex disease	Neutrophils	Vasculitis Dermatitis herpetiformis Serum sickness
IV	Cell-mediated immunity	Lymphocytes Monocytes	Contact dermatitis Photoallergic dermatitis Skin test reaction Skin graft rejection

chial constriction, hypotension due to decreased intravascular volume, severe gastrointestinal cramping, urticaria or angioedema, and laryngeal edema. Anaphylaxis is caused by generalized mast cell degranulation releasing histamine and other vasoactive substances and is initiated by antigens binding to mast cell surface IgE, by degranulating drugs, and by complement fragments (C3a and C5a) that can directly induce mast cell degranulation. Clinically, anaphylaxis is most commonly caused by drugs or other injections (*e.g.,* penicillin, sulfonamides, salicylates, local anesthetics, vaccines, hyperimmune sera, or allergen extracts), diagnostic compounds (radiocontrast media), foods (legumes, nuts, berries, seafood, eggs), or the stings of insects (bees, wasps, fire ants). Therapy must be rapid and must include drugs that block histamine release from mast cells (sympathomimetics, such as epinephrine and terbutaline, and methylxanthines, such as aminophylline), drugs that block histamine effect (antihistamines), and intravascular volume replacement.

Urticaria

Most cases of *acute urticaria* are mediated by IgE mast cell degranulation after ingestion of certain foods and drugs or following insect bites or infections such as hepatitis. The mast cell products cause localized vessel wall leakage and edema, producing the well-known hive or wheal.

Chronic urticaria is a more difficult problem. The cause of chronic urticaria in any individual patient is usually not identifiable. Occult infections (dental, gastrointestinal, sinus, and genitourinary), over-the-counter medications, foods, or psychogenic causes are frequently cited. Whether the mechanism of disease is purely IgE-induced mast cell degranulation is not clear. The variable response to antihistamines suggests that other pathomechanisms are involved. Evidence of mild necrotizing vasculitis in some cases (*urticarial vasculitis*) suggests that immune complexes, complement, and neutrophils can be important components of this process.

Physical urticarias are another group of poorly understood entities whose relationships to type I disease is not clear. *Symptomatic dermographism* can be passively transferred (*i.e.,* transferred by serum from affected persons) and may be IgE mediated. *Solar urticaria* can also be passively transferred, and there is inferential evidence that the active molecule is IgE. *Cholinergic urticaria* represents hypersensitivity of mast cells or vessels to cholinergic stimuli. *Cold urticaria* is a composite of familial cold urticaria, which is not histamine mediated, and acquired cold urticaria, which is histamine mediated; it is induced by IgE or IgM triggering of mast cells. *Pressure urticaria* is responsive to corticosteroids and apparently not caused by histamine.

Atopic Disease

Patients with atopic dermatitis have a strong personal or family history of allergic rhinitis and asthma, both of which are type I immunologic diseases. However, the precise mechanism of skin disease in atopic persons is not well understood. Peripheral blood eosinophilia, elevated serum IgE levels, and aberrant histamine and cholinergic responses in the skin suggest type I reactivity, but the injection of histamine into the skin of atopic patients does not produce dermatitis and the serum IgE does not follow the course of the skin disease. In addition, atopic persons are susceptible to recurrent cutaneous bacterial infections and severe generalized viral exanthems (Kaposi's varicelliform eruption) and also exhibit defects in T-cell function. Thus, the basic immunologic defect in atopic dermatitis remains elusive.

Mast Cell Disease

There are a variety of patients with increased numbers of cutaneous mast cells. These may be solitary tumors (mastocytoma) or widespread infiltrates (urticaria pigmentosa). When the skin is stroked, there is often mast cell degranulation with pruritus and edema. When enough mast cell degranulation occurs, systemic symptoms such as bronchospasm or gastrointestinal cramping may occur.

Diseases Characterized by Type II Injury

Bullous Pemphigoid

Clinically, bullous pemphigoid is characterized by large, flaccid, often intact blisters on an erythematous base. The immunologic findings explain this clinical picture. Histologically, bullous pemphigoid displays a subepidermal blister and a dermal neutrophilic infiltrate, often with eosinophils. Direct immunofluorescent staining of skin from these patients shows "linear or tubular" IgG (sometimes IgA or IgM) and complement deposited at the basement membrane. Serum from 80% of these patients contains IgG, which forms a linear pattern in the basement membrane.

This linear pattern suggests that a specific IgG antibody combines with a specific basement membrane antigen (known as the bullous pemphigoid antigen), fixes complement by the classic pathway, and generates C3a and C5a, which attract neutrophils to the dermal-epidermal junction, generating both release of proteolytic enzymes and tissue destruction. Activation of mast cells by C5a also appears to be very important in blister formation.

The blister is stable and intact because the separation occurs beneath the epidermis, so the blister roof is "almost normal" epidermis. The activation of complement may be responsible for the associated erythema and dermal infiltrate.

Pemphigus Vulgaris

The flaccid bullae and erosions of pemphigus are caused by an intraepidermal blister associated with a neutrophilic infiltrate. Direct immunofluorescence of involved skin demonstrates IgG and complement components in the intercellular spaces surrounding the cells of the epidermis. Over 90% of patients have a serum IgG antibody directed against the intercellular cement substance of the epidermis, and increases in the level of this antibody may precede clinical flare-ups of the disease. It is believed that the combination of antigen and antibody at the site of the intercellular cement fixes complement by the classic pathway and causes acantholysis and cell separation. There is also considerable evidence that antibody alone releases epidermal proteases, which cause acantholysis with or without complement. Direct epidermal cell destruction by antibody or antibody plus complement is probably not a primary mechanism of acantholysis.

Diseases Characterized by Type III Injury (Immune Complex Disease)

Necrotizing Vasculitis

Necrotizing vasculitis is a histologic diagnosis based on vessel wall necrosis, with invasion of the vessel wall with neutrophils, nuclear fragmentation ("leukocytoclasis") of neutrophils, fibrinoid deposits in the vessel wall, and often thrombosis, perivascular hemorrhage, and chronic granulomatous inflammation. The following list outlines one classification of necrotizing vasculitis:

I. **Leukocytoclastic Vasculitis (Hypersensitivity Angiitis, Allergic Vasculitis)**
   A. Henoch-Schönlein purpura
   B. Hypocomplementemic vasculitis
   C. Mixed cryoglobulinemia
   D. Disease-related vasculitis (*e.g.*, subacute bacterial endocarditis, ulcerative colitis)
   E. Drug-induced vasculitis
II. **Rheumatic Vasculitis**
   A. Systemic lupus erythematosus
   B. Rheumatoid vasculitis
   C. Scleroderma
   D. Dermatomyositis
   E. Acute rheumatic fever
III. **Granulomatous Vasculitis**
   A. Allergic granulomatosis (Churg and Strauss)
   B. Wegener's granulomatosis
IV. **Polyarteritis Nodosa—Classic, Limited, Hepatitis-associated**
V. **Giant Cell Arteritis**

The role of immune complexes in inducing necrotizing vasculitis is widely accepted for many diseases characterized by these histologic findings but has been most clearly demonstrated in hypersensitivity angiitis and rheumatic vasculitis. These two forms of necrotizing vasculitis are characterized by discrete palpable purpuric lesions or sometimes by local tissue infarcts, caused by immune complex deposition in superficial dermal postcapillary venules and small arterioles. Larger subcutaneous vessels, as well as dermal arterioles, are involved in granulomatous vasculitis and polyarteritis nodosa, producing dermal and subcutaneous nodules, livedo reticularis, or larger segmental infarcts. In addition, the joints, the gastrointestinal tract, and other organs such as the kidney, brain, and lungs can be involved in these varying types of vasculitis.

Dermatitis Herpetiformis

Dermatitis herpetiformis is an intensely pruritic eruption consisting of grouped tiny vesicles. In this disease, IgA is deposited in the dermal papillae, complement is locally activated by way of the alternative pathway, and neutrophils and eosinophils are attracted to the dermal papillae. The tissue damage induced by their proteolytic enzymes produces subepidermal blister formation, associated clinically with intense pruritus. Immunofluorescent staining for IgA, C3, or properdin is positive in the dermal papillae. Dermatitis herpetiformis and gluten-sensitive enteropathy are believed to be clinically related and are both improved by gluten-free diet. One current hypothesis is that the IgA is complexed with gluten protein, which binds nonspecifically in the dermis.

Serum Sickness

Serum sickness is the prototype of an immune complex–mediated disease. When large doses of foreign serum (usually horse serum) are injected into a patient, often the humoral immune response may start producing antibodies while the horse antigens are still in the body. Circulating complexes are produced that cause fever, lymphadenopathy, arthritis, and urticarial skin lesions, particularly on the soles. The risk of such a severe reaction greatly limits the present-day use of such antibodies.

Diseases Characterized by Type IV Injury

Contact Dermatitis

Contact dermatitis occurs in patients sensitized to one of a group of chemicals or metals that bind covalently to protein in skin to produce complete antigens. These compounds are usually of low molecular weight, lipid soluble, highly reactive with protein, and able to penetrate the skin well. The antigen processing cell in the skin is the dendritic Langerhans' cell, which takes up the antigen and then presents it to a T_H cell. Application on thin skin (*e.g.*, scrotum or eyelids), on areas of inflammation (as in diaper dermatitis), or

over abrasions will increase the likelihood of sensitization. Once the patient is sensitized to the material, subsequent exposure to even small amounts of the compound will produce (after a 12- to 24-hour delay) acute dermatitis associated with a lymphocytic dermal infiltrate. This type of reaction may persist for 2 to 4 weeks after discontinuing the allergen.

Photoallergic Dermatitis

An exogenous antigen may react with the skin under the stimulation of ultraviolet light to produce a substance capable of stimulating cellular immune response. The eliciting agent can be applied topically (many plant products such as celery or grasses) or taken systemically (thiazide derivatives). In contrast, in a phototoxic reaction, the exogenous chemical is turned into a toxic substance by interaction with ultraviolet light without evoking a T-cell response.

Diseases with Multiple Defects

Many diseases defy simple categorization in the Gell and Coombs' scheme. We will discuss two of particular interest to dermatologists.

Lupus Erythematosus

Lupus erythematosus is a polysystemic disorder involving skin, kidneys, pleura, pericardium, joints, and central nervous system. Patients have a variety of cutaneous manifestations, including photosensitivity, scarring erythematous rash, and hair loss. Different immunologic mechanisms seem to be involved. Although there is immune complex–mediated renal disease in lupus erythematosus, the skin lesions are not typically type III. The epidermis shows damage by lymphocytic attack, but immunoglobulins are deposited in a band at the epidermal-dermal junction or diffusely in the epidermis. The hair loss is associated with a lymphocytic infiltrate penetrating the follicle. Patients with lupus erythematosus also have a wide variety of circulating antinuclear antibodies, which are of great diagnostic value but have unclear pathologic roles. These antibodies can be identified either by their pattern of binding to a substrate cell or on the basis of their reactions to particular antigens (Table 10–3).

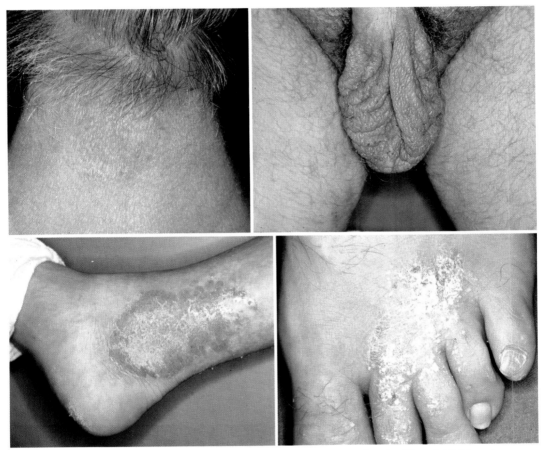

Plate 16. **Localized neurodermatitis.** (*Top, left*) In occipital area of scalp. (*Top, right*) Of scrotum, with marked lichenification and thickening of the skin. (*Bottom, left*) Of medial aspect of ankle, following lichen planus of this area. (*Bottom, right*) On dorsum of foot. (*Duke Labs, Inc.*)

Neurodermatitis is a common skin condition characterized by the occurrence of single or, less frequently, multiple patches of chronic, itching, thickened, scaly, dry skin in one or more of several classic locations (see Plate 16). It is unrelated to atopic eczema, which unfortunately has the synonym *disseminated neurodermatitis,* a term that should be abandoned.

PRIMARY LESIONS. This disease begins as a small, localized, pruritic patch of dermatitis that might have been an insect bite, a chigger bite, contact dermatitis, or other minor irritation, which may or may not be remembered by the patient. Because of various etiologic factors mentioned, a cycle of itching, scratching, more itching, and more scratching supervenes, and the chronic dermatosis develops.

SECONDARY LESIONS. These include excoriations, lichenification, and, in severe cases, marked verrucous thickening of the skin, with pigmentary changes. In these severe cases healing is bound to be followed by some scarring.

DISTRIBUTION. This condition is seen most commonly at the hairline of the nape of the neck and on the wrists, the ankles, the ears (see external otitis), anal area (see pruritus ani), and so on.

COURSE. The disease is quite chronic and recurrent. The majority of cases respond quickly to correct treatment, but some can last for years and defy all forms of therapy.

SUBJECTIVE COMPLAINTS. Intense itching, usually worse at night, occurs even during sleep.

ETIOLOGY. The initial cause (a bite, stasis dermatitis, contact dermatitis, seborrheic dermatitis, tinea cruris, psoriasis) may be very evanescent, but it is generally agreed that the chronicity of the lesion is due to the nervous habit of scratching. It is a rare patient who will not volunteer the information or admit, if questioned, that the itching is worse when he or she is upset, nervous, or tired. Why some persons with a minor skin injury respond with the development of a lichenified patch of skin and others do not is due to the personality makeup of that patient.

AGE-GROUP. It is very common to see localized neurodermatitis of the posterior neck in menopausal women. Other clinical types of neurodermatitis are seen in any age.

FAMILY INCIDENCE. This disorder is unrelated to allergies in patient or family, thus differing from atopic eczema. Atopic persons are "more itchy" persons, however.

RELATED TO EMPLOYMENT. Recurrent exposure and contact to irritating agents at work can lead to neurodermatitis.

Differential Diagnosis

Psoriasis: several patches on the body in classic areas of distribution; family history of disease; classic whitish scales; sharply circumscribed patch (see Chap. 14).

Atopic eczema: allergic history in patient or family; multiple lesions; classically seen in cubital and popliteal areas and face (see Chap. 9).

Contact dermatitis: acute onset; contact history positive; usually red, vesicular, and oozing; may be acute contact dermatitis overlying neurodermatitis, due to overzealous therapy (see Chap. 9).

Lichen planus, hypertrophic form on anterior tibial area: lichen planus in mouth and on other body areas; biopsy specimen usually characteristic (see Chap. 14).

Seborrheic dermatitis of scalp: does not itch as much; is better in summer; a diffuse, scaly, greasy eruption (see Chap. 13).

Treatment

A 45-year-old female patient presents with a severely itching, scaly, red, lichenified patch on back of the neck at the hairline.

1. Explain the condition to the patient and tell her that your medicine will be directed toward stopping the itching. If this can be done, and if she will cooperate by keeping her hands off the area, the disease will disappear. Emphasize the effect of scratching by stating that if both arms were broken, the eruption would be gone when the casts were removed. However, this is not a recommended form of therapy.
2. For severe bouts of intractable itching:
   Ice cold Burow's Solution packs
   Sig: 1 packet of Domeboro Powder to 1 quart of ice cold water. Apply cloth wet with this solution for 15 minutes p.r.n.
3. A moderate-potency corticosteroid ointment or emollient cream   15.0
   Sig: Apply q.i.d., or more often, as itching requires.

   The moderate-potency fluorinated corticosteroid creams (Synalar, Cordran, Lidex, Diprosone, Topicort, see p. 40) can be used under an occlusive dressing of Saran Wrap or Jiffy Wrap on lesions on an extremity. The dressing can be left on overnight. *Warning:* Long-continued occlusive dressing therapy with corticosteroids can cause atrophy of the skin.

TREATMENT ON RETURN VISIT
1. Add menthol (0.25%) or coal-tar solution (3% to 10%) to above ointment or cream for greater antipruritic effect.
2. Intralesional corticosteroid therapy. This is a very effective and safe treatment. The technique is as follows. Use a 1-inch long No. 26 needle and a Luer-Lok type syringe. Inject 5 or 10 mg of triamcinolone parenteral solution (Kenalog-10 or Aristocort Intralesional Suspension) intradermally or subcutaneously, directly under the skin lesion. An equal amount of saline should be mixed with the solution in the syringe. Do not inject all the solution in one area, but spread it around as you advance the needle. The injection can be repeated every 2 or 3 weeks as necessary to eliminate the patch of dermatitis.

   Warning: A complication of an atrophic depression at the injection site can occur. This usually can be avoided if the concentration of triamcinolone in one area is kept low.

TREATMENT OF RESISTANT CASES

1. A tranquilizer
   Sig: 1 tablet q.i.d., a.c. and h.s.
2. Prednisone   10 mg.
   Sig: 1 tablet q.i.d. for 3 days, then 2 tablets every morning for 7 days.
3. Dome-Paste Boot or Coban Wrap. Apply in office for cases of neurodermatitis localized to arms and legs. This is a physical deterrent to scratching. Leave on for a week at a time.
4. Psychotherapy is of questionable value.

External Otitis

External otitis is a descriptive term for a common and persistent dermatitis of the ears, due to several causes. The agent most frequently blamed for this condition is "fungus," but pathogenic fungi are rarely found in the external ear. The true causes of external otitis, in order of frequency, are as follows: seborrheic dermatitis, neurodermatitis, contact dermatitis, atopic eczema, psoriasis, *Pseudomonas* bacterial infection (which is usually secondary to other causes) and, lastly, fungal infection, which also can be primary or secondary to other factors. For further information on the specific processes, refer to each of the diseases mentioned.

Treatment

Primarily, treatment should be directed toward the specific cause, such as care of the scalp for seborrheic cases or avoidance of jewelry for contact cases. However, when this is done, certain special techniques and medicines must be used, in addition, to clear up this troublesome area.

An elderly woman comes in with an oozing, red, crusted, swollen left external ear, with a wet canal but an intact drum. A considerable amount of seborrheic dermatitis of the scalp is confluent with the acutely inflamed ear area. The patient has had itching ear trouble off and on for 10 years, but in the past month it has become most severe.

1. Always inspect the canal and the drum with an otoscope. If excessive wax and debris are present in the canal, or if the drum is involved in the process, the patient should be treated for these problems or referred to an ear specialist. Salves should not be placed in the ear canal. An effective liquid to dry up the oozing canal is as follows:
   Hydrocortisone powder   1%
   Burow's Solution, 1:10 strength, q.s. 15.0
   Sig: 2 drops in ear t.i.d.
2. Burow's Solution wet packs
   Sig: 1 packet of Domeboro Powder to 1 quart of cool water. Apply wet cloths to external ear for 15 minutes three times a day.
3. A corticosteroid ointment   15.0
   Sig: Apply locally to external ear t.i.d., not in canal.

SAUER NOTES:

1. Many cases of acute ear dermatitis are aggravated by an allergy to the therapeutic cream, such as Neosporin, or the ingredients in the base.
2. A corticosteroid in a petrolatum base eliminates this problem.
3. Use 1% Hytone Ointment, Des-Owen Ointment, or Tridesilon Ointment.

SUBSEQUENT THERAPY

Several days later, following decreased swelling, cessation of oozing, and lessening of itching, institute the following changes in therapy:

1. Decrease the soaks to once a day.
2. Sulfur, ppt.   5%
   A corticosteroid ointment q.s.   15.0
   Sig: Apply locally t.i.d. to ear with the little finger, *not* down in the canal with a cotton-tipped applicator.

For persistent cases, a short course of oral corticosteroid or antibiotic therapy often removes the "fire," so that local remedies will be effective.

Pruritus Ani

Itching of the anal area is a common malady that can vary in severity from mild to marked. The patient with this very annoying symptom is apt to resort to self-treatment and therefore delay the visit to the physician. Usually, the patient has overtreated the sensitive area, and the immediate problem of the physician is to quiet the acute contact dermatitis. The original cause of the pruritus ani is often difficult to ascertain.

PRIMARY LESIONS. These can range from slight redness confined to a very small area to an extensive contact dermatitis with redness, vesicles, and oozing of the entire buttock.

SECONDARY LESIONS. Excoriations from the intense itching are very common, and after a prolonged time they progress toward lichenification. A generalized papulovesicular id eruption can develop from an acute flare-up of this entity.

COURSE. The majority of cases of pruritus ani respond rapidly and completely to proper management, especially if the cause can be ascertained and eliminated. However, every physician will have a patient who will continue to scratch and defy all therapy.

ETIOLOGY. The proper management of this socially unacceptable form of pruritus consists in searching for and eliminating the several factors that contribute to the persistence of this symptom-complex. These factors can be divided into general and specific etiologic factors.

GENERAL FACTORS

Diet. The following irritating foods should be removed from the diet: chocolate, nuts, cheese, and spicy foods. Coffee, because of its stimulating effect on any form of itching, should be limited to 1 cup a day. Rarely, certain other foods will be noted by the patient to aggravate the pruritus.

Bathing. Many patients have the misconception that the itching is due to uncleanliness. Therefore, they resort to excessive bathing and scrubbing of the anal area. This is harmful and irritating and must be stopped.

Toilet Care. Harsh toilet paper contributes greatly to the continuance of this condition. Cotton or a proprietary cleansing cloth called "Tucks" must be used for wiping. Mineral oil can be added to the cotton if necessary.

Rarely, an allergy to the pastel tint in colored toilet tissues is a factor causing the pruritus.

Scratching. As with all of the diseases of this group, chronic scratching leads to a vicious cycle. The chief aim of the physician is to give relief from this itching, but a gentle admonishment to the patient to keep hands off is indicated. With the physician's help, the itch-and-scratch habit can be broken. The emotional and mental personality of the patient regulates the effectiveness of this suggestion.

SPECIFIC ETIOLOGIC FACTORS

Oral Antibiotics. Pruritus ani from oral antibiotic therapy is seen frequently. It may or may not be due to an overgrowth of candidal organisms. The physician who automatically questions patients about recent drug ingestion will not miss this diagnosis.

Localized Neurodermatitis. It is always a problem to know which comes first, the itching or the "nervousness." In most instances the itching comes first, but there is no denying that once pruritus ani has developed, it is aggravated by emotional tensions and "nerves." However, it is a rare case that has a "deep-seated" psychological problem.

Psoriasis. In this area, psoriasis is common. Usually, other skin surfaces are also involved.

Atopic Eczema. Atopic eczema of this site in adults is rather unusual. A history of atopy in the patient or family is helpful in establishing this cause.

Fungal Infection. Contrary to old beliefs, this cause is quite rare. Clinically, a raised, sharp, papulovesicular border is seen that commonly is confluent with tinea of the crural area. If a scraping or a culture reveals fungi, then stronger local therapy than usual is indicated for cure.

Worm Infestation. In children, pinworms can usually be implicated. A diagnosis is made by finding eggs on morning anal smears or by seeing the small white worms when the child is sleeping. Worms are a rare cause of adult pruritus ani.

Hemorrhoids. In the lay person's mind this is undoubtedly the most common cause. Actually, it is an unimportant primary factor but may be a contributing factor. Hemorrhoidectomy alone is rarely successful as a cure for pruritus ani.

Cancer. This is a very rare cause of anal itching, but a rectal or proctoscopic examination may be indicated.

Treatment

FIRST VISIT

A patient states that he has had anal itching for 4 months. It followed a 5-day course of an antibiotic for the flu. Many local remedies have been used; the latest, a supposed remedy for athlete's foot, aggravated the condition. Examination reveals an oozing, macerated, red area around the anus.

1. Initial therapy should include removal of the general factors listed under "etiology," above, and giving instructions as to diet, bathing, toilet care, and scratching. Use the noncarbon form (see Fig. 4–1) for these instructions.
2. Burow's solution wet packs.
    Sig: 1 packet of Bluboro or Domeboro to 1 quart of cool water. Apply wet cloths to the area b.i.d. while lying in bed for 20 minutes, or more often if necessary for severe itching. Ice cubes may be added to the solution for more anti-itching effect.
3. Low-potency corticosteroid cream or ointment q.s.   15.0
    Sig: Apply to area b.i.d.
4. Benadryl, 50 mg
    Sig: 1 capsule h.s. (for itching and sedation). (Available over-the-counter.)

SAUER NOTES:

1. Do not prescribe a fluorinated corticosteroid salve for the anal area. It can cause telangiectasia and atrophy of the skin after long-term use.
2. One of my favorite medications for pruritus ani is 1% Hytone Ointment applied sparingly locally two to three times a day. The petrolatum base is well tolerated.

SUBSEQUENT VISITS
1. As tolerated, add increasing strengths of sulfur, coal-tar solution, or menthol (0.25%) or phenol (0.5%) to the above cream, or change to Vioform ointment with hydrocortisone 1%.
2. Intralesional corticosteroid injection therapy. This is very effective. Usually the minor discomfort of the injection is quite well tolerated because of the patient's desire to "get cured." The technique is given under "Neurodermatitis" on page 106.

Genital Pruritus

Itching of the female vulva or the male scrotum can be treated in much the same way as pruritus ani if these special considerations are borne in mind.

VULVAR PRURITUS. Etiologically, vulvar pruritus is due to *Candida* or *Trichomonas* infection; contact dermatitis from underwear, douche chemicals, contraceptive jellies and diaphragms; chronic cervicitis; neurodermatitis; menopausal or senile atrophic changes; lichen sclerosus et atrophicus; or leukoplakia. Pruritus vulvae is frequently seen in patients with diabetes mellitus and during pregnancy.

Treatment can be adapted from that for pruritus ani (see preceding section) with the addition of a daily douche, such as vinegar, 2 tablespoons to 1 quart of warm water.

Vulvodynia is a difficult problem to manage. The sensation of burning and pain in the vulvar area is not uncommon and requires careful etiologic evaluation from a patient physician and a patient patient. Most cases can be managed as a contact dermatitis, but there is a strong psychic element. A minimal dose of haloperidol (Haldol), 1 mg, b.i.d. is occasionally indicated and effective. Larger doses may be necessary.

SCROTAL PRURITUS (see Plate 16). Etiologically, scrotal pruritus is due to tinea infection; contact dermatitis from soaps, powders, or clothing; or neurodermatitis.

Treatment is similar to that given for pruritus ani in the preceding section.

Notalgia Parasthetica

Notalgia parasthetica is a moderately common localized pruritic dermatosis usually confined to the mid upper back or scapular area. A pigmented patch is formed by the chronic rubbing. There is no effective therapy. Some evidence exists for a hereditary factor.

BIBLIOGRAPHY

Denman ST: A review of pruritus. J Am Acad Dermatol 14:375, 1986

Van Scott EJ, Yu RJ: Hyperkeratinization: Corneocyte cohesion and alpha hydroxy acids. J Am Acad Dermatol 11:867, 1984

Weber PJ, Poulos EG: Notalgia paresthetica. J Am Acad Dermatol 18:25, 1988

12

Vascular Dermatoses

Urticaria, erythema multiforme and its variants, and erythema nodosum are included under the heading of vascular dermatoses because of their vascular reaction patterns. Stasis dermatitis is included because it is a dermatosis due to venous insufficiency in the legs.

URTICARIA
(Plate 17)

The commonly seen entity of urticaria, or hives, can be acute or chronic and due to known or unknown causes. Numerous factors, both *immunologic* and *nonimmunologic*, can be involved in its pathogenesis. The urticarial wheal results from liberation of histamine from tissue mast cells and from circulating basal cells.

Nonimmunologic factors that can release histamine from these cells include chemicals, various drugs (including morphine and codeine), principles in lobster, crayfish, and other lower animals, bacterial toxins, and physical agents. Examples of the type caused by physical agents are the linear wheals that are produced by light stroking of the skin, known as *dermographism*. (Consult the Dictionary-Index for the triple response of Lewis reaction.)

Immunologic mechanisms are probably involved more often in acute, than in chronic urticaria. The most commonly considered of these mechanisms is the type I hypersensitivity state that is triggered by polyvalent antigen bridging two specific IgE molecules that

are bound to the mast cell or basal cell surface (see Chap. 10).

LESIONS. Pea-sized red papules to large circinate patterns with red borders and white centers that can cover an entire side of the trunk or the thigh may be noted. Vesicles and bullae are seen in severe cases, along with hemorrhagic effusions. Edema of the glottis is a serious complication that can occur in the severe form of urticaria labeled *angioneurotic edema*.

COURSE. Acute cases may be mild or explosive but usually disappear with or without treatment in a few hours or days. The chronic form has remissions and exacerbations for months and years.

ETIOLOGY. Many cases of hives, particularly of the chronic type, are concluded after careful questioning and investigation to result from no apparent causative agent. Other cases, mainly the acute ones, have been found to result from the following factors or agents:

Drugs or Chemicals. Penicillin and derivatives are probably the most common cause of acute hives, but any other drug, whether ingested, injected, inhaled, or, rarely, applied on the skin, can cause the reaction. (See Drug Eruption, Chap. 9.)

Foods. Foods are a common cause of acute hives. The main offenders are seafood, strawberries, chocolate, nuts, cheeses, pork, eggs, wheat, and milk. Chronic hives can be caused by traces of penicillin in milk products.

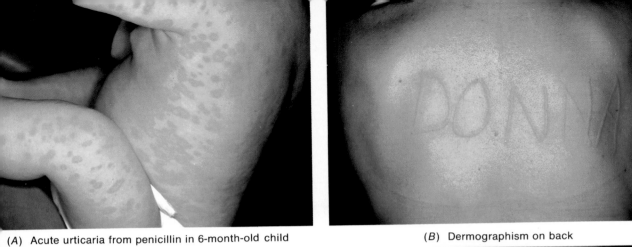

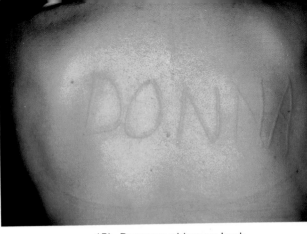

(A) Acute urticaria from penicillin in 6-month-old child

(B) Dermographism on back

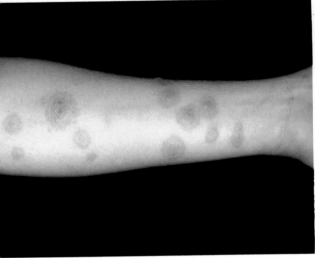

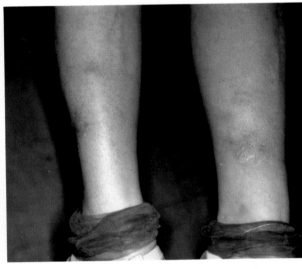

(C) Erythema-multiforme–like eruption on arm during pregnancy

(D) Erythema nodusum on legs

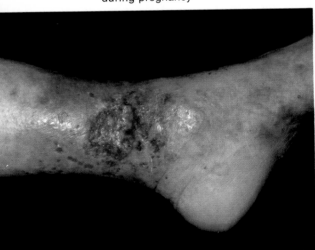

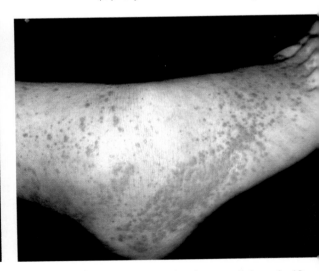

(E) Stasis dermatitis

(F) Acute purpura, of unknown etiology, in 12-year-old boy

Plate 17. **Vascular dermatoses.** (*Dermik Laboratories, Inc.*)

Insect Bites and Stings. Insect bites and stings from mosquitos, fleas, spiders, and contact with certain moths, leeches, and jellyfish cause hives.

Physical Agents. Hives result from heat, cold, radiant energy, and physical injury. *Dermographism* is a term applied to a localized urticarial wheal produced by scratching the skin of certain persons (see Plate 17).

SAUER NOTE:

Dermographism is commonly overlooked as a cause of the patient's "welts" or vague itching.

Inhalants. Nasal sprays, insect sprays, dust, feathers, pollens, and animal danders are some offenders.

Infections. A focus of infection is always considered, sooner or later, in chronic cases of hives, and in unusual instances it is causative. The sinuses, the teeth, the tonsils, the gallbladder, and the genitourinary tract should be checked.

Internal Disease. Urticaria has been seen with liver disease, intestinal parasites, cancer, and rheumatic fever.

"Nerves." After all other causes of chronic urticaria have been ruled out, there remain a substantial number of cases that appear to be related to nervous stress, worry, or fatigue. These cases benefit most from the establishment of good rapport between the patient and the physician.

Contact Urticaria Syndrome. This uncommon response can be incited from the local contact on the skin of drugs and chemicals, foods, insects, and plants.

Differential Diagnosis

Hebra's erythema multiforme: systemic fever, malaise, and mouth lesions are noted in children and young adults (see the next section of this chapter).
Dermographism: a *common* finding in young adults, especially who present complaining of "welts" on their skin or vague itching of the skin with no residual lesions. To make the diagnosis, stroke the skin firmly to see if an urticarial response develops. The course can be chronic, but hydroxyzine, 10 mg, b.i.d. or t.i.d. is quite helpful. (Warn the patient about the possibility of drowsiness.)

Treatment

For a case of *acute* hives due to penicillin injection 1 week previously for a "cold":

1. Colloidal bath
   Sig: 1 cup of starch or oatmeal (Aveeno) to 6 to 8 inches of lukewarm water in the tub. Bathe for 15 minutes once or twice a day.
2. Camphor   1%
   Alcoholic white shake lotion q.s.   120.0
   Sig: Apply b.i.d. locally for itching.
3. Hydroxyzine (Atarax or Durrax),
   10 mg   #30
   Sig: 1 tab t.i.d., a.c. (drowsiness warning)
4. Diphenhydramine (Benadryl),
   50 mg   OTC
5. Betamethasone sodium phosphate. (Celestone), 3 mg/ml. Dose: 1 to 1.5 ml subcutaneously.

For a more severe case of acute hives:

1. Benadryl injection. Give 2 ml (20 mg) subcutaneously, or
2. Epinephrine hydrochloride. Give 0.3 to 0.5 ml of 1 : 1,000 solution subcutaneously, or
3. Prednisone tablets, 10 mg   #30
   Sig: 1 tab q.i.d. for 3 days, then 1 tablet in AM.

For treatment of patient with *chronic* hives of 6 months' duration when cause is undetermined after careful history and examination:

1. Hydroxyzine (Atarax or Durrax), 10 to 25 mg   #60
   Sig: 1 tablet t.i.d. depending on drowsiness and effectiveness. Continue for weeks or months.
2. Terfenadine (Seldane), 60 mg   #60
   Sig: 1 tablet b.i.d., or
   Astemizole (Hismanal), 10 mg   #30
   Sig: 1 tablet h.s. 2 hours after food.
   These two H1 blockers can be used alone or in conjunction with the older antihistamines for chronic urticaria.

3. Cimetidine (Tagamet), 300 mg   #60
   Sig: 1 tab t.i.d. This H2 blocker is of benefit in some cases.
4. Diet. Suggest avoidance of chocolate, nuts, cheese and other milk products, seafood, strawberries, pork, excess spicy foods, and excess of coffee or tea.
5. A mild sedative or tranquilizer such as meprobamate, 400 mg, t.i.d. or chlordiazepoxide (Librium), 5 mg, t.i.d. may help.

ERYTHEMA MULTIFORME
(Plate 17)

The term *erythema multiforme* introduces a flurry of confusion in the mind of any student of medicine. It will be my purpose in this section to attempt to dispel that confusion. Erythema multiforme, as originally described by Hebra, is an uncommon distinct disease of unknown cause characterized by red iris-shaped or bull's-eye–like macules, papules, or bullae confined mainly to the extremities, the face, and the lips. It is accompanied by mild fever, malaise, and arthralgia. It occurs usually in children and young adults in the spring and the fall, has a duration of 2 to 4 weeks, and frequently is recurrent for several years.

The only relationship between Hebra's erythema multiforme and the following diseases or syndromes is the clinical appearance of the eruption.

Stevens-Johnson syndrome is a very severe and often fatal variant of erythema multiforme. It is characterized by high fever, extensive purpura, bullae, ulcers of the mucous membranes, and, after 2 to 3 days, ulcers of the skin. Eye involvement can result in blindness.

Erythema multiforme bullosum is a severe, chronic, bullous disease of adults. (See Chap. 22.)

Erythema-multiforme–like drug eruption is frequently due to phenacetin, quinine, penicillin, mercury, arsenic, phenylbutazone, barbiturates, trimethadione, phenytoin, sulfonamides, and antitoxins. (See Chap. 9.)

Erythema-multiforme–like eruption is seen rather commonly as part of a herpes simplex outbreak and also in conjunction with rheumatic fever, pneumonia, meningitis, measles, herpes simplex, coxsackievirus infection, pregnancy, and cancer, following deep x-ray therapy, and as an allergic reaction to foods.

Erythema perstans group of diseases (see Fig. DI-7) includes over a dozen clinical entities with impossible-to-remember names. (See Dictionary-Index under "Erythema perstans.") All have varying sized erythematous patches, papules, or plaques with a definite red border and a less active center, forming circles, half circles, groups of circles, and linear bands. Multiple causes have been ascribed, including tick bites, allergic reactions, fungal, bacterial, viral, and spirochetal infections, and internal cancer. The duration of and the response to therapy varies with each individual case.

Erythema chronicum migrans is the distinctive cutaneous eruption of the multisystem tick-borne spirochetosis Lyme disease. The deer tick, *Ixodes dammini*, is the vector for the spirochete. Early therapy with tetracycline or penicillin can prevent late manifestations of the disease (see p. 180).

Reiter's syndrome is a triad of conjunctivitis, urethritis, and, most important, arthritis, occurring predominantly in males, which lasts approximately 6 months.

Behçet's syndrome consists of a triad of genital, oral, and ophthalmic ulcerations seen most commonly in males; it can last for years, with recurrences.

Differential Diagnosis

Urticaria: clinically, it may resemble erythema multiforme, but hives are associated with only mild systemic symptoms; it can occur in any age-group; iris lesions are unusual; usually it can be attributed to penicillin or other drug therapy; and it responds rapidly but often not completely to antihistamine therapy (see first part of this chapter).

Treatment

A 12-year-old child presents with bull's eye–like lesions on hands, arms, and feet, erosions of the lips and mucous membranes of the mouth, malaise, and temperature of 101° F (38.3° C) orally. He had a similar eruption last spring.

1. Order bed rest and increased oral fluid intake.

2. Acetaminophen (Tylenol) 325 mg OTC
Sig: 1 to 2 tablets q.i.d.
or
Prednisone, 10 mg #16
Sig: 2 tablets stat. and then 2 every morning for 7 days.

3. For severe cases, such as the Stevens-Johnson form, hospitalization will be indicated, where intravenous corticosteroid therapy, intravenous infusions, γ-globulin, and other supportive measures can be administered.

ERYTHEMA NODOSUM
(Plate 17)

Erythema nodosum is an uncommon reaction pattern seen mainly on the anterior tibial areas of the legs. It appears as erythematous nodules in successive crops and is preceded by fever, malaise, and arthralgia.

PRIMARY LESIONS. Bilateral red, tender, rather well-circumscribed nodules are seen mainly on the pretibial surface of the legs but also on the arms and the body. Later, the flat lesions may become raised, confluent, and purpuric. Only a few lesions develop at one time.

SECONDARY LESIONS. They never suppurate or form ulcers.

COURSE. The lesions last several weeks, but the duration can be affected by therapy directed to the cause, if it is known. Relapses are related to the cause.

ETIOLOGY. Careful clinical and laboratory examination is necessary to determine the cause of this toxic reaction pattern. The following tests should be performed: complete blood cell count, erythrocyte sedimentation rate, urinalysis, serologic test for syphilis, chest roentgenogram, and specific skin tests, as indicated. The causes of erythema nodosum are streptococcal infection (rheumatic fever, pharyngitis, scarlet fever, arthritis), fungal infection (coccidioidomycosis, *Trichophyton* infection), pregnancy, lymphogranuloma venereum, syphilis, chancroid, drugs (contraceptive pills, sulfonamides, iodides, bromides) and, rarely, tuberculosis.

AGE AND SEX INCIDENCE. The disorder occurs predominantly in adolescent and young women.

LABORATORY FINDINGS. Histopathologic examination will reveal a nonspecific but characteristically localized inflammatory infiltrate in the subcutaneous tissue and in and around the veins.

Differential Diagnosis

Erythema induratum: chronic vasculitis of young women that occurs on the posterior calf area and often suppurates; biopsy will show a tuberculoid-type infiltrate, usually with caseation.

Necrobiosis lipoidica diabeticorum: an uncommon cutaneous manifestation of diabetes mellitus, characterized by well-defined patches of reddish yellow atrophic skin, primarily on anterior areas of legs; the lesions can ulcerate; biopsy results are characteristic, but biopsy is usually not necessary or indicated because of the possibility of poor healing (see Chapter 26).

Periarteritis nodosa: a rare, usually fatal arteritis that most often occurs in males; 25% of patients show painful subcutaneous nodules and purpura, mainly of the lower extremities.

Nodular vasculitis: chronic, painful nodules of the calves of middle-aged women, which rarely ulcerate but recur commonly; biopsy is of value; this disorder may be a variant of erythema nodosum.

Superficial thrombophlebitis migrans of Buerger's disease: an early venous change of Buerger's disease commonly seen in male patients, with painful nodules of the anterior tibial area; biopsy is of value.

Nodular panniculitis or Weber-Christian disease: occurs mainly in obese middle-aged women; tender, indurated, subcutaneous nodules and plaques are seen, usually on the thighs and the buttocks; each crop is preceded by fever and malaise; residual atrophy and hyperpigmentation occur.

Leukocytoclastic vasculitis: includes a constellation of diseases, such as allergic angiitis, allergic vasculitis, necrotizing vasculitis, or cutaneous-systemic vasculitis. Clinically, one sees palpable purpuric lesions, most commonly on the lower part of the legs. In later stages the lesions may become nodular, bullous, infarctive, and ulcerative. Various etiologic agents have been implicated, such as infection, drugs, and foreign proteins. Treatment includes bed rest, pentoxifylline (Trental), and corticosteroids (see Chap. 10).

For completeness, the following five very rare syndromes with *inflammatory nodules of the legs* are defined in the Dictionary-Index: (1) subcutaneous fat necrosis with pancreatic disease, (2) migratory panniculitis, (3) allergic granulomatosis, (4) necrobiosis granulomatosis, and (5) embolic nodules from several sources.

Treatment

1. Treat the cause, if possible.
2. Rest, local heat, and aspirin are valuable. The eruption is self-limited if the cause can be eliminated.
3. Chronic cases can be disabling enough to warrant a short course of corticosteroid therapy. Some cases have benefited from naproxen (Naprosyn), 250 mg, b.i.d. (or other nonsteroidal anti-inflammatory drugs) for 2 to 4 weeks.

STASIS (VENOUS) DERMATITIS AND ULCERS
(Plates 17 and 97)

Stasis dermatitis is a common condition due to impaired venous circulation in the legs of older patients. Almost all cases are associated with varicose veins, and since the tendency to develop varicosities is a familial characteristic, stasis dermatitis is also familial. Stasis ulcers can develop in the impaired skin.

PRIMARY LESIONS. Early cases of stasis dermatitis begin as a red, scaly, pruritic patch that rapidly becomes vesicular and crusted, owing to scratching and subsequent secondary infection. The bacterial infection is responsible for the spread of the patch and the chronicity of the eruption. Edema of the affected ankle area results in a further decrease in circulation and, consequently, more infection. The lesions may be unilateral or bilateral.

SECONDARY LESIONS. Three secondary conditions can arise from untreated stasis dermatitis:

1. *Hyperpigmentation* is inevitable following the healing of either simple or severe stasis dermatitis of the legs. This increase in pigmentation is slow to disappear, and in many elderly patients it never does.
2. *Stasis ulcers* can occur as the result of edema, deeper bacterial infection, or improper care of the primary dermatitis.
3. *Infectious eczematoid dermatitis* (see Chap. 15) may develop on the legs, the arms, and even the entire body, either slowly, or as an explosive, rapidly spreading eruption.

COURSE. The rapidity of healing of stasis dermatitis depends on the age of the patient, and on other factors listed under Etiology. In elderly patients who have untreated varicose veins, stasis dermatitis can persist for years with remissions and exacerbations. If stasis dermatitis develops in a patient in the 40- to 50-year age-group, the prognosis is particularly bad for future recurrences and possible ulcers, unless the varicosities are removed. Once stasis ulcers develop, they can rapidly expand in size and depth. Healing of the ulcer, if possible for a given patient, depends on many factors.

ETIOLOGY. Poor venous circulation, due to the sluggish blood flow in tortuous, dilated varicose veins, is the primary cause. If the factors of obesity, lack of proper rest or care of the legs, pruritus, secondary infection, low protein diet, and old age are added to the circulation problem, the result can be a chronic, disabling disease.

Differential Diagnosis

Contact dermatitis: history is important, especially regarding nylon hose, new socks, contact with ragweed, high-top shoes, and so on; no venous insufficiency is noted (see Chap. 9).

Neurodermatitis: thickened, dry, very pruritic patch; no venous insufficiency is found (see Chap. 11).

Atrophie blanche: characterized by small ulcers that heal with irregular white scars; seen mainly over the ankles and legs. Telangiectasis and hyperpigmentation surround the scars. This arterial vasculitis responds to pentoxifylline (Trental).

Differential diagnosis for stasis ulcers includes *pyodermic ulcers, arterial ulcers* (such as mal perforans of diabetes), *necrobiosis lipoidica* ulcers, *pyoderma gangrenosum, malignancies*, and ulcers from hematologic and other internal problems. Blood tests, cultures, and biopsies help to establish the type of ulcer.

Treatment of Stasis Dermatitis

A 55-year-old laborer presents with scaly, reddish, slightly edematous, excoriated dermatitis on the medial aspect of the left ankle and leg of 6 weeks' duration.

1. Prescribe rest and elevation of the leg as much as possible by lying in bed. The foot of the bed should be elevated 4 inches by placing two bricks under the legs. Sitting in a chair with the leg propped on a stool is of very little value.
2. Burow's solution wet packs
   Sig: 1 packet of powder to 1 quart of warm water. Apply cloths wet with this solution for 30 minutes, b.i.d.
3. An antibiotic-corticosteroid
   ointment qs.   15.0
   Sig: Apply to leg t.i.d.
4. Surgical removal of varicose veins. This should be strongly recommended, particularly in younger patients, to prevent recurrences and eventual irreversible changes, including ulcers.

For the more *severe case* of stasis dermatitis with oozing, cellulitis, and 3-plus pitting edema, the following treatment should be ordered, in addition:

1. Hospitalization or enforced bed rest at home for the purpose of (a) applying the wet packs for longer periods of time and (b) strict rest and elevation of the leg
2. A course of an oral antibiotic
3. Prednisone, 10 mg   #36
   Sig: 2 tablets b.i.d. for 4 days then 2 tabs in AM for 10 days
4. Ace elastic bandage, 4 inches wide, No. 8

After the patient is dismissed from the hospital and will be ambulatory, give instructions for the correct application of this bandage to the leg before arising in the morning. This helps to reduce the edema that could cause a recrudescence of the dermatitis.

Treatment of Stasis Ulcer

As for any chronic difficult medical problem there are many methods touted for successful management.

Consider a 75-year-old obese woman on a low income who has a 5 × 4-cm ulcer on her medial right ankle area with surrounding dermatitis, edema, and pigmentation.

1. Manage the primary problem or problems. Attempt to remedy the obesity, make sure there is adequate nutrition, and treat systemic or other causes of the ulcer.
2. Correct the physiologic alterations. Control the edema with elastic Ace-type bandages of adequate width (4 inches wide usually), and with correct application from foot up to knee.
3. Treat contributing factors. Control the dermatitis, itching, and infection.
4. Promote healing. Occlusion of the ulcer has been proved to accelerate healing. Unna boots, Coban and Ace-type elastic dressings, and polyurethane-type films have been used with success. Enzymatic granules have their proponents.

Here is the technique I would use for this case. The diagnosis is stasis or venous ulcer.

1. Advise a multiple vitamin and mineral supplement tablet once a day.
2. Elevate leg as much as possible lying down prone.
3. Erythromycin, 250 mg   #100
   Sig: 2 to 3 tablets a day until ulcer is healed. Every ulcer is infected.
4. Prednisone, 10 mg   #60
   Sig: 1 tablet every morning.
   Actions: Antipruritic and anti-inflammatory
5. Occlusive dressing. This is to be applied in the office. If there is a lot of drainage and debris, the frequency of dressing should be every 3 to 4 days at first, then weekly. Use a foot-rest stand for the leg. Keep a record on the size of the ulcer.
   Procedure:
   A. Apply Bactroban Ointment to a Telfa dressing.
   B. Place gauze squares in four layers over the Telfa dressing.
   C. Coban Self-adherent Wrap is applied over the gauze, down to the foot arch and up to below the knee. Do not apply too tightly at first.
   D. Ace Elastic Bandage, 4 inches wide, is wrapped over the Coban.
   E. The dressing is left on for 3 to 7 days and then reapplied.

No management of a venous stasis ulcer is 100% effective, but this routine with modifications is the one I use.

After the ulcer has healed, which will take many weeks, advise the patient to wear an elastic bandage or support hose *constantly* during the day, primarily as protection against injury of the damaged and scarred skin.

PURPURIC DERMATOSES
(Plate 17)

Purpuric lesions are caused by an extravasation of red blood cells into the skin or mucous membranes. The lesions can be distinguished from erythema and telangiectasia by the fact that purpuric lesions do not blanch under pressure applied by the finger or by diascopy.

Petechiae are small, superficial purpuric lesions. *Ecchymoses*, or bruises, are more extensive, round or irregularly shaped purpuric lesions. *Hematomas* are large, deep, fluctuant, tumor-like hemorrhages into the skin.

The purpuras can be divided into the *thrombocytopenic* forms and the *nonthrombocytopenic* forms.

Thrombocytopenic purpura may be idiopathic or secondary to various chronic diseases or to a drug sensitivity. The platelet count is below normal, the bleeding time is prolonged, and the clotting time is normal, but the clot does not retract normally. This form of purpura is rare.

Nonthrombocytopenic purpura is more commonly seen. *Henoch-Schönlein purpura* is a form of nonthrombocytopenic purpura most commonly seen in children that is characterized by recurrent attacks of purpura accompanied by arthritis, hematuria, and gastrointestinal disorders.

The ecchymoses, or *senile purpura*, seen in elderly patients following minor injury are very common. Ecchymoses are also seen in patients who have been on long-term systemic corticosteroid therapy, such as occurs following prolonged use of the high potency corticosteroids *locally* and from corticosteroid nasal inhalers.

Another common purpuric eruption is that known as *stasis purpura*. These lesions are associated with vascular insufficiency of the legs and occur as the early sign of this change, or they are seen around areas of stasis dermatitis or stasis ulcers.

Quite frequently seen is a petechial *drug eruption* due to the chlorothiazide diuretics.

Pigmented Purpuric Eruptions

A less common group of cases are those seen in middle-aged adults, classified under the name of *pigmented purpuric eruptions*. Some cases of pigmented purpuric eruptions itch severely. The cause is unknown; the majority of cases have a positive tourniquet test, but other bleeding tests are normal. Clinically these patients have grouped petechial lesions that begin on the legs and extend up to the thighs, and occasionally up to the waist and on to the arms.

Some clinicians are able to separate these pigmented purpuric eruptions into *purpura annularis telangiectodes (Majocchi), progressive pigmentary dermatosis (Schamberg),* and *pigmented purpuric lichenoid dermatitis (Gougerot-Blum). Majocchi's disease* commonly begins on the legs but slowly spreads, to become generalized. Telangiectatic capillaries become confluent and produce annular or serpiginous lesions. The capillaries break down, causing purpuric lesions. *Schamberg's disease* is a slowly progressive pigmentary condition of the lower part of the legs that fades after a period of months. The *Gougerot-Blum form* is accompanied by severe itching; otherwise it resembles Schamberg's disease.

Treatment

For these pigmented purpuric eruptions, therapy with a combination of hesperidin complex, 200 mg, t.i.d. and vitamin C, 500 mg, t.i.d. is occasionally effective. Occlusive dressing therapy with a corticosteroid cream is also beneficial.

For resistant cases, prednisone, 10 mg, 1 to 2 tablets in the morning for 3 to 6 weeks is indicated.

TELANGIECTASES

Telangiectases are abnormal dilated small blood vessels. Telangiectases are divided into *primary forms*, in which the causes are unknown, and *secondary forms*, in which they are related to some known disturbance.

The primary telangiectases include the simple and compound hemangiomas of infants and the spider hemangiomas (see Chap. 33).

Secondary telangiectasia is very commonly seen on the fair-skinned person as a result of aging and chronic sun exposure. X-ray therapy and burns can also cause dilated vessels.

Treatment for the secondary telangiectasias can be accomplished quite adequately with very light electrosurgery to the vessels, which is usually tolerated without anesthesia. Injectable sclerosing agents are available for therapy.

BIBLIOGRAPHY

Berger BW: Treating erythema chronicum migrans of Lyme disease. J Am Acad Dermatol 15:459, 1986

Centers for Disease Control: Henoch-Schönlein purpura—Connecticut. Arch Dermatol 124:639, 1988

Eaglstein WH: Experiences with biosynthetic dressings. J Am Acad Dermatol 12:434, 1985

Ekenstam E, Callen JP: Cutaneous leukocytoclastic vasculitis. Arch Dermatol 120:484, 1984

Falanga V, Eaglstein WH: A therapeutic approach to venous ulcers. J Am Acad Dermatol 14:777, 1986

Goldman MP, Bennett RG: Treatment of telangiectasia: A review. J Am Acad Dermatol 17:167, 1987

Jacobson KW et al: Laboratory tests in chronic urticaria. JAMA 243:1644, 1980

Krull EA: Chronic cutaneous ulcerations and impaired healing in human skin. J Am Acad Dermatol 12:394, 1985

Monroe EW: Chronic urticaria: Review of nonsedating H1 antihistamines in treatment. J Am Acad Dermatol 19:842, 1988

13

Seborrheic Dermatitis, Acne, and Rosacea

SEBORRHEIC DERMATITIS
(Plates 18 through 20)

Seborrheic dermatitis, in my opinion, is a synonym for dandruff. The former is the more severe manifestation of this dermatosis.

Seborrheic dermatitis is exceedingly common on the scalp but less common on the other areas of predilection: ears, face, sternal area, axillae, and pubic area. It is well to consider seborrheic dermatitis as a "condition" of the skin and not as a "disease." It occurs as part of the "acne seborrhea complex," most commonly seen in the brown-eyed brunette who has a family history of these conditions. Dandruff is spoken of as oily or dry, but it is all basically oily. If dandruff scales are pressed between two pieces of tissue paper, an oily residue is expressed, leaving its mark on the tissue.

Certain misconceptions that have arisen concerning this common dermatosis need to be corrected. Seborrheic dermatitis cannot be cured, but remissions for varying amounts of time do occur naturally or as the result of treatment. Seborrheic dermatitis does not cause permanent hair loss or baldness unless it becomes grossly infected. Seborrheic dermatitis is not contagious. The cause is unknown but an important etiologic factor is the fungus *Pityrosporum ovale*.

PRIMARY LESIONS. Redness and scaling appear in varying degrees. The scale may be of the "dry" type or the "greasy" type (see Plate 18).

SECONDARY LESIONS. Rarely seen are excoriations from severe itching and secondary bacterial infection. Neurodermatitis with lichenification can follow a chronic itching and scratching habit.

COURSE. Exacerbations and remissions are common, depending on the season, treatment, and the age and general health of the patient. Since this is a condition of the skin, and not a disease, a true cure is impossible.

SEASONAL INCIDENCE. This condition is worse in colder weather, presumably due to lower indoor humidity and lack of summer sunlight.

Differential Diagnosis

SCALP LESIONS

Psoriasis: sharply defined, whitish, dry, scaly patches; typical psoriasis lesions on elbows, knees, nails, or elsewhere (see Chap. 14).

Neurodermatitis: usually a single patch on the posterior scalp area or around the ears; intense itching; excoriation; and thickening of the skin (see Chap. 11).

Tinea capitis: usually occurs in a child; broken-off hairs, with or without pustular reaction are seen. Some types fluoresce under Wood's light. Culture is positive (see Chap. 19).

Atopic eczema: usually occurs in infants or children; diffuse dry scaliness; eczema also on face, arms, and legs (see Chap. 9).

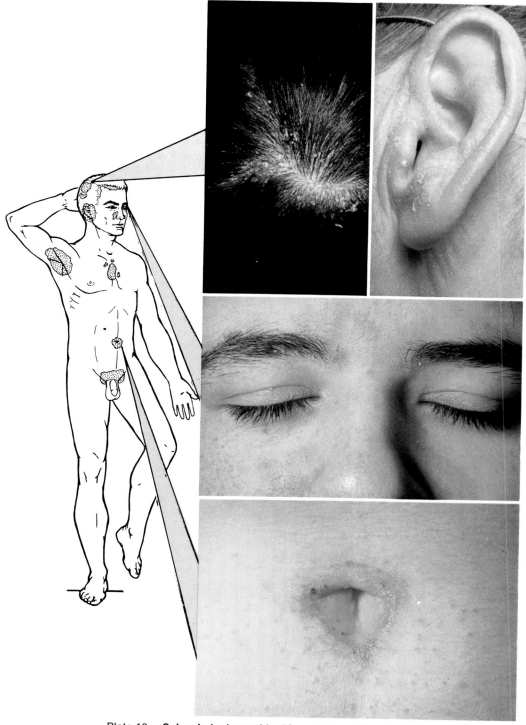

Plate 18. **Seborrheic dermatitis.** (*Owen Laboratories, Inc.*)

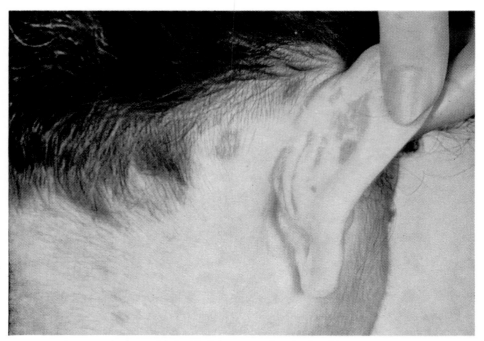

Plate 19. **Seborrheic dermatitis behind the ear and at the border of the scalp.** (*Smith Kline & French Laboratories*)

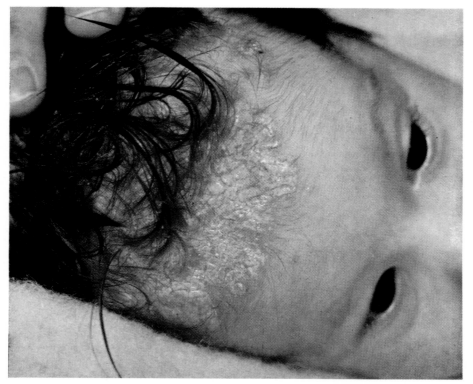

Plate 20. **Seborrheic dermatitis of infancy.** This is one of the causes of "cradle cap." (*Smith Kline & French Laboratories*)

FACE LESIONS

Systemic lupus erythematosus: faint, reddish, slightly scaly "butterfly" eruption, aggravated by sunlight, with fever, malaise, and positive antinuclear antibody test (see Chap. 25).

Chronic discoid lupus erythematosus: sharply defined, red, scaly, atrophic areas with large follicular openings, resistant to local therapy (see Chap. 25).

BODY LESIONS

Tinea corporis (see Chap. 19).
Psoriasis (see Chap. 14).
Pityriasis rosea (see Chap. 14).
Tinea versicolor (see Chap. 14).

Treatment

A young man presents with recurrent red, scaly lesions at the border of the scalp and forehead and diffuse, mild, whitish scaling throughout the scalp.

1. Management of cases of dandruff must include explaining about the disease, stating that it is not contagious, that there is no true cure, that it will not cause baldness, and that there are seasonal variations. Therapy can be very effective, but only for keeping the dandruff under control.

2. Shampooing. With the above information in mind, tell the patient that shampooing offers the best management. There are several shampoos available, and the patient may have to experiment to find the one most suitable. The following types can be suggested:

   A. Selenium sulfide 2½% suspension (Selsun, Exsel)   120.0
      Sig: Shampoo as frequently as necessary to alleviate itching and scaling. Use no other soap. Refill prescription p.r.n.

   B. Additional Shampoos:
      Tar shampoos, such as Ionil T, Sebutone, X-Seb T, Vanseb-T, and T-Gel; or
      Zinc pyrthione shampoos such as Zincon, Head & Shoulders, DHS-Zinc; or
      Salicylic acid-sulfur shampoos such as Sebulex, Vanseb, Ionil, and X-Seb
      Sig: Shampoo as frequently as necessary to keep scaling and itching to a minimum.

3. Triamcinolone (Kenalog) Spray,   63 ml
   Sig: Apply sparingly to scalp at night. Squirt the spray through a plastic tube that is supplied.
   Comment: A spray is less messy on the scalp than a corticosteroid solution, but solutions are available.

4. A low-potency corticosteroid cream   15.0
   Sig: Apply b.i.d. locally to body lesions.

5. Ketoconazole (Nizoral) 2% cream   15.0
   Sig: Apply b.i.d. on scalp or body lesions. This is a corticosteroid-sparing agent.

SAUER NOTES:

1. Do not prescribe a fluorinated corticosteroid cream for long-term use on the face or in intertriginous areas.

2. Reiterate that there is no cure for seborrheic dermatitis; long-term management is necessary.

3. Reassure the patient that seborrheic dermatitis does not cause hair loss.

ACNE
(Plate 21)

Acne vulgaris is a very common skin condition of adolescents and young adults. It is characterized by any combination of comedones (blackheads), pustules, cysts, and scarring of varying severity (Figs. 13–1 and 13–2).

PRIMARY LESIONS. Comedones, papules, pustules, and, in severe cases, cysts occur.

SECONDARY LESIONS. Pits and scars are evident in severe cases. Excoriations of the papules are seen in some adolescents, but most often they appear as part of the acne of women in their 20s and 30s.

DISTRIBUTION. Acne occurs on the face and neck and, less commonly, on the back, the chest, and the arms.

COURSE. The condition begins at ages 9 to 12, or later, and lasts, with new outbreaks, for months or years. It subsides in the majority of cases by the age of 18 to 19, but occasional flare-ups may occur for years. The residual scarring varies with severity of the case and response to treatment.

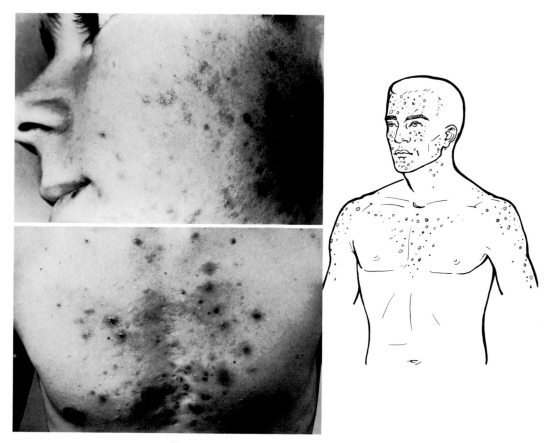

Figure 13–1. **Acne of face and chest.**

SUBJECTIVE COMPLAINT. Tenderness of the large pustules and itching may be reported (rarely). Emotional upset is common as a result of the unattractive appearance.

ETIOLOGY. These factors are important: heredity, hormonal balance, diet, cleanliness, and general health.

In a case of severe adult acne, one should rule out an endocrine disorder. Hirsutism in women is a clue.

SEASON. Most cases are better during the summer.

CONTAGIOUSNESS. Acne is not contagious.

Differential Diagnosis

Drug eruption: note history of ingestion of lithium, corticosteroids, iodides, bromides, trimethadione, or testosterone and ACTH by injection (see Chap. 9).

Contact dermatitis from industrial oils (see Chap. 9).

Perioral dermatitis (see Plate 21): red papules, small pustules, and some scaling on chin, upper lip, and nasolabial fold. The cause is unknown, but formaldehyde in the Kleenex-type tissues, toothpastes, and new clothes may be a factor; acne and seborrhea may also be factors. *Corticosteroid creams, locally, eventually aggravate the eruption and usually should not be prescribed.* Tetracycline, orally, as for acne, is the therapy of choice.

Adenoma sebaceum: rare; see papular lesions; associated with epilepsy and mental deficiency (see Fig. 33–3).

Management

FIRST VISIT

A 14-year old patient presents with moderate amount of facial blackheads and pustules.

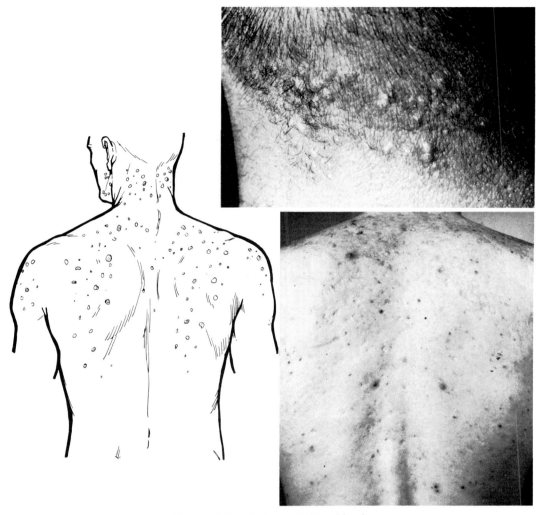

Figure 13–2. **Acne of neck and back.**

1. Give instructions regarding skin care (see sheet that can be given to patient, "What You Should Know About Acne," later in this chapter).

   Stress the fact to the patient and the parent that not one factor but several factors (heredity, hormones, diet, stress, season of the year, greasy cosmetics, cleanliness, and general health) influence acne breakouts. Some of these factors cannot be altered.

2. Bar soap. The affected areas should be washed twice a day with a washcloth and a noncreamy soap, such as Dial, Neutragena for acne-prone skin, and Purpose Soaps.

3. Sulfur, ppt.   6%
   Resorcinol   4%
   Colored alcoholic shake lotion
      (See in Formulary, p. 38) q.s.   60.0
   Sig: Apply locally at bedtime with fingers.
   Proprietary products for the above lotion include Sulfacet-R, Komed lotion, Acno lotion, Sebasorb liquid, and Rezamid lotion.

4. Benzoyl peroxide preparations.
   Benzoyl peroxide gel (5% or 10%) as in Benzagel, Desquam X, Benzac-W, Panoxyl, Persa-Gel, and others. Some of these are also available as emollient gels. Benzamycin Lotion is a combination of benzoyl peroxide and erythromycin.

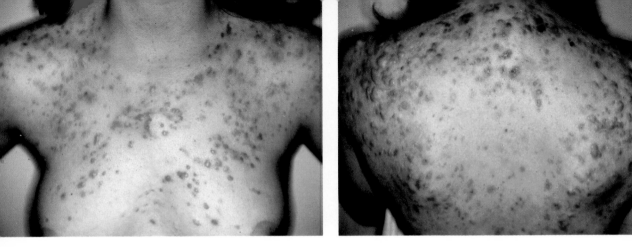

(*A* and *B*) Severe acne of chest and back of a 15-year-old girl

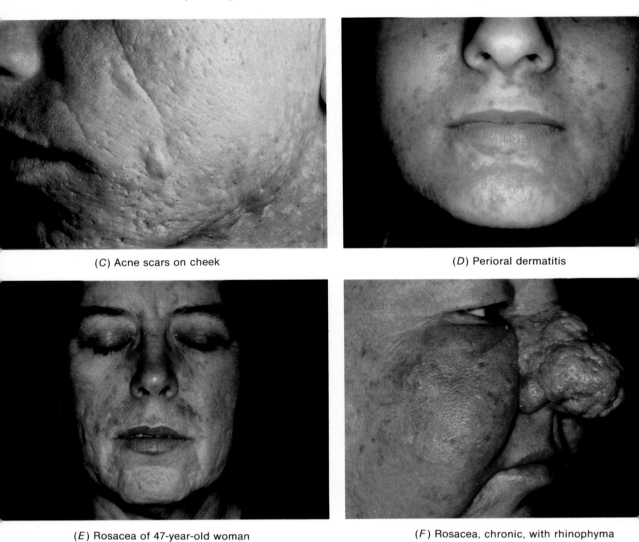

(*C*) Acne scars on cheek

(*D*) Perioral dermatitis

(*E*) Rosacea of 47-year-old woman

(*F*) Rosacea, chronic, with rhinophyma

Plate 21. **Severe acne vulgaris, perioral dermatitis, and rosacea.** (*Hoechst-Roussel Pharmaceuticals, Inc.*)

Sig: Apply locally once a day. Some dryness of skin is to be expected.
5. Tretinoin gel (0.01% or 0.025%)
(Retin A) q.s.   15.0
Sig: Apply locally once a day. Patient toleration varies considerably. Especially valuable for comedome acne.
6. Local antibiotic solutions.
Clindamycin 1% or erythromycin 2% lotion q.s.   30.0
Sig: Apply locally once or twice a day.
Many proprietary antibiotic products are available, some in pledgets.

SAUER NOTES:

1. For local acne medications, one product can be applied in the morning and a different product at night.
2. To ensure compliance, start with milder agents, increasing the strength as indicated and tolerated.

---

7. Remove the blackheads with a comedone extractor (Fig. 13–3) in the office.

SUBSEQUENT VISITS
1. Ultraviolet therapy with increasing suberythema doses once or twice a week can be used. Treat both sides of the face, back, or chest as indicated.
2. Increase the strengths of local medications as tolerated.

SAUER NOTES:

1. Acne flare-ups occur in cycles—hormonal (both females and males) and seasonal (fall and spring). Keep reminding your patient of these natural flare-ups.
2. "Prom pills." The high school prom (or a wedding or a job interview) is in one week.
Prednisone, 10-mg tablets   #14
Sig: 2 tablets q. AM for 7 days will clear much of that inflammatory acne.
3. Unfortunately, an appreciable number of men and women continue to have acne into the 20s, 30s, and even later years. Explain this fact to your patient.

TREATMENT FOR A CASE OF SCARRING ACNE
1. Tetracycline, or similar antibiotic,
250 mg   #100
Sig: 1 capsule q.i.d. for 3 days, then 1 capsule b.i.d. This dose can be continued for weeks, months, or years, or the dose can be lowered to 1 capsule a day for maintenance, depending, of course, on the extent of the involvement. Severe cases respond to 3 to 6 capsules a day.
Tetracycline should be taken 30 minutes before meals or 2 hours after a meal, and not concurrently with iron or calcium for optimal absorption.
Other effective antibiotics include erythromycin, 250 mg, b.i.d. or t.i.d., and minocycline, 100 mg/day.

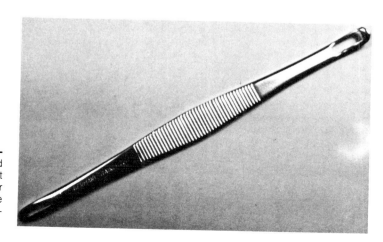

Figure 13–3. **Comedone extractor.** The most frequently used instrument in my office. Firm but gentle pressure with the smaller end over a comedone will force the comedone out of the sebaceous gland opening.

2. Other treatments:
   A. Vitamin A (water-soluble synthetic A) 50,000 U.　　　#100
      Sig: 1 capsule b.i.d. for 4 months.
   B. Abrasive cleansers are somewhat effective in removing comedones. These include Brasivol, Pernox, and Sastid.
   C. Large papules or early cysts. Intralesional corticosteroid can be injected with care. Dilute Kenalog Suspension (10 mg/ml) with equal part of saline, and inject approximately 0.1 ml into the lesion. Atrophy can result if too large a quantity is injected.
   D. Incision of fluctuant acne cysts. *Never incise these widely*, but if you believe the pus must be drained, do it through a very small incision.
   E. Short-term prednisone systemic therapy is effective for severe cystic acne, especially for *acne fulminans*, an acute, disabling form of acne.
   F. Isotretinoin (Accutane). For severe, scarring, cystic acne this therapy has proved very beneficial. The usual dosage is 1.0 mg/kg/day given for 4 to 5 months. There are many minor and major side effects with this therapy (notably *teratogenic effects on pregnant women*) so that isotretinoin should *only* be prescribed by those knowledgeable in its use.
3. The residual scarring of severe acne (see Plate 21) can be lessened by surgical dermabrasion, using a rapidly rotating wire brush or diamond fraise. This procedure is being done by many dermatologists and plastic surgeons. Some scars can be injected with silicone or collagen.

WHAT YOU SHOULD KNOW ABOUT ACNE*

Acne is a disorder in which the oil glands of the skin are overactive. It usually involves the face and, frequently, the chest and the back, since these areas are the richest in oil glands. When an oil gland opening becomes plugged, a blackhead is formed and irritates the skin in exactly the same way as any other foreign body, such as a sliver of wood. This irritation takes the form of red pimples or deep painful cysts. These infections destroy the tissues and, when healed, may result in permanent scars.

The tendency to develop acne runs in families, especially those in which one or both parents have an oily skin. Acne is aggravated by certain foods, improper care of the skin, lack of adequate sleep, and nervous tension. In girls, acne is usually worse before a menstrual period. Even in boys, acne flares on a cyclic basis. Any or all of these factors may exaggerate the tendency of the oily skin to develop acne. Therefore, the prevention of acne depends on correcting not one but several of these factors.

Because acne is so common, is not contagious, and does not cause loss of time from school or work, many persons tend to ignore it or regard it as a necessary part of growing up. Actually, the old statement, "You'll be all right when you're married," has little or no significance. Marriage itself has no relationship to acne, except that ordinarily by the time a person is ready to get married, he or she usually is past the acne age and the acne would have cleared anyway.

Reasons for Treating Acne

There are at least two very important reasons for seeking medical care for acne. The first is to prevent the scarring mentioned previously. Once scarring has occurred, it is permanent. Then a patient must go through the rest of life being embarrassed and annoyed by the scars, even though active pimples are no longer present. This scarring may vary from tiny little pits, which are frequently mistaken for "enlarged pores," to deep, large, disfiguring pockmarks.

* This information is from an instruction sheet that I give to my acne patients. I am well aware of differences of opinion regarding the role of diet in acne, but I am presenting my belief.

continued

14

Papulosquamous Dermatoses

The papulosquamous dermatoses include several specific entities that predominantly affect the chest and the back with clinically similar macular, papular, and scaly lesions (see Fig. 3–5). The most common diseases in the group are psoriasis, pityriasis rosea, tinea versicolor, lichen planus, seborrheic dermatitis, secondary syphilis, and drug eruptions. The last three conditions are considered elsewhere in this book. To be complete with regard to the differential diagnoses of this group, the following rarer diseases can also be included: parapsoriasis and its variants, lichen nitidus, and pityriasis rubra pilaris.

PSORIASIS
(Plates 22 through 25)

Psoriasis is a common, chronically recurring, papulosquamous disease, characterized by varying sized whitish, scaly patches seen most commonly on the elbows, the knees, and the scalp.

PRIMARY LESIONS. Erythematous, papulosquamous lesions vary in shapes and sizes from drop size to large circinate areas, which can become generalized. The scale is usually thick and silvery and bleeds from minute points when it is removed by the fingernail (Auspitz's sign).

Pustular psoriasis is a severe type of psoriasis involving the palms and soles, or it can be generalized on the body.

SECONDARY LESIONS. Although unusual, excoriations, thickening (lichenification), and oozing can be found.

DISTRIBUTION. Psoriasis most commonly occurs on the scalp, the elbows, and the knees, but it can involve any area of the body, including the nails.

COURSE. Psoriasis is notoriously chronic and recurrent. However, cases have been known to clear and not recur.

ETIOLOGY. The cause of psoriasis is unknown. Approximately 30% of patients with psoriasis have a family history of the disease.

There is an acute form of psoriasis, called *guttate psoriasis*, that very frequently develops following a streptococcal throat infection. The scaly lesions are the size of drops, hence guttate. This form of psoriasis is usually seen in children.

SUBJECTIVE COMPLAINTS. Fortunately, only 30% of patients with psoriasis itch.

SEASON. Psoriasis is usually worse in winter, probably because of low indoor humidity and relative lack of sunlight.

AGE-GROUP. The disease may affect a person of any age but is unusual in children.

CONTAGIOUSNESS. Psoriasis is not contagious.

RELATIONSHIP TO EMPLOYMENT. Psoriatic lesions can develop or flare up in areas of skin injury (Koebner phenomenon).

LABORATORY FINDINGS. Microscopic section is characteristic in typical cases.

(text continues on page 138)

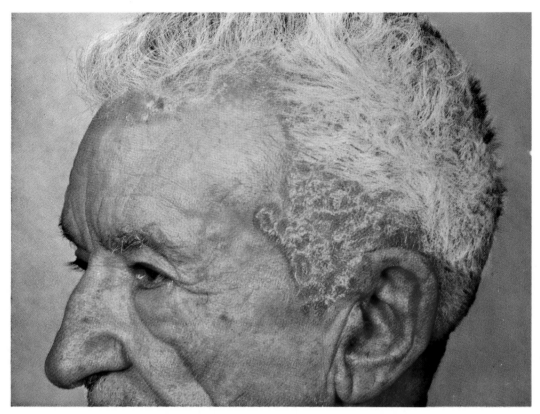

Plate 22. **Psoriasis of the border of the scalp.** Psoriasis in this location is often difficult to distinguish from seborrheic dermatitis. (*Smith Kline & French Laboratories*).

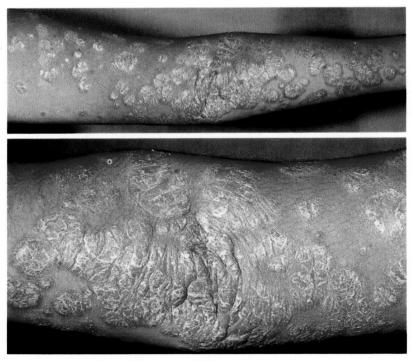

Plate 23. **Psoriasis on elbows of a 17-year-old girl.** (Continued on facing page.)

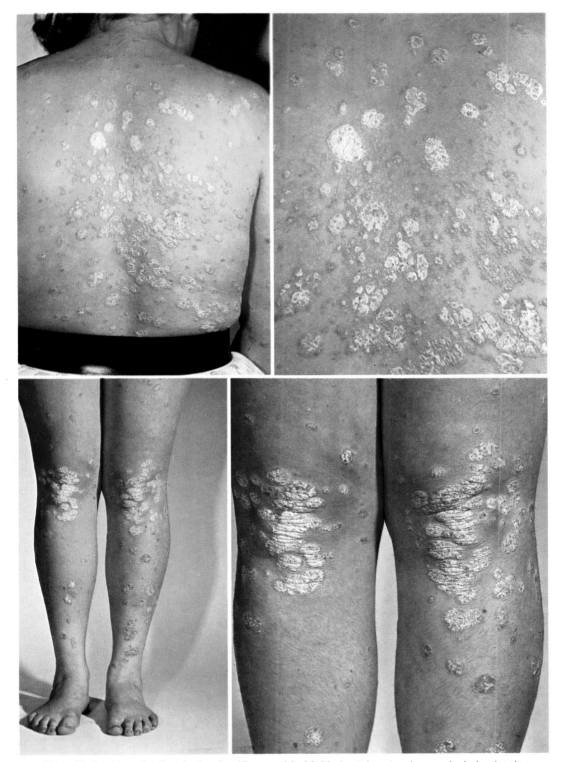

Plate 23. (continued)   **Psoriasis of a 17-year-old girl.** Moderately extensive psoriasis in classic distribution on back and knees. (*K.U.M.C.*) (*Roche Laboratories*).

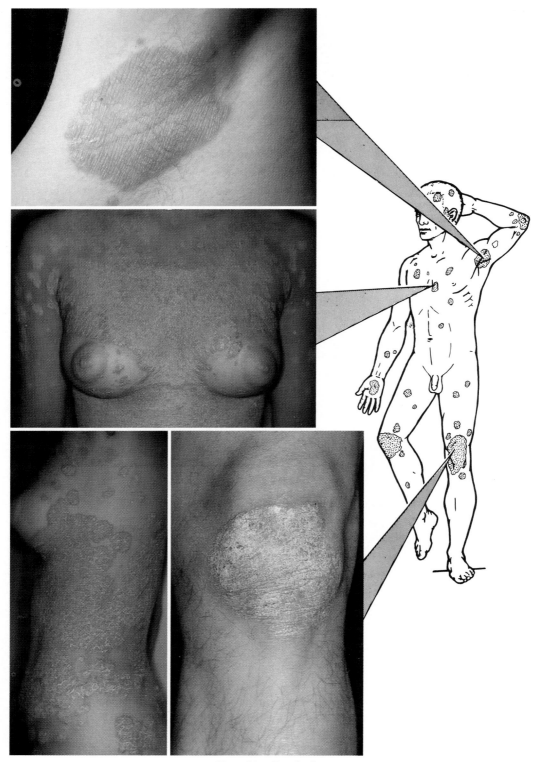

Plate 24. **Psoriasis.**

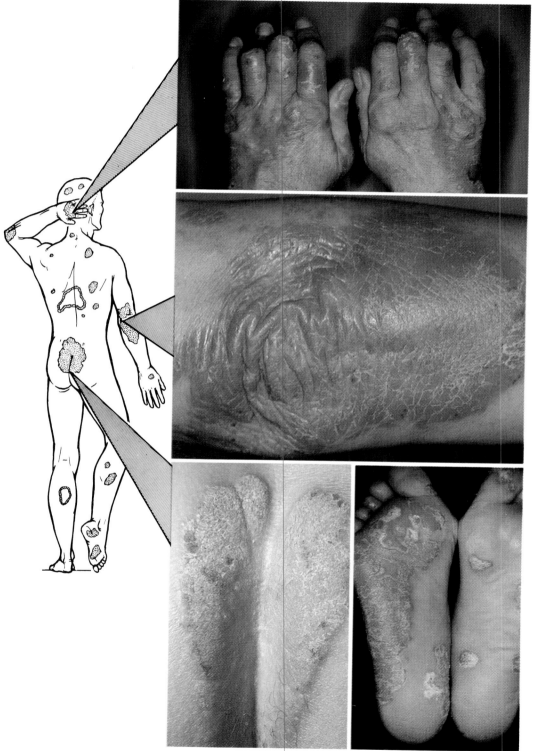

Plate 25. **Psoriasis.**

Differential Diagnosis

Tinea corporis: single lesion, usually round with healing in center; scraping and culture positive for fungi (see Chap. 20).

Seborrheic dermatitis: lesions more greasy and occur in hairy areas; scalp lesions are often impossible to differentiate from psoriasis (see Chap. 13).

Pityriasis rosea: "herald patch"; acute onset (see this chapter).

Atopic eczema: patches on flexural surfaces; allergic history (see Chap. 9).

Secondary or tertiary syphilis: can be psoriasiform; blood serology positive; local therapy is of little value (see Chap. 16).

Lichen planus: lesions violaceous; small papules; very little scaling (see this chapter).

A single lesion of psoriasis may resemble *neurodermatitis.*

Psoriasis of nails (see Plate 76) is similar to *tinea of nails.*

Management

It is most important in the management of patients with psoriasis that you be frank with them regarding the prognosis and "cure." Reassure them that it is not contagious, that the disease disappears in many cases, and that you can help them manage the disease. But be straightforward in saying that no physician at this moment knows a "cure" for psoriasis. It might help the patient (or it might not) for you to say that psoriasis should not be considered a disease but should be thought of as a hobby.

FIRST VISIT OF PATIENT WITH RED SCALY LESIONS ON SCALP AND ELBOWS ONLY

1. For body lesions:
   A. Medium-Potency Fluorinated Corticosteroid Cream or Ointment   30.0
      q.s.,
      or
   B. Coal tar solution (L.C.D.)   5%
      Sulfur, ppt.   5%
      White petrolatum q.s.   30.0
      Sig: Apply locally b.i.d. to body lesions.
   This treatment has the added value of being inexpensive.
2. For scalp lesions:
   A. Tar Shampoo (see list in Formulary, Chap. 5).
      Sig: Shampoo scalp frequently.

Use without any other soap; also useful in relieving itching.
   B. Triamcinolone (Kenalog) Spray, 63 g
      Sig: Apply to scalp at night with plastic tube applicator.
   C. Derma-Smoothe FS with or without L.C.D., 5%, is effective when applied at night.

SUBSEQUENT VISITS OF PATIENT WITH LOCALIZED CASE

1. For body lesions, gradually increase the strength of the medicines in the above salves.
2. Occlusive dressing—corticosteroid therapy. For localized areas of psoriasis, especially on the extremities, a fluorinated corticosteroid cream can be applied at night and covered with an occlusive plastic dressing such as Saran Wrap. This wrapping should be left on overnight. If the lesions of psoriasis are small, the cream can be covered with Blenderm Tape or Actiderm Patch for occlusion.

   For greater therapeutic effectiveness, on subsequent visits, coal tar solution (3% to 6%) can be incorporated in the corticosteroid cream.
3. Intralesional corticosteroid therapy. For localized patches of psoriasis, parenteral triamcinolone can be injected under the lesions. This is a very effective treatment for small lesions. The technique is given on page 106.

FIRST VISIT OF PATIENT WITH PSORIASIS ON 65% OF THE BODY SURFACE

1. Coal tar solution (L.C.D.)   120.0
   Sig: 2 tablespoons to the bathtub, with 6 to 8 inches of warm water. Soak for 15 minutes once a day. Soap may be used, unless there is much itching.
2. Prescribe a mild body salve:
   Coal tar solution (L.C.D.)   3%
   White petrolatum q.s.   120.0
   Sig: Apply locally b.i.d.
      Later the concentration of the coal tar solution (L.C.D.) can be slowly increased.
3. Ultraviolet therapy (UVB), in increasing suberythema doses, once or twice a week can be used following a daily thin application of a tar salve, similar to the Goeckerman regimen.

   The combination of oral psoralen and ultraviolet A therapy (PUVA) for extensive

SAUER NOTES:

Here are some of my thoughts on the management of psoriasis.

1. Use the noncarbon form shown in Chapter 4 to give written information to the patient on the diagnosis, whether it can be cured or not (there is no cure, but there is help available). Tell the patient that the cause of psoriasis is unknown, that it is cyclic and seasonal, and that it is aggravated by stress. Provide an outline of your proposed therapy.

2. I rarely prescribe a silver or plastic tube of **single** medication salve for psoriasis. My prescriptions are compounded with L.C.D., 3% to 10%, sulfur, ppt 3% to 10%, salicylic acid, 3% to 6%, singly or in combination, in a base of corticosteroid ointment, or in Unibase or white petrolatum. I am aware of the pros and cons on mixing locally applied salves, but this is what I do.

3. I begin with lower concentrations of any medication and increase or further modify the mixtures according to the patient's individual response.

4. There is evidence that β-blocking drugs can aggravate psoriasis.

or persistent psoriasis is being used with definite benefit. This therapy requires special UVA light sources, equipment, timers, and trained personnel. Many precautions must be observed with PUVA therapy.

4. Methotrexate therapy. In cases of severe psoriasis, dermatologists occasionally use this oral method of therapy with good results. Since methotrexate is a potent and dangerous drug, those wishing to use it must consult recently published papers on the subject to become thoroughly familiar with the effects of the drug.

5. Etretinate (Tegison) therapy. For a severe case of psoriasis in a man (or in a postmenopausal woman) this therapy is effective, but there are many side effects. The long terminal elimination half-life of up to 6 months is a major problem. Acitretin, not yet released in the United States, has a half-life of 50 hours, so this drug may prove more useful and safer for severe psoriasis cases.

SUBSEQUENT VISITS OF PATIENT WITH RATHER GENERALIZED CASE

1. Increase the concentrations of medicines used locally or use:

Anthralin USP (or Drithocreme)   0.1%
q.s.   60.0

Sig: Apply locally b.i.d. Avoid getting salve near the eyes.

There is also a technique of applying anthralin and removing it in 30 minutes, done once a day (short contact therapy). The concentration of the anthralin can be increased cautiously, as necessary up to 1.0%. Anthralin stains the skin and clothing.

2. Systemic corticosteroids are of some value. Prednisone, 10-mg tablets in a low dosage of 2 tablets in the morning, is beneficial. Given in this manner one rarely sees side-effects. If conjunctive local therapy is not effective, relapses are the rule after corticosteroid therapy and may be difficult to handle. This is not a recommended form of therapy for general use.

PITYRIASIS ROSEA
(Plates 26 through 28)

Pityriasis rosea is a moderately common papulosquamous eruption, mainly of the trunk of young adults. It is mildly pruritic and occurs most often in the spring and the fall.

PRIMARY LESIONS. Papulosquamous, oval erythematous discrete lesions are seen. A larger "herald patch" resembling a patch of "ringworm" may precede the general rash by 2 to 10 days.

SECONDARY LESIONS. Excoriations are rare. The effects of overtreatment or contact dermatitis are commonly seen.

DISTRIBUTION. The lesions appear mainly on the chest and trunk along the lines of cleavage. Many cases have the oval lesions in a "Christmas tree branches" pattern. In atypical cases the lesions are seen in the axillae and the groin only. Face lesions are rare in white adults but are rather commonly seen in children and blacks.

(text continues on page 143)

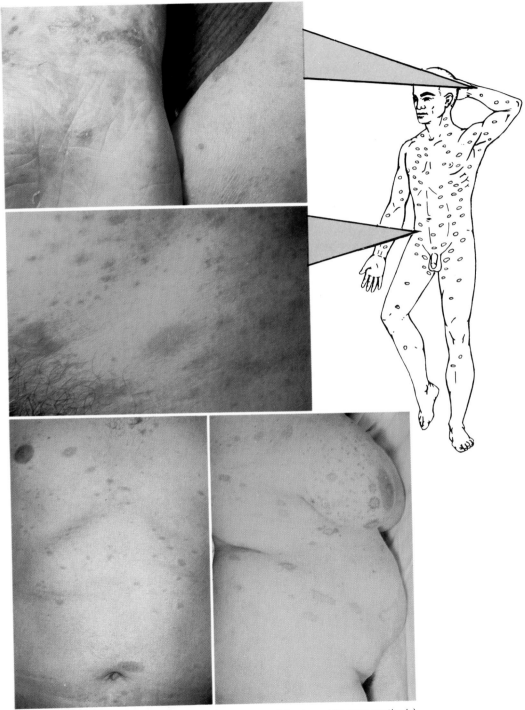

Plate 26. **Pityriasis rosea.** (*Westwood Pharmaceuticals*)

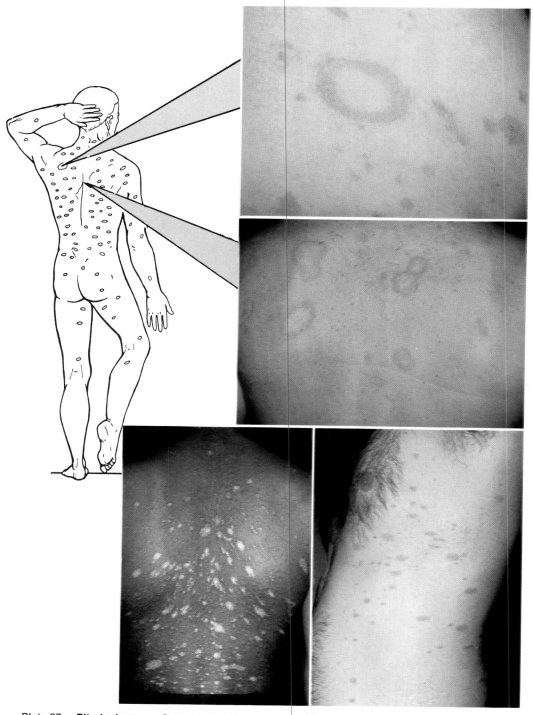

Plate 27. **Pityriasis rosea.** Bottom left photograph is of a black man. (*Westwood Pharmaceuticals*)

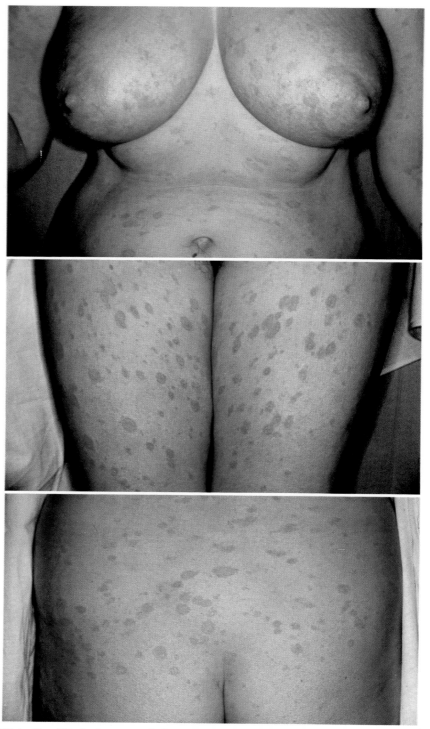

Plate 28. **Pityriasis rosea of chest, thighs, and buttocks of one patient.** (*Syntex Laboratories, Inc.*)

COURSE. Following the development of the "herald patch," new generalized lesions continue to appear for 2 to 3 weeks. The entire rash commonly disappears within 6 weeks. Recurrences are rare.

SUBJECTIVE COMPLAINTS. Itching varies from none to severe.

ETIOLOGY. The cause is unknown.

SEASON. Spring and fall "epidemics" are common.

AGE GROUP. Young adults are mainly affected.

CONTAGIOUSNESS. The disease is not contagious.

Differential Diagnosis

Tinea versicolor: lesions tannish and irregularly shaped; fungi seen on scraping (see this chapter).

Drug eruption: no "herald patch"; positive drug history for bismuth or sulfa (see Chap. 9).

Secondary syphilis: no itching (99% true); history or presence of genital lesions; positive blood serology (see Chap. 16).

Psoriasis: also usually on elbows, knees, and scalp; lesions have whitish scale (see this chapter).

Seborrheic dermatitis: greasy, irregular, scaly lesions on sternal and other hairy areas (see Chap. 13).

Lichen planus: lesions more papular and violaceous; on mucous membranes of mouth and lip (see this chapter).

Parapsoriasis: rare, very chronic.

SAUER NOTE:

If the pityriasis rosea–like rash does not itch, obtain blood serologic test for syphilis.

Treatment

FIRST VISIT

1. Reassure the patient that he does not have a "blood disease," that the eruption is not contagious, and that it would be rare to get it again. (Active treatment is preferred to saying, "Go home, it will disappear in 6 weeks." There are three reasons for this: (a) treatment *may* shorten the duration of the disease; (b) the usual itching must be alleviated; and (c) if you do not treat these patients, they might go to someone else less qualified. If the eruption does not itch and the patient can be reassured of the mild nature of the disease, then no treatment is necessary.)

2. Colloidal bath.
   Sig: Use 1 packet of Aveeno oatmeal preparation to the tub containing 6 to 8 inches of lukewarm water. Bathe for 10 to 15 minutes every day or every other day. Avoid soap as much as possible to reduce any itching.

3. Nonalcoholic white shake lotion or Calamine lotion q.s.   120.0
   (See Formulary, Chap. 5.)
   Sig: Apply b.i.d. locally to affected areas.

4. If there is itching, prescribe an antihistamine drug, such as:
   Cyproheptadine (Periactin), 4 mg   #60
   Sig: 1 tablet a.c. and h.s.

5. Ultraviolet B therapy in increasing suberythema doses once or twice a week may be given. The entire body is treated with two front and two back exposures.

SUBSEQUENT VISITS

1. If the skin becomes too dry from the colloidal bath and the lotion, stop the lotion or alternate it with the following:
   Hydrocortisone Cream, 1% q.s.   60.0
   Sig: Apply b.i.d. locally to dry areas.

2. Continue the ultraviolet treatments.

SEVERELY PRURITIC CASES

In addition to the above, add:
Prednisone, 5 mg   #40
Sig: 1 tablet q.i.d. for 3 days, then 1 tablet t.i.d. for 4 days, then 2 tablets every morning for 1 to 2 weeks, as symptom of itching demands.

TINEA VERSICOLOR
(Plate 29)

Tinea versicolor is a moderately common skin eruption with characteristics of tannish colored, irregularly shaped scaly patches causing no discomfort that are usually located on the upper chest and back. It is caused by a lipophilic yeast. (See Chap. 19.)

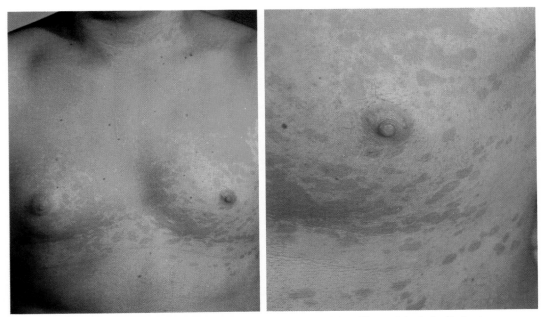

Plate 29. **Tinea versicolor on the chest.** The dark areas of the skin are infected with the fungus. (*K.U.M.C.*) (*Sandoz Pharmaceuticals*)

PRIMARY LESIONS. Papulosquamous or maculosquamous, tan, and irregularly shaped lesions occur.

SECONDARY LESIONS. Relative depigmentation results because the involved skin does not tan when exposed to sunlight. This cosmetic defect, obvious in the summer, often brings the patient to the office.

DISTRIBUTION. The upper part of the chest and the back, neck, and arms are affected. Rarely are the lesions on the face or generalized.

COURSE. The eruption can persist for years unnoticed. Correct treatment is readily effective, but, if treatment is not thorough, the tinea can recur.

ETIOLOGY. The causative agent is a lipophilic yeast, *Pityrosporum orbiculare*, which has a hyphae form called *Pityrosporum* or *Malassezia furfur*.

CONTAGIOUSNESS. The disease is rarely contagious.

LABORATORY FINDINGS. A scraping of the scale placed on a microscopic slide, covered with a 20% solution of potassium hydroxide (see p. 11) and a coverslip will show the hyphae. Under the low-power lens of the microscope, very thin mycelial filaments are seen. Diagnostic grapelike clusters of spores are seen best with the high-power lens. This dimorphic organism does not grow on routine culture media.

Differential Diagnosis

Pityriasis rosea: acute onset; lesions oval with definite border (see earlier in this Chapter).

Seborrheic dermatitis: greasy scales in hairy areas, mainly (see Chap. 13).

Mild psoriasis: thicker scaly lesions on trunk and elsewhere (see earlier in this chapter).

Vitiligo: since tinea versicolor commonly manifests with depigmentation of the skin, many cases have been called vitiligo. This is indeed unfortunate because tinea versicolor is quite easy to treat and has a much better prognosis than vitiligo (see Chap. 24).

Secondary syphilis: lesions are more widely distributed and rarely only scaly (see Chap. 16).

Treatment

Selenium (Selsun or Exsel) Suspension
2½% 120.0
Sig: Bathe and dry completely. Then apply medicine as a lotion to all the involved areas, usually from neck down to pubic area. Let it dry. Bathe again in 24 hours and wash off the medicine. Repeat procedure again at weekly intervals for four treatments. Recurrences are rather common and can be easily re-treated.

SAUER NOTES:

1. It is important to tell the patient that depigmented spots may remain after the tinea versicolor is cured. These can be tanned by gradual exposure to sunlight or ultraviolet light.

2. There are other local therapies for tinea versicolor, but I prefer the weekly selenium routine. It is simple and effective.

3. Ketoconazole (Nizoral) orally is effective, but I rarely use it. Anaphylactic-type reactions have occurred.

LICHEN PLANUS
(Plates 1 and 30 through 33)

Lichen planus is an uncommon, chronic, pruritic disease characterized by violaceous flat-topped papules that are usually seen on the wrists and the legs. Mucous membrane lesions on the cheeks or lips are whitish.

PRIMARY LESIONS. Flat-topped, violaceous papules and papulosquamous lesions appear. On close examination of a papule, preferably after the lesion has been wet with an alcohol swipe, intersecting small white lines (Wickham's striae) can be seen. These confirm the diagnosis. Uncommonly, the lesions may assume a ring-shaped configuration or may be atrophic or bullous. On the mucous membranes the lesions appear as a whitish, lacy network.

SECONDARY LESIONS. Excoriations and, on the legs, thick, scaly, lichenified patches have been noted.

DISTRIBUTION. Most commonly the lesions appear on the flexural aspects of the wrists and the ankles, the penis, and the oral

(text continues on page 149)

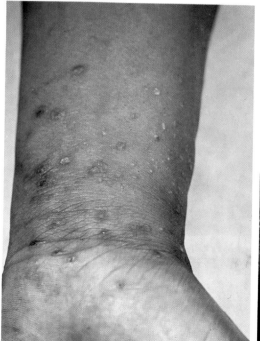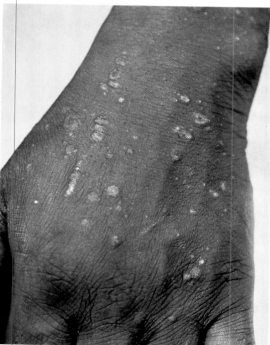

Plate 30. **Lichen planus on the wrist and the dorsum of the hand in a black patient.** Note the violaceous color of the papules and the linear Koebner phenomenon on the dorsum of the hand. *(E. R. Squibb)*

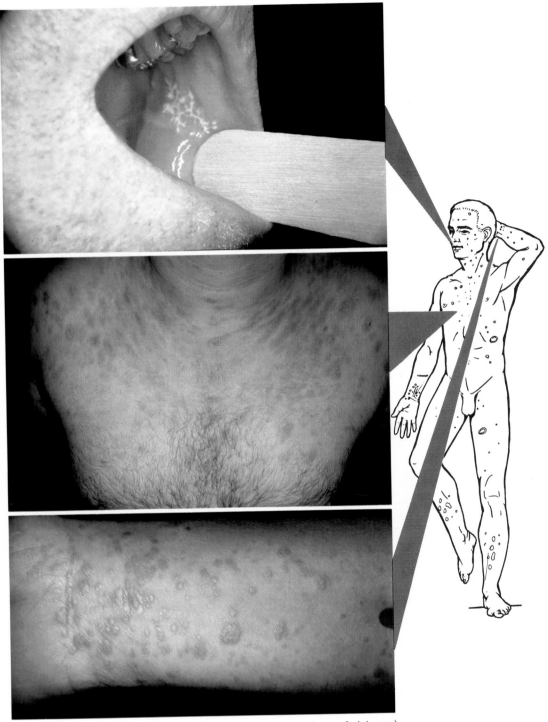

Plate 31. **Lichen planus.** (*Johnson & Johnson*)

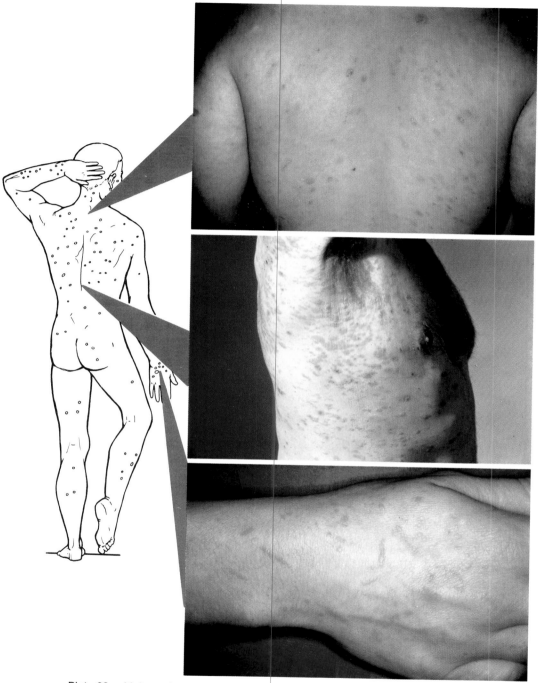

Plate 32.   **Lichen planus.** Note the Koebner reaction in the lower photograph.

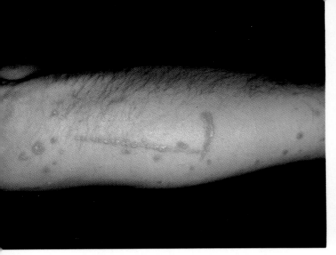

(A) Koebner reaction in scratched areas on arm

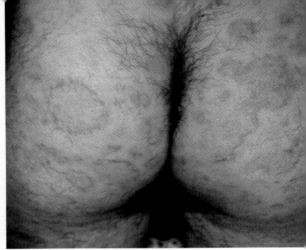

(B) Atrophic scarring lesions on buttocks

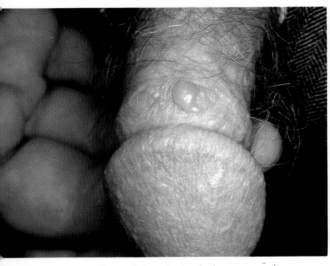

(C) Bullous and vesicular lesions on penis

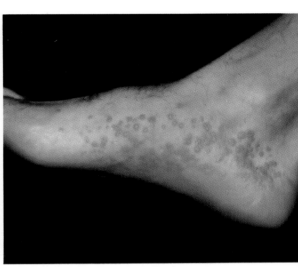

(D) Lichen planus on sole of foot

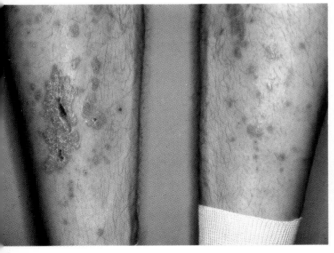

(E) Hypertrophic lesions on anterior tibial area of legs

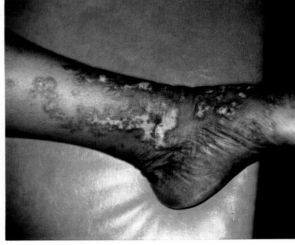

(F) Hypertrophic lesions on leg of a black woman

Plate 33.   **Lichen planus, unusual variations.**   (*Neutrogena Corp.*)

mucous membranes, but they can be anywhere on the body or become generalized.

COURSE. The outbreak is rather sudden with the chronic course averaging 9 months' duration. Some cases last several years. There is no effect on the general health except for itching. Recurrences are moderately common.

ETIOLOGY. The cause is unknown. The disorder is rather frequently associated with nervous or emotional upsets.

SUBJECTIVE COMPLAINTS. Itching varies from mild to severe.

CONTAGIOUSNESS. Lichen planus is not contagious.

RELATED TO EMPLOYMENT. As in psoriasis, the lichen planus lesions can develop in scratches or skin injuries (Koebner phenomenon).

LABORATORY FINDINGS. Microscopic section is quite characteristic.

Differential Diagnosis

Secondary syphilis: no itching; blood serology positive (see Chap. 16).
Drug eruption: history of taking atabrine, arsenic, or gold (see Chap. 9).
Psoriasis: lesions more scaly, whitish on knees and elbows (see earlier in this chapter).
Pityriasis rosea: "herald patch," on trunk, mainly (see earlier in this chapter).
Lichen planus on leg may resemble *neurodermatitis* (usually one patch only; intensely pruritic; no mucous membrane lesions; see Chap. 11).

Treatment

FIRST VISIT

A patient presents with generalized papular eruption and moderate itching.

1. Assure the patient that the disease is not contagious, is not a blood disease, and is chronic but not serious.

2. Avoid excess bathing with soap.
3. Low-potency corticosteroid cream   60.0
   Sig: Apply locally b.i.d.
4. Antihistamine such as chlorpheniramine, 8 mg   #60
   Sig: (over-the-counter) 1 tablet b.i.d. for itching (warn of drowsiness at onset of therapy).

SUBSEQUENT VISITS
1. Occlusive dressing—corticosteroid therapy. This is quite effective for localized cases. I have also found that if occlusive dressings are applied only to the lichen planus on the legs, the rest of the body lesions improve. For technique see p. 106.
2. Meprobamate, 400 mg, or   #100
   chlordiazepoxide (Librium), 5 mg
   Sig: 1 tab t.i.d.
3. It is important in some resistant cases to rule out a focus of infection in teeth, tonsils, gallbladder, genitourinary system, and so on.
4. Corticosteroids orally or by injection are of definite value for temporarily relieving the acute cases that have severe itching or a generalized eruption.

BIBLIOGRAPHY

Faergemann J, Fredriksson T: Tinea versicolor: Some new aspects on etiology, pathogenesis, and treatment. Int J Dermatol 21:8, 1982

Fox BJ, Odum RB: Papulosquamous diseases: A review. J Am Acad Dermatol 12:597, 1985

Gold MH, Holy AK, Roenigk HH: Beta-blocking drugs and psoriasis. J Acad Dermatol 19:837, 1988

Gupta AK, Goldfarb MT, Ellis CN et al: Side-effect profile of acitretin therapy in psoriasis. J Am Acad Dermatol 20:1088, 1989

Kingston TP, Matt LH, Lowe NJ: Etretin therapy for severe psoriasis. Arch Dermatol 123:55, 1987

Kofoed ML, Wantzin GL: Familial lichen planus. J Am Acad Dermatol 13:50, 1985

Stern RS, Armstrong RB, Anderson TF et al: Effect of continued ultraviolet B phototherapy on the duration of remission of psoriasis. J Am Acad Dermatol 15:546, 1986

15

Dermatologic Bacteriology

Bacteria exist on the skin as normal non-pathogenic resident flora or as pathogenic organisms. The pathogenic bacteria cause primary, secondary, and systemic infections. For clinical purposes it is justifiable to divide the problem of bacterial infection into these three classifications.

I. **Primary Bacterial Infections**
   A. Impetigo
   B. Ecthyma
   C. Folliculitis
      1. Superficial folliculitis
      2. Folliculitis of the scalp
         Superficial—acne necrotica miliaris
         Deep—folliculitis decalvans
      3. Folliculitis of the beard
      4. Stye
   D. Furuncle
   E. Carbuncle
   F. Sweat gland infections
   G. Erysipelas
II. **Secondary Bacterial Infections**
   A. Cutaneous diseases with secondary infection
   B. Infected ulcers
   C. Infectious eczematoid dermatitis
   D. Bacterial intertrigo
III. **Systemic Bacterial Infections**
   A. Scarlet fever
   B. Granuloma inguinale
   C. Chancroid
   D. Myocobacterial infections
      1. Tuberculosis of the skin
      2. Leprosy
   E. Gonorrhea
   F. Rickettsial diseases
   G. Actinomycosis

With an alteration in immune capabilities in a person, bacteria and other infectious agents can have erratic behavior. Ordinary nonpathogens can act as pathogens, and pathogenic agents can act more aggressively.

PRIMARY BACTERIAL INFECTIONS (PYODERMAS)

The most common causative agents of the primary skin infections are the coagulase-positive micrococci (staphylococci) and the β-hemolytic streptococci. Superficial or deep bacterial lesions can be produced by these organisms.

In managing the pyodermas certain *general principles of treatment* must be initiated.

1. *Improve the bathing habits.* More frequent bathing and the use of bactericidal soap, such as Dial soap, is indicated. Any pustules or crusts should be removed during the bathing to facilitate penetration of the local medications.
2. *General isolation procedures.* Clothing and bedding should be changed frequently and cleaned. The patient should have a separate towel and washcloth.
3. *Systemic drugs.* The patient should be questioned regarding ingestion of drugs that can cause lesions that mimic or cause pyodermas, such as iodides, bromides, testosterone, and lithium.
4. *Diabetes.* In chronic skin infections, particularly recurrent boils, rule out diabetes by history and laboratory examination.
5. *Immunosuppressed patients.* A good history of abnormal laboratory tests should

alert the physician to the many patients now who are on chemotherapy for cancer or are post-transplant patients or have the acquired immunodeficiency syndrome.

Impetigo
(Plates 1 G, 34, and 35)

Impetigo is a very common superficial bacterial infection seen most often in children. This is the "infantigo" every mother respects.

PRIMARY LESIONS. The lesions vary from small vesicles to large bullae that rupture and discharge a honey-colored serous liquid. New lesions can develop in a matter of hours.

SECONDARY LESIONS. Crusts form from the discharge and appear to be lightly stuck on the skin surface. When removed, a superficial erosion remains, which may be the only evidence of the disease. In debilitated infants the bullae may coalesce to form an exfoliative type of infection called *Ritter's disease* or *pemphigus neonatorum.*

DISTRIBUTION. The lesions occur most commonly on the face but may be anywhere.

CONTAGIOUSNESS. It is not unusual to see brothers or sisters of the patient and, rarely, the parents similarly infected.

Differential Diagnosis

Contact dermatitis due to poison ivy or oak: linear blisters; does not spread as rapidly; itches (see Chap. 9).
Tinea of smooth skin: fewer lesions; spread slowly; small vesicles in annular configuration, which is an unusual form for impetigo; fungi found on scraping (see Chap. 19).
Bullous impetigo: in infants, massive bullae (see Plate 39) can develop rapidly, particularly with staphylococcal infection. The severe but not too serious form of this infection is known as the *staphylococcal scalded skin syndrome* (see Chap. 22).

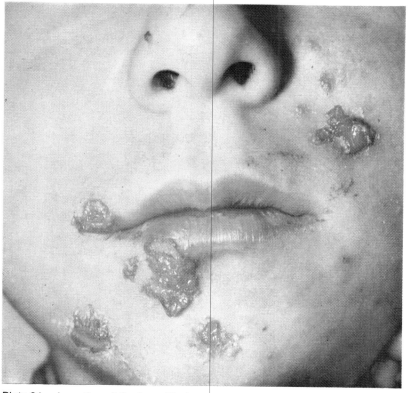

Plate 34. **Impetigo of the face.** The honey-colored crusts are very typical. (*Abner Kurtin: Folia Dermatologica, No. 2. Geigy Pharmaceuticals*)

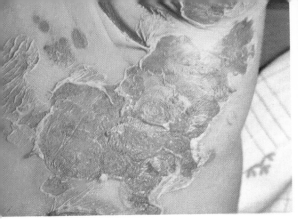

(A) Bullous impetigo of axillae in 1-year-old child

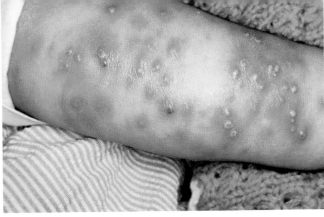

(B) Folliculitis of forearm in 7-month-old infant

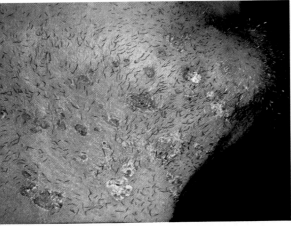

(C) Folliculitis of the beard area

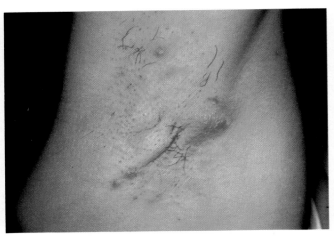

(D) Hidradenitis suppurativa of axilla of 6 years' duration

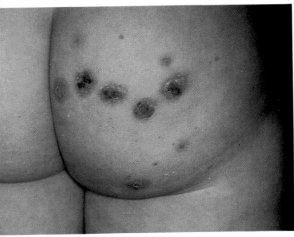

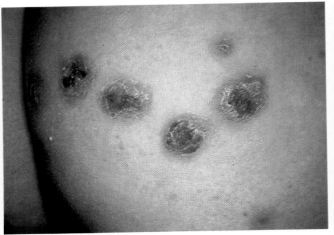

(E) Ecthyma of buttocks of 13-year-old boy with (F) close-up of lesions

Plate 35. **Primary bacterial infections.** (*Burroughs Wellcome Co.*)

Treatment

1. Outline the general principles of treatment. Emphasize the removal of the crusts once or twice a day during bathing with an antibacterial soap or chlorhexidine (Hibiclens) skin cleanser.
2. Mupirocin (Bactroban), or gentamicin (Garamycin) ointment q.s.   15.0
   Sig: Apply t.i.d. locally.

SAUER NOTES:

1. I routinely add sulfur 5% and hydrocortisone 1% to 2% to the antibiotic cream or ointment for treatment of impetigo and other superficial pyodermas. Many patients with impetigo whom I see have been using a plain antibiotic salve with an oral antibiotic, and the impetigo persists. With this compound salve the impetigo heals.
2. Advise the patient that the local treatment be continued for 5 days after the lesions apparently have disappeared to prevent recurrences—"therapy-plus."

---

3. Systemic antibiotic therapy. Some physicians believe that every patient with impetigo should be treated with systemic antibiotic therapy to heal these lesions and also to prevent chronic glomerulonephritis. Oral penicillin or erythromycin in appropriate dosages for 10 days would be effective.

Ecthyma
(Plate 35)

Ecthyma is another superficial bacterial infection, but it is seen less commonly and is deeper than impetigo. It is usually caused by β-hemolytic streptococci and occurs on the buttocks and the thighs of children.

PRIMARY LESION. A vesicle or vesicopustule appears and rapidly changes into the secondary lesion.

SECONDARY LESION. This is a piled-up crust, 1 to 3 cm in diameter, overlying a superficial erosion or ulcer. In neglected cases scarring can occur as a result of extension of the infection into the dermis.

DISTRIBUTION. Most commonly the disease is seen on the posterior aspect of the thighs and the buttocks, from which areas it can spread. Ecthyma commonly follows the scratching of chigger bites.

AGE GROUP. Children are affected mainly.

CONTAGIOUSNESS. Ecthyma is rarely found in other members of the family.

Differential Diagnosis

Psoriasis: unusual in children; whitish, firmly attached scaly lesion, also in scalp, on knees, and elbows (see Chap. 14).
Impetigo: much smaller crusted lesions, not as deep (see preceding section).

Treatment

1. Outline the general principles of treatment listed on p. 150. The crusts must be removed daily. Response to therapy is slower than with impetigo, but the treatment is the same for both conditions.
2. Systemic antibiotics. Commonly with extensive ecthyma in children, but only rarely with impetigo, there is a low-grade fever and evidence of bacterial infection in other organs, such as the kidney. If so, give one of the antibiotic syrups or tablets orally q.i.d. for 6 to 10 days.

Folliculitis
(Plate 35)

Folliculitis is a very common pyogenic infection of the hair follicles, usually caused by coagulase-positive staphylococci. Seldom does a patient consult the physician for a single outbreak of folliculitis. The physician is consulted because of recurrent and chronic pustular lesions. The patient realizes that the present acute episode will clear up with the help of nature but seeks the medicine and the advice that will prevent recurrences. For this reason the *general principles of treatment* listed on page 150, particularly the drug history and the diabetes investigation, are important. Some physicians believe that a focus of infection in the teeth, tonsils, gallbladder, or genitourinary tract should be ruled out when pyodermas are recurrent.

The folliculitis may invade only the superficial part of the hair follicle, or it may extend down to the hair bulb. Many variously named clinical entities based on the location and the chronicity of the lesions have been carried down through the years. A few of these entities bear presentation here, but the majority are defined in the Dictionary-Index.

Superficial Folliculitis

The physician is rarely consulted for this minor problem, which is most commonly seen on the arms, the face, and the buttocks of children and adults with the "acne-seborrhea complex." A history of excessive use of hair oils, bath oils, or suntan oils can often be obtained. The use of these oily agents should be avoided.

Folliculitis of the Scalp (Superficial Form)

A *superficial form* has the appellation *acne necrotica miliaris*. This is an annoying, pruritic, chronic, recurrent folliculitis of the scalp in adults. The scratching of the crusted lesions occupies the patient's evening hours.

Treatment

1. General principles
2. Selenium sulfide (Selsun,
   Exsel) suspension shampoo   120.0
   Sig: Shampoo twice a week as directed on the label. Use no other shampoo or rinse.
3. Antibiotic-corticosteroid cream
   q.s.   15.0
   Sig: Apply to scalp h.s.

Folliculitis of the Scalp (Deep Form)

The *deep form* of scalp folliculitis is called *folliculitis decalvans*. This is a chronic, slowly progressive folliculitis with an active border and scarred atrophic center. The end result, after years of progression, is patchy, scarred areas of alopecia, with eventual burning out of the infection.

Differential Diagnosis

Chronic discoid lupus erythematosus: redness; enlarged hair follicles (see Chap. 25).
Alopecia cicatrisata: rare, no evidence of infection (see Chap. 27).
Tinea of the scalp: it is important to culture the hair for fungi in any chronic infection of the scalp; *Trichophyton tonsurans* group can cause a similar clinical picture (see Chap. 19).

Treatment

Results of treatment are very disappointing. Follow the routine for the superficial form of folliculitis and give oral antibiotics.

Folliculitis of the Beard (Plate 35)

This is the familiar "barber's itch," which in the days prior to antibiotics was very resistant to therapy. This bacterial infection of the hair follicles is spread rather rapidly by shaving, but after treatment is begun, shaving should be continued.

Differential Diagnosis

Contact dermatitis due to shaving lotions: history of new lotion applied, general redness of the area with some vesicles (see Chap. 9).

Tinea of the beard: very slowly spreading infection; hairs broken off; usually a deeper nodular type of inflammation; culture of hair produces fungi (see p. 220).

Ingrown beard hairs: hair circling back into the skin with resultant chronic infection; a hereditary trait, especially in blacks. Close shaving aggravates the condition. Local antibiotics rarely help, but locally applied depilatories do help.

Treatment

1. General principles, stressing the use of Dial or other antibacterial soap for washing of the face.
2. Shaving instructions:
   A. Change the razor blade daily or sterilize the head of the electric razor by placing it in 70% alcohol for 1 hour.
   B. Apply the following salve very lightly to the face before shaving and again after shaving. *Do not shave closely.*
3. An antibiotic-hydrocortisone cream
   q.s.   15.0
   Sig: Apply to face before shaving, after shaving, and at bedtime.
   For stubborn cases, add sulfur 5% to the cream.
4. Oral erythromycin therapy. Erythromycin, 250 mg, 1 capsule q.i.d. for 7 days, then 1 capsule b.i.d. for 7 days.

Stye (Hordeolum)

A stye is a deep folliculitis of the stiff eyelid hairs. A single lesion is treated with hot-packs of 1% boric acid solution and an ophthalmic antibiotic ointment. Recurrent lesions may be linked with the blepharitis of *seborrheic dermatitis* (dandruff). For this type, cleansing the eyelashes with Johnson Baby Shampoo is indicated.

Furuncle
(Plate 36)

A furuncle, or boil, is a more extensive infection of the hair follicle, usually due to *Staphylococcus*. A boil can occur in any person at any age, but certain predisposing factors account for most outbreaks. An important factor is the "acne-seborrhea complex" (oily skin, dark complexion, and history of acne and dandruff). Other factors include poor hygiene, a diet rich in sugars and fats, diabetes, local skin trauma from friction of clothing, and maceration, in obese persons. One boil usually does not bring the patient to the physician, but recurrent boils do.

Differential Diagnosis

Single Lesion: *primary chancre-type diseases* (see list in Dictionary-Index).

Multiple Lesion: *drug eruption from iodides or bromides* (see Chap. 9).

Treatment

A young man has had recurrent boils for 6 months. He does not have diabetes, is not obese, is taking no drugs, and bathes daily. He now has a large boil on his buttocks.

1. Burow's solution hot packs.
   Sig: 1 packet of Domeboro powder to 1 quart of hot water. Apply hot wet packs for 30 minutes twice a day.
2. Incision and drainage. This should be done only on "ripe" lesions where a necrotic white area appears at the top of the nodule. Drains are not necessary unless the lesion has extended deep enough to form a fluctuant *abscess*.
3. Oral antistaphylococcal penicillin, such as dicloxacillin, should be prescribed for 5 to 10 days. (Bacteriologic culture and sensitivity studies are helpful in determining which antibiotic to use.)
4. For recurrent form:
   A. General principles of treatment, stressing low-carbohydrate diet and use of an antibacterial soap.
   B. Rule out focus of infection in teeth, tonsils, genitourinary tract, and so on.
   C. Bacterial Vaccine injections as outlined under folliculitis of the scalp (see earlier in this chapter).

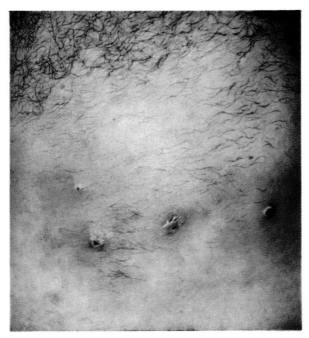

Plate 36. **Multiple furuncles (boils) on the chest.** (*Abner Kurtin: Folia Dermatologica, No. 2. Geigy Pharmaceuticals*)

D. Oral erythromycin therapy. Erythromycin, 250 mg, in a dose of 4 capsules a day for 4 days, then 1 capsule b.i.d. for weeks, is very effective in breaking the cycle of recurrent cases.

Carbuncle
(Plates 37 and 38)

A carbuncle is an extensive infection of several adjoining hair follicles that drains with multiple openings onto the skin surface. Fatal cases were not unusual in the preantibiotic days. A common location for a carbuncle is the posterior neck region. Large, ugly, crisscross scars in this area in an older patient demonstrate the outdated treatment for this disease, namely, multiple bold incisions. Since a carbuncle is, in reality, a multiple furuncle, the same etiologic factors apply. Recurrences are uncommon.

Treatment

Treatment is the same as that for a boil (see preceding section) but with greater emphasis on systemic antibiotic therapy and physical rest.

Sweat Gland Infections
(Plate 39)

Primary *eccrine* sweat gland or duct infections are very rare. However, *prickly heat*, a sweat-retention disease, very frequently develops secondary bacterial infection.

Primary *apocrine* gland infection is rather common. Two types of infection exist:

Apocrinitis denotes infection of a single apocrine gland, usually in the axilla, and is commonly associated with a change in deodorant. It responds to the therapy listed under furuncles. In addition, a lotion containing an antibiotic aids in keeping the area dry, such as an erythromycin solution (A/T/S, Erymax, EryDerm, Erycette, T-Stat, Staticin).

The second form of apocrine gland infection is *hidradenitis suppurativa*. This chronic, recurring, pyogenic infection is characterized by the development of multiple nodules, abscesses, draining sinuses, and eventual hypertrophic bands of scars. The most common location is in the axillae, but it can also occur in the groin, perianal, and suprapubic regions. It does not occur before puberty. Etiologically, there appears to be a hereditary tendency in these patients toward occlusion of the follicular orifice, and subse-

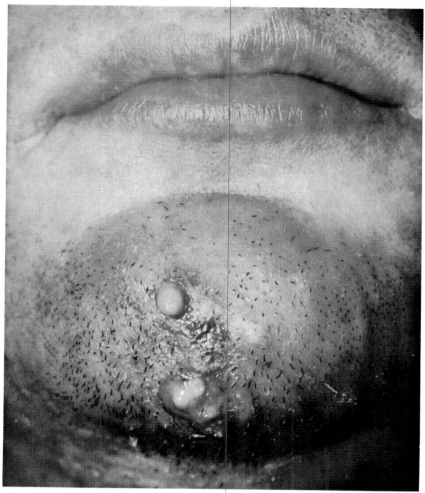

Plate 37. **Carbuncle on the chin.** Notice the multiple openings. (*Abner Kurtin: Folia Dermatologica, No. 2. Geigy Pharmaceuticals*)

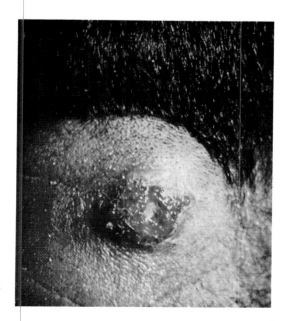

Plate 38. **Carbuncle on the back of the neck.** (*J. Lamar Callaway: Folia Dermatologica, No. 4. Geigy Pharmaceuticals*)

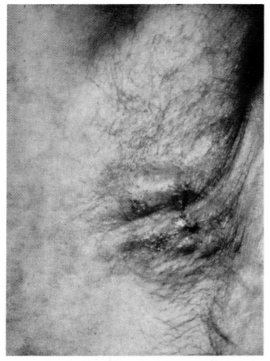

Plate 39. **Sweat gland infection of the axilla (hidradenitis suppurativa).** (*Abner Kurtin: Folia Dermatologica, No. 2. Geigy Pharmaceuticals*)

quent retention of the secretory products. Two other diseases are related to hidradenitis suppurativa and may be present in the same patient: (1) a severe form of acne called *acne conglobata* and (2) *dissecting cellulitis of the scalp.*

Treatment

The management of these cases is difficult. In addition to the general principles mentioned previously, one should use hot packs locally and an oral antibiotic for several weeks.

Plastic surgery or a marsupialization operation is indicated in severe cases. When draining canals or sinuses are present, the marsupialization operation is very curative and can be done in the office. After the bridge over the canal has been trimmed away, bleeding is controlled by electrosurgery.

Erysipelas
(Plate 40)

Erysipelas is an uncommon β-hemolytic streptococcal infection of the subcutaneous tissue that produces a characteristic type of cellulitis, with fever and malaise. Recurrences are frequent.

PRIMARY LESION. A red, warm, raised, brawny, sharply bordered plaque enlarges peripherally. Vesicles and bullae may form on the surface of the plaque. Usually a preexisting skin wound or pyoderma will be found that initiated the acute infection. Multiple lesions of erysipelas are rare.

DISTRIBUTION. Most commonly lesions occur on the face and around the ears (following ear piercing), but no area is exempt.

COURSE. When treated with systemic antibiotics, the response is rapid. Recurrences are common in the same location and may lead to *lymphedema* of that area, which eventually can become irreversible. The lip, the cheek, and the legs are particularly prone to this chronic change, which is called *elephantiasis nostras* (Fig. DI-5).

SUBJECTIVE COMPLAINTS. Fever and general malaise can precede the development of the skin lesion and persist until therapy is instituted. Pain at the site of the infection can be severe.

Differential Diagnosis

Cellulitis: lacks a sharp border; recurrences are rare.
Contact dermatitis: sharp border absent; fever and malaise absent; eruption predominantly vesicular (see Chap. 9).

Treatment

1. Bed rest is instituted and therapy is directed toward reducing the fever. If the patient is hospitalized, semi-isolation procedures should be initiated.
2. Give appropriate systemic antibiotic, such as erythromycin or a penicillin derivative, for 10 days.
3. Apply local cool wet dressing, as necessary for comfort.

Erythrasma
(Plate 40)

Erythrasma is a rather uncommon bacterial infection of the skin that clinically resembles regular tinea or tinea versicolor. It affects the

velops after a day of rapidly rising fever, head-ache, sore throat, and various other symptoms. The rash begins first on the neck and the chest but rapidly spreads over the entire body, except for the area around the mouth. Close examination of the pale scarlet eruption reveals it to be made up of diffuse pinhead-sized, or larger macules. In untreated cases the rash reaches its peak on the fourth day, and scaling commences around the seventh day and continues for 1 or 2 weeks. The "strawberry tongue" is seen at the height of the eruption.

The presence of petechiae on the body is a grave prognostic sign. Complications are numerous and common in untreated cases. Nephritis, in mild or severe form, is a serious complication.

Differential Diagnosis

Measles: early rash on face and forehead; larger macular rash; running eyes; cough (see Chap. 17).

Drug eruption: lack of high fever and other constitutional signs; atropine and quinine can cause eruption clinically similar to scarlet fever (see Chap. 9).

Treatment

Penicillin or a similar systemic antibiotic is the therapy of choice. Complications should be watched for and should be treated early.

Granuloma Inguinale
(Plate 41)

Prior to the use of antibiotics, particularly streptomycin and tetracycline, this disease was one of the most chronic and resistant afflictions of humans. Formerly, it was a rather common disease in the South, particularly among blacks. Granuloma inguinale should be considered a venereal disease, although other factors may have to be present to initiate infection.

PRIMARY LESION. An irregularly shaped, bright red, velvety appearing, flat ulcer with rolled border is seen.

SECONDARY LESIONS. Scarring may lead to complications similar to those seen with lymphogranuloma venereum. A *squamous cell carcinoma* can develop in old, chronic lesions.

DISTRIBUTION. Genital lesions are most common on the penis, the scrotum, the labia, the cervix, or the inguinal region.

COURSE. Without therapy, the granuloma grows slowly and persists for years, causing marked scarring and mutilation. Under modern therapy, healing is rather rapid, but recurrences are not unusual.

ETIOLOGY. Granuloma inguinale is due to *Calymmatobacterium granulomatis*, which can be cultured on special media.

LABORATORY FINDINGS. Scrapings of the lesion reveal Donovan bodies, which are dark-staining, intracytoplasmic, cigar-shaped bacilli found in large macrophages. The material for the smear can be obtained best by snipping off a piece of the lesion with a small scissors and rubbing the tissue on several slides. Wright or Giemsa stains can be used.

Differential Diagnosis

Granuloma pyogenicum: small lesion; history of injury, usually; short duration; rarely on genitalia; no Donovan bodies.

Primary syphilis: short duration, inguinal adenopathy, serology may be positive, find spirochetes (see Chap. 16).

Chancroid: short duration, lesion small, not red and velvety, no Donovan bodies (see next section).

Squamous cell carcinoma: more indurated lesion with nodule, may coexist with granuloma inguinale, biopsy specific.

Treatment

Tetracycline, 500 mg, q.i.d. is continued until all the lesions are healed.

Chancroid
(Plate 41)

Chancroid is a venereal disease with a very short incubation period of 1 to 5 days. It is caused by *Hemophilus ducreyi*.

PRIMARY LESION. A small, superficial or deep erosion occurs with surrounding redness and edema. Multiple genital or distant lesions can be produced by autoinoculation.

SECONDARY LESIONS. Deep, destructive ulcers form in chronic cases, which may lead

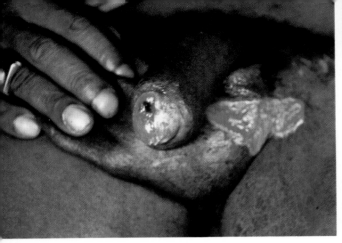

(A) Granuloma inguinale of penis and crural area

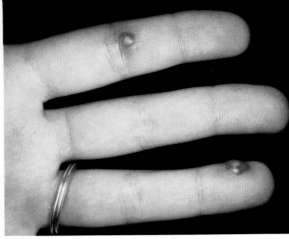

(B) Gonococcal septicemia with hemorrhagic vesicles

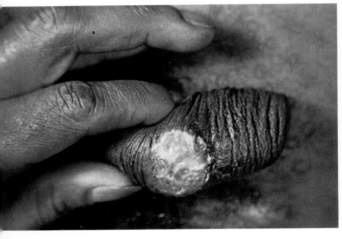

(C) Chancroid of penis

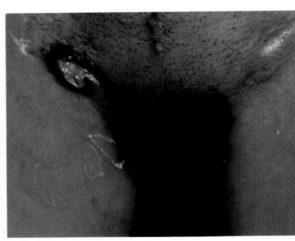

(D) Chancroid buboes in inguinal area

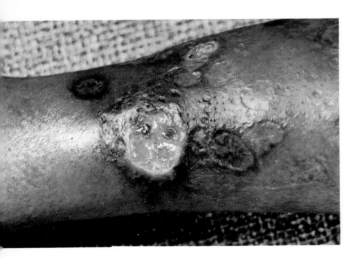

(E) Tuberculosis ulcer of leg

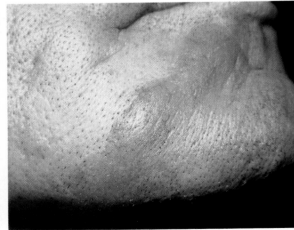

(F) Tuberculoid leprosy of the chin (Drs. W. Schorr and F. Kerdel-Vegas)

Plate 41. **Systemic bacterial infections.** (Derm-Arts Laboratories)

to gangrene. Marked regional adenopathy, usually unilateral, is common and eventually suppurates in untreated cases.

COURSE. Without therapy most cases heal within 1 to 2 weeks. In rare cases, severe local destruction and draining lymph nodes (buboes) result. Early therapy is quite effective.

LABORATORY FINDINGS. The organisms arranged in "schools of fish" can often be demonstrated in smears of clean lesions.

Differential Diagnosis

SAUER NOTE:

Syphilis must be considered in any patient with a penile lesion. It can be ruled out by darkfield examination or blood serology tests.

Primary or secondary syphilis genital lesions: longer incubation period; more induration; *Treponema pallidum* found on darkfield examination; serology positive in late primary and secondary stage (see Chap. 16).

Herpes simplex progenitalis: recurrent multiple blisters or erosions; mild inguinal adenopathy (see Chap. 17).

Lymphogranuloma venereum: primary lesion is rare; Frei test is positive (see Chap. 17).

Granuloma inguinale: chronic, red velvety plaque; Donovan bodies seen on tissue smear (see preceding section).

Treatment

The therapy for chancroid is a sulfonamide such as sulfisoxazole, 1 g, q.i.d. for 2 weeks, or erythromycin, 2 g/day for 10 to 15 days. Third-generation cephalosporins are effective also. A fluctuant bubo should never be incised but should be aspirated with a large needle.

Tuberculosis
(Plates 2B and 41)

Skin tuberculosis is rare in the United States. However, a text on dermatology would not be complete without some consideration of this infection. For this purpose the most common tuberculosis infection, lupus vulgaris, will be discussed. A classification of skin tuberculosis follows this section.

Lupus vulgaris is a chronic, granulomatous disease characterized by the development of nodules, ulcers, and plaques arranged in any conceivable configuration. Scarring in the center of active lesions or at the edge, in severe, untreated cases, leads to atrophy and contraction, resulting in mutilating changes.

DISTRIBUTION. Facial involvement is most common.

COURSE. The course is often slow and progressive, in spite of therapy.

LABORATORY FINDINGS. The histopathology shows typical tubercle formation with epithelioid cells, giant cells, and peripheral zone of lymphocytes. The causative organism, *Mycobacterium tuberculosis,* is not abundant in the lesions. The 48-hour tuberculin test is usually positive.

Differential Diagnosis

Other granulomas, such as those associated with *syphilis, leprosy, sarcoidosis, deep fungus disease,* and *neoplasm,* are to be ruled out by appropriate studies (see also Chap. 20).

Treatment

Early localized lesions can be treated by surgical excision. For more widespread cases, long-term systemic therapy offers high hopes for cure. Isonicotinic acid hydrazide is usually prescribed along with other antituberculous drugs, such as rifampin and ethambutol (Myambutol).

Classification of Cutaneous Tuberculosis

I. True Cutaneous Tuberculosis (Lesions contain tubercle bacilli.)
   A. *Primary tuberculosis* (no previous infection; tuberculin-negative in initial stages)
      1. Primary inoculation tuberculosis. Tuberculosis chancre (exogenous implantation into skin producing the primary complex)

2. Miliary tuberculosis of the skin (hematogenous dispersion)

B. *Secondary tuberculosis* (lesions develop in person already sensitive to tuberculin as result of prior tuberculous lesion; tubercle bacilli difficult or impossible to demonstrate.)

1. Lupus vulgaris (inoculation of tubercle bacilli into the skin from external or internal sources)
2. Tuberculosis verrucosa cutis (inoculation of tubercle bacilli into the skin from external or internal sources)
3. Scrofulderma (extension to skin from underlying focus in bones or glands)
4. Tuberculosis cutis orificialis (mucous membrane lesions and extension onto the skin near mucocutaneous junctions)

II. Tuberculids (Allergic origin; no tubercle bacilli in lesions.)

A. *Papular forms*

1. Lupus miliaris disseminatus faciei (purely papular)
2. Papulonecrotic tuberculid (papules with necrosis)
3. Lichen scrofulosorum (follicular papules or lichenoid papules)

B. *Granulomatous, ulceronodular forms*

1. Erythema induratum (nodules or plaques subsequently ulcerating; may be a nonspecific vasculitis)

Leprosy
(Plates 41 and 101)

Leprosy or Hansen's disease is to be considered in the differential diagnosis of any skin granulomas. It is endemic in the southern part of the United States and in semitropical and tropical areas the world over.

Two definite types of leprosy are recognized: lepromatous and tuberculoid. In addition, there are cases that cannot presently be classified in either of these two categories but eventually develop either lepromatous or tuberculoid leprosy.

Lepromatous leprosy is the malignant form, which represents minimal resistance to the disease, with a negative lepromin reaction, characteristic histology, infiltrated cutaneous lesions with ill-defined borders, and progression to death from tuberculosis and secondary amyloidosis.

Tuberculoid leprosy is generally benign in its course because of considerable resistance to the disease on the part of the host. This is manifested by a positive lepromin test, histology that is not diagnostic, cutaneous lesions that are frequently erythematous with elevated borders, and minimal effect of the disease on the general health.

Early lesions of the lepromatous type include reddish macules with an indefinite border, nasal obstruction, and nosebleeds. Erythema nodosum–like lesions occur commonly. The tuberculoid type of leprosy is diagnosed early by the presence of an area of skin with impaired sensation, polyneuritis, and skin lesions with a sharp border and central atrophy.

ETIOLOGY. The causative organism is *Mycobacterium leprae.*

CONTAGIOUSNESS. The source of infection is believed to be from patients with the lepromatous form. Infectiousness is of a low order.

LABORATORY FINDINGS. The bacilli are usually uncovered in the lepromatous type but seldom in the tuberculoid type. Smears should be obtained from the tissue exposed by a small incision made into the dermis through an infiltrated lesion.

The lepromin reaction, a delayed reaction test similar to the tuberculin test, is of value in differentiating the lepromatous form from the tuberculoid form of leprosy, as stated previously. False-positive reactions do occur.

Biologic false-positive tests for syphilis are common in patients with the lepromatous type of leprosy.

Differential Diagnosis

Consider any of the granulomatous diseases, such as *syphilis, tuberculosis, sarcoidosis,* and *deep fungal infections* (see also Chapter 20).

Treatment

Dapsone (diaminodiphenyl sulfone [DDS]), rifampin, and isoniazid are all quite effective.

Other Mycobacterial Dermatoses

Mycobacteria are pathogenic and saprophytic. *Mycobacterium marinum* can cause the *swimming pool granuloma* and also granulomas in fisherman and those involved with fish tanks.

Gonorrhea
(Plate 41)

Gonorrhea is considerably more prevalent than syphilis. Skin lesions with gonorrheal infection are rare. But a statement is due here on the therapy for uncomplicated gonorrhea.

The therapy suggested by the Centers for Disease Control is ceftriaxone, 250 mg, intramuscularly, one dose, or spectinomycin, 2 g, intramuscularly, one dose.

Untreated or inadequately treated infection due to *Neisseria gonorrhoeae* can involve the skin through metastatic spread. *Primary cutaneous infection* with multiple erosions at the site of the purulent discharge is very rare.

Metastatic complications include a *bacteremia*, in which there is an intermittent high fever, arthralgia, and skin lesions. The skin lesions (see Plate 41) are quite characteristic hemorrhagic vesicopustules, most commonly seen on the fingers. Treatment with intravenous penicillin for 10 days with 5 to 10 million units/day is indicated.

The rarer *septicemic form*, with very high fever and meningitis or endocarditis, may have purpuric skin lesions similar to those seen in *meningococcemia*.

Rickettsial Diseases

The most common rickettsial disease in the United States is *Rocky Mountain spotted fever*, which is spread by ticks of various types. The skin eruption occurs after 3 to 7 days of fever and other toxic signs and is characterized by purpuric lesions on the extremities, mainly the wrists and the ankles, which then become generalized. The Weil-Felix test using *Proteus* OX19 and OX2 is positive. Tetracycline and chloramphenical are effective.

The typhus group of rickettsial diseases includes *epidemic* or *louse-born typhus, Brill's disease,* and *endemic murine* or *flea-borne typhus.* Less common forms include *scrub typhus* (tsutsugamushi disease), *trench fever,* and *rickettsialpox.* The last-named rickettsial disease is produced by a mite bite. The mite ordinarily lives on rodents. Approximately 10 days after the bite a primary lesion develops in the form of a papule that becomes vesicular. After a few days fever and other toxic signs are accompanied by a generalized eruption that resembles chickenpox. The disease subsides without therapy.

Ehrlichiosis is another rickettsial disease well known in dogs and now seen in humans. It is transmitted by tick bite. The nonspecific symptoms are similar to those of *Rocky Mountain spotted fever,* but only 20% of the patients have a rash.

Actinomycosis

Actinomycosis is a chronic, granulomatous, suppurative infection that characteristically causes the formation of a draining sinus. The most common location of the draining sinus is in the jaw region, but thoracic and abdominal sinuses do occur.

PRIMARY LESION. A red, firm, nontender tumor in the jaw area slowly extends locally to form a "lumpy jaw."

SECONDARY LESIONS. Discharging sinuses become infected with other bacteria and, if untreated, may develop into osteomyelitis.

COURSE. General health is usually unaffected unless extension occurs into bone or deeper neck tissues. Recurrence is unusual if treatment is continued long enough.

ETIOLOGY. *Actinomyces israelii,* which is an anaerobic bacterium that lives as a normal inhabitant of the mouth, particularly in persons who have poor dental hygiene, is the causative agent. Injury to the jaw or a tooth extraction usually precedes the development of the infection. Infected cattle are not the source of human infection. The disease is twice as frequent in men as in women.

LABORATORY FINDINGS. Pinpoint-sized "sulfur" granules, which are colonies of the organism, can be seen grossly and microscopically in the draining pus. A Gram stain of the pus will show masses of interlacing gram-positive fibers with or without club-shaped processes at the tips of these fibers. The organism can be cultured anaerobically on special media.

Differential Diagnosis

Consider *pyodermas, tuberculosis,* and *neoplasm.*

Treatment

1. Penicillin, 2.4 million units intramuscularly, is given daily, until definite improvement is noted. Then oral penicillin in the same dosage should be continued for 3 weeks after the infection apparently has been cured. In severe cases, 10 million or more units of penicillin given intravenously, daily, may be necessary.
2. Incision and drainage is performed of the lumps and the sinuses.
3. Good oral hygiene is required.
4. In resistant cases, broad-spectrum antibiotics can be used alone or in combination with the penicillin.

BIBLIOGRAPHY

Boyd AS: Clinical efficacy of antimicrobial therapy in *Haemophilus ducreyi* infections. Arch Dermatol 125:1399, 1989

Feingold DS, Hirschmann JV, Leyden JJ: Bacterial infections of the skin. J Am Acad Dermatol 20:469, 1989

Hirschmann JV: Topical antibiotics in dermatology. Arch Dermatol 124:1691, 1988

Johnson JD: The cephalosporins in dermatologic practice. Int J Dermatol 25:427, 1986

Modlin RL, Rea TH: Leprosy: New insight into an ancient disease. J Am Acad Dermatol 17:1, 1987

Parish LC, Witkowski JA: The decubitus ulcer. Int J Dermatol 26:639, 1987

Prystowsky JH, Kahn SN, Lazarus GS: Present status of pyoderma gangrenosum. Arch Dermatol 125:57, 1989

Roth RR, James WD: Microbiology of the skin: Resident flora, ecology, infection. J Am Acad Dermatol 20:367, 1989

Sehgal VN, Jain MK, Srivastava G: Evolution of the classification of leprosy. Int J Dermatol 28:161, 1989

Sehgal VN, Jain MK, Srivastava G: Changing pattern of cutaneous tuberculosis. Int J Dermatol 28:231, 1989

Van Scoy RE, Wilkowske CJ: Antituberculous agents. Mayo Clin Proc 62:1129, 1987

16

Spirochetal Infections

Two spirochetal diseases will be presented in this chapter, syphilis and Lyme disease.

SYPHILIS

When I was stationed at the West Virginia State Rapid Treatment Center, from 1946 to 1948, our average admittance was 30 patients a day with venereal disease. Approximately one third of these patients had infectious syphilis. In 1949 the center was closed because of the low patient census. The incidence of reported syphilis has risen again to alarming heights. Many patients with acquired immunodeficiency syndrome (AIDS) also have syphilis. Because of this resurgence, it is imperative for all physicians to have a basic understanding of this polymorphous disease.

SAUER NOTES:

1. In order to diagnose syphilis, the physician must have a high index of suspicion for it.
2. Syphilis is the great imitator and can mimic many other conditions.

Cutaneous lesions of syphilis occur in all three stages of the disease.

Under what circumstances will the present-day physician be called on to diagnose, evaluate, or manage a patient with syph-ilis? (1) The cutaneous manifestations, such as a penile lesion or a rash that could be secondary syphilis, may bring a patient to the office. (2) A positive blood test found on a premarital examination or as part of a routine physical examination may be responsible for a patient's being seen by the physician. (3) Syphilis may be seen in conjunction with AIDS. The problem becomes complicated because the serologic test for syphilis may not be positive in patients with AIDS. (4) Cardiac, central nervous system, or other organ disease may be a reason for a patient's consulting a physician.

To manage these patients properly a thorough knowledge of the natural *untreated* course of the disease is essential.

Primary Syphilis
(Plates 42 and 43)

The first stage of acquired syphilis usually develops within 2 to 6 weeks (average 3 weeks) after exposure. The *primary chancre* most commonly occurs on the genitalia, but extragenital chancres are not rare and are often misdiagnosed. Without treatment the chancre heals within 1 to 4 weeks, depending on the location, the amount of secondary infection, and host resistance.

The blood serologic test for syphilis (STS) may be negative in the early days of the chancre but eventually becomes positive. A cerebrospinal fluid examination during the primary stage reveals invasion of the spirochete in approximately 25% of cases.

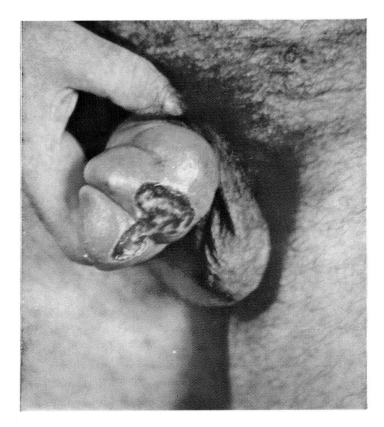

Plate 42. Primary syphilis with a chancre of the penis. This chancre is accompanied by marked edema of the penis. (*J. E. Moore and The Upjohn Company*)

Clinically, the chancre may vary in appearance from a single small erosion to multiple indurated ulcers of the genitalia. Primary syphilis commonly goes unnoticed in the female patient. Bilateral or unilateral regional lymphadneopathy is common. Malaise and fever may be present.

Early Latent Stage

Latency, manifested by a positive serology and no other subjective or objective evidence of syphilis, may occur between the primary and the secondary stages.

Secondary Syphilis
(Plates 44 through 46)

Early secondary lesions may develop before the primary chancre has healed or after latency of a few weeks.

Late secondary lesions are more rare and usually are seen after the early secondary lesions have healed.

Both types of secondary lesions contain the spirochete *Treponema pallidum*, which can be easily seen with the darkfield microscope. The STS is positive (an exception is in a patient with AIDS), and approximately 30% of the cases have abnormal cerebrospinal fluid findings.

Clinically, the early secondary rash can consist of macular, papular, pustular, squamous, or eroded lesions or combinations of any of these lesions. The entire body may be involved or only the palms and the soles, the mouth, or the genitalia.

Condylomata lata is the name applied to the flat, moist, warty lesions teeming with spirochetes found in the groin and the axillae (see Plates 45 and 46).

The late secondary lesions are nodular, squamous, and ulcerative and are to be distinguished from the tertiary lesions only by the time interval after the onset of the infection and by the finding of the spirochete in superficial smears of serum from the lesions. Annular and semiannular configurations of late secondary lesions are common.

(text continues on page 174)

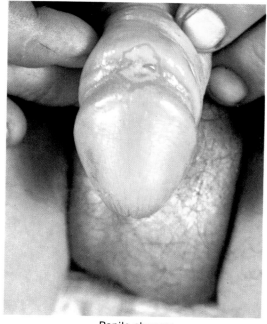

Penile chancre

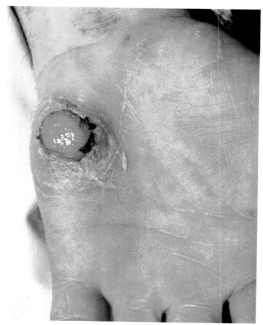

Chancre of the palm

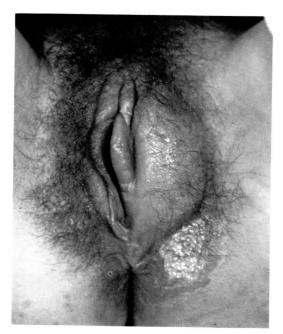

Vulvar chancre with edema of the labia majora

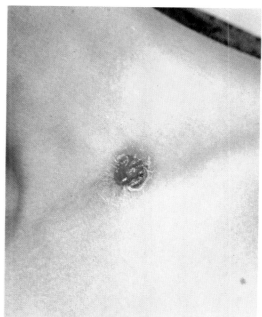

Chancre over the clavicle

Plate 43. **Primary syphilis.** (*The Upjohn Company*)

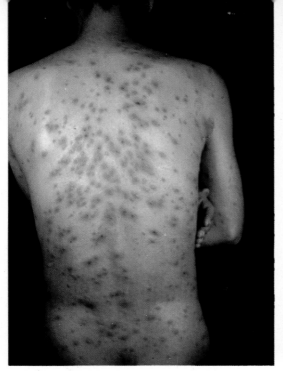

(A) Secondary papulosquamous lesions on the back

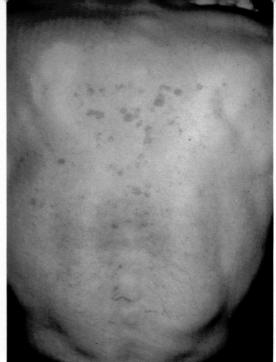

(B) Papulosquamous lesions on the back

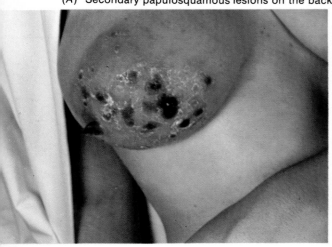

(C) Crusted lesions on the breast

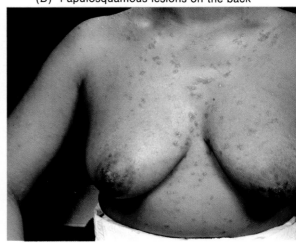

(D) Papular lesions on the chest (*K.U.M.C.*)

Plate 44. **Secondary syphilis.**

(E) Papulosquamous lesions on the palms

(F) Late secondary annular lesions on penis and scro

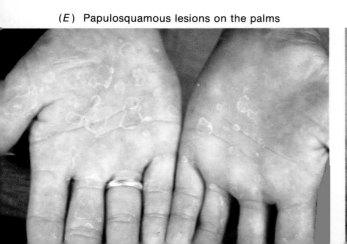

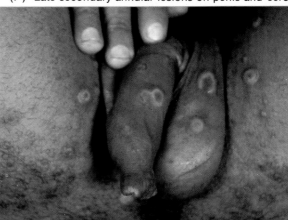

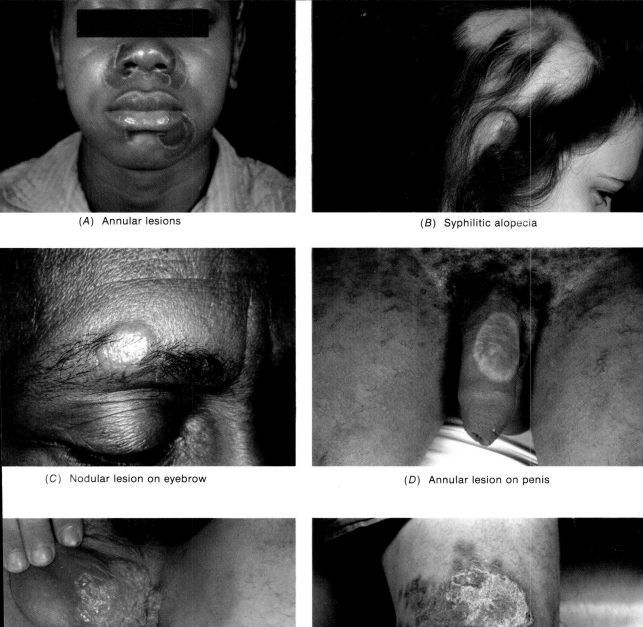

(A) Annular lesions

(B) Syphilitic alopecia

(C) Nodular lesion on eyebrow

(D) Annular lesion on penis

(E) Condylomata lata in groin area

(F) Psoriatic-type lesion on leg

Plate 45. **Late secondary syphilis.**

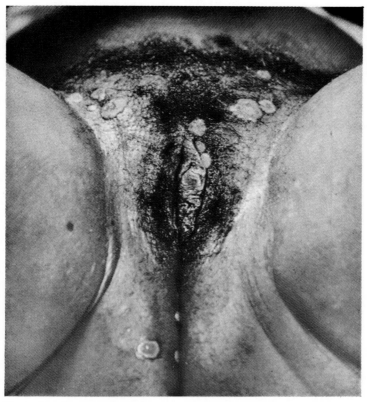

Plate 46. **Secondary syphilis with condylomata lata of the vulva.**
(*J. E. Moore and The Upjohn Company*)

Generalized lymphadenopathy, malaise, fever, and arthralgia occur in many patients with secondary syphilis.

Early Latent Stage

Following the secondary stage, many patients with untreated syphilis have only a positive STS. After 4 years of infection, the patient enters the late latent stage.

Late Latent Stage

This time span of 4 years arbitrarily divides the early infectious stages from the later noninfectious stages, which may or may not develop.

Tertiary Syphilis
(Plates 47 and 48)

This late stage is manifested by subjective or objective involvement of any of the organs of the body, including the skin. Tertiary changes may be precocious but most often develop 5 to 20 years after the onset of the primary stage. Clinically, the skin lesions are characterized by nodular and gummatous ulcerations (see Plate 48). Solitary or multiple annular and nodular lesions are common. Subjective complaints are rare unless considerable secondary bacterial infection is present in a gumma. Scarring, on healing, is inevitable in the majority of the tertiary skin lesions. Larger texts should be consulted for the late changes seen in the central nervous system, the cardiovascular system, the bones, the eyes, and the viscera. Approximately 15% of the patients who acquire syphilis and receive no treatment die of the disease.

Late Latent Stage

Another latent period may occur after natural healing of some types of benign tertiary syphilis.

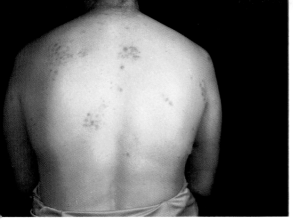

(A) Tertiary grouped papular lesions on the back

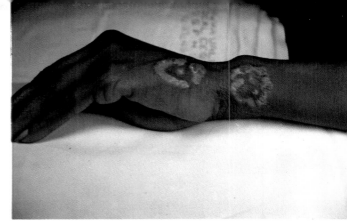

(B) Tertiary annular nodular lesions on hand

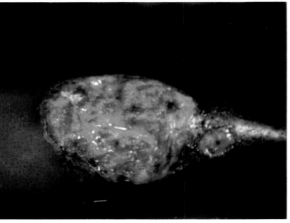

(C) Tertiary gumma on the leg

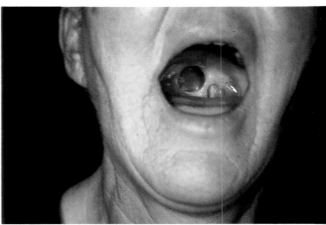

(D) Tertiary perforation from old gumma of soft palate

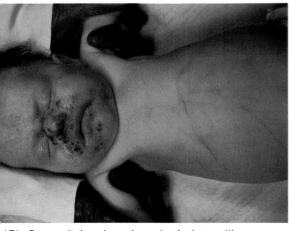

(E) Congenital scaly and erosive lesions with large liver (fatal)

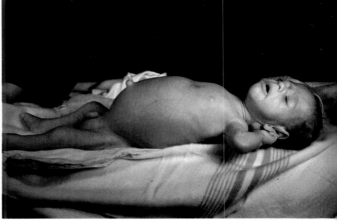

(F) Congenital syphilis with massively enlarged liver and spleen

Plate 47. **Tertiary and congenital syphilis.**

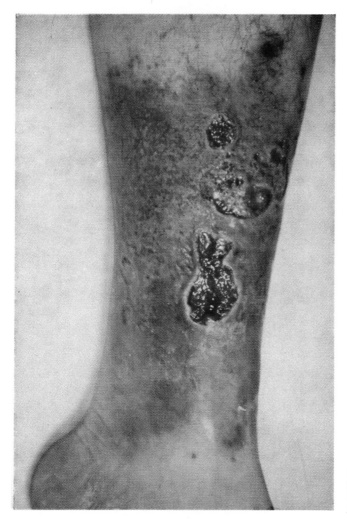

Plate 48. **Tertiary syphilis with a gumma of the leg.** This resembles a stasis ulcer. (*J. E. Moore and The Upjohn Company*)

Congenital Syphilis

Congenital syphilis is acquired *in utero* from an infectious mother (see Plates 47 and 89). The STS required of pregnant women by most states has lowered the incidence of this unfortunate disease. Stillbirths are not uncommon from mothers who are untreated. After the birth of a live infected child, the mortality rate depends on the duration of the infection, the natural host resistance, and the rapidity of initiating correct treatment. Early and late lesions are seen in these children, similar to those found in the adult cases of acquired syphilis.

Laboratory Findings

Darkfield Examination

The etiologic agent, *Treponema pallidum*, can be found in the serum from the primary or secondary lesions. However, a darkfield microscope is necessary, and very few physician's offices or laboratories have this instrument. A considerable amount of experience is necessary to distinguish *T. pallidum* from other *Treponema* species.

Serologic Test for Syphilis

A rather simple and readily available test is the serologic test for syphilis (STS), of which there are several modifications. The rapid plasma reagin (RPR) test and the VDRL flocculation test are used most commonly. The fluorescent treponemal antibody absorption (FTA-ABS) test and modifications are more difficult to perform in the laboratory and therefore are used primarily when the RPR and VDRL tests are "reactive."

When a report is received from the laboratory that the STS is positive (RPR or VDRL reactive), a second blood specimen should be submitted to obtain a *quantitative* report. In many laboratories this repeat test is not necessary, since a quantitative test is run routinely on all positive blood specimens. A dilution of 1:2 is only weakly positive and might be a biologic false-positive reaction. A test positive in a dilution of 1:32 is strongly positive. In evaluating the response of the STS to treatment, remember that a change in titer from 1:2 to 1:4 to 1:16 to 1:32 to 1:64, or downward in the same gradations, is only a change in one tube, in each instance. Thus a change from 1:2 to 1:4 is of the same magnitude as a change from 1:32 to 1:64. Quantitative tests enable the physician to (1) evaluate the efficacy of the treatment, (2) discover a relapse before it becomes infectious, (3) differentiate between a relapse and a reinfection, (4) establish a reaction as a seroresistant type, and (5) differentiate between true and biologic false-positive serologic reactions.

In most laboratories it is now routine to do an FTA-ABS test on all patients with reactive RPR and VDRL tests. With rare exceptions, a positive FTA-ABS test means that the patient has or had syphilis and is not a biologic false-positive reactor.

The serologic test for syphilis may not be positive in patients with AIDS.

Tissue Examination

A direct fluorescent antibody test for *T. pallidum* (DFA-TP) can be performed on lesion exudate or on biopsy tissue.

Cerebrospinal Fluid Test

As has been stated, the cerebrospinal fluid is frequently positive in the primary and the secondary stages of the disease. Invasion of the central nervous system is an early manifestation, even though the perceptible clinical effects are a late manifestation. The cerebrospinal fluid should be examined at least once during the course of the disease. Cerebrospinal fluid examination is appropriate for all patients with syphilis who are at a high risk for human immunodeficiency virus (HIV) infection. The best routine is to perform a cerebrospinal fluid test before treatment is initiated and repeat the test as indicated. If the cerebrospinal fluid is negative in a patient who has had syphilis for 4 years, central nervous system syphilis will not occur, and future cerebrospinal fluid tests are not necessary. If the test is positive, repeat tests should be done every 6 months for 4 years.

The following three tests are run on the cerebrospinal fluid:

1. *Cell Count.* The finding of four or more lymphocytes or polymorphonuclear leukocytes per cubic millimeter is positive. The cell count is the most labile of the tests. It becomes increased early in the infection and responds fastest to therapy. Therefore, it is a good index to activity of the disease. The cell count must be done within an hour after the fluid is withdrawn.

2. *Total Protein.* When measured in milligrams per deciliter, it normally should be below 40.

3. *Nontreponemal Flocculation Test.* Presently, the most common test performed is the qualitative and quantitative VDRL. This test is the last to turn positive and the slowest to return to negativity. In some cases therapy causes a decrease in the titer, but slight positivity or "fastness" can remain for the lifetime of the patient.

Differential Diagnosis

Primary syphilis: from chancroid, herpes simplex, fusospirochetal balanitis, granuloma inguinale, and any of the *primary chancre-type diseases* (see Dictionary-Index).

Secondary syphilis: from any of the papulosquamous diseases, fungal diseases, drug eruption, and alopecia areata.

Tertiary skin syphilis: from any of the granulomatous diseases, particularly tuberculosis, leprosy, sarcoidosis, deep mycoses, and lymphoblastomas.

Congenital syphilis: from atopic eczema, diseases with lymphadenopathy, hepatomegaly, and splenomegaly.

A *true positive syphilitic serology* is to be differentiated from a biologic false-positive reaction. This serologic differentiation is accomplished best by using the FTA-ABS test, or its modifications, along with a good history and a thorough examination of the patient. Many patients with biologic false-positive reactions develop one of the collagen diseases at a later date.

Treatment

A 22-year-old married man presents with a 1-cm-diameter sore on his glans penis of 5 days' duration. Three weeks previously he had extramarital intercourse, and 10 days prior to this office visit he had marital intercourse.

FIRST VISIT
1. Perform a darkfield examination of the penile lesion. Treatment can be started if *T. pallidum* is found. If you cannot perform a darkfield examination, then refer the patient to the local health department.
2. Obtain a blood specimen for a serologic test for syphilis (STS).
3. While waiting for the STS report, advise the patient to soak the site in saline solution for 15 minutes twice a day. The solution is made by placing ¼ teaspoon of salt in a glass of water.
4. Advise against sexual intercourse until the reports are completed.
5. Explain to the patient the seriousness of treating him for syphilis if he does not have it. The "syphilitic" label is one he should not want, if it is at all possible to avoid.

SECOND VISIT
Three days later the lesion is larger and the STS report is "nonreactive."

1. Obtain blood specimen for a second STS.
2. Antibiotic ointment   15.0
   Sig: Apply t.i.d. locally after soaking in saline solution.
3. Explain again why you are delaying therapy until a definite diagnosis is made.

THIRD VISIT
Three days later the sore is smaller but the STS report is "reactive." The diagnosis is now known to be "primary syphilis."

1. Reassure the patient that present-day therapy is highly successful, but he must follow your instructions closely.
2. His wife should be brought in for examination and a blood test. If the blood test is negative, it should be repeated weekly for 1 month. However, some syphilologists believe that therapy is indicated for the marital partner in the face of a negative STS if the husband has infectious syphilis and is being treated. A single injection of 2.4 million units of a long-acting type of penicillin is used. This will prevent "ping-pong" syphilis, which is a cycle of reinfection from one marital partner to another.
3. The patient's contact should be found. The patient knows her only as "Jane," and he cannot remember over which bar she presided. Report these findings to the local health department.
4. A cerebrospinal fluid specimen should be obtained. (The report was returned as normal for all three tests.)
5. Penicillin therapy should be begun. Here, two factors are important: (1) the dose must be adequate and (2) the duration of effective blood levels of medication must be maintained over a period of 10 to 14 days.

DOSAGE
Primary and Secondary Syphilis. Administer 2.4 million units of benzathine penicillin G, half in each buttock, single session. Consult larger texts or relevant literature for other treatment schedules.

Latent (Both Early and Late) Syphilis. If no cerebrospinal fluid examination: 7.2 million units benzathine penicillin G divided into three weekly injections.

If cerebrospinal fluid examination is non-reactive: 2.4 million units in single dose.

Neurosyphilis or Cardiovascular Syphilis. 9 to 12 millions units of a long-acting penicillin. For other routines or complicated cases, consult larger texts for therapy and care. HIV-infected patients with neurosyphilis should be treated for 10 days at least with aqueous crystalline penicillin G in a dosage of 2 to 4 million units intravenously every 4 hours.

Benign Late Syphilis: Same as neurosyphilis.

Congenital Syphilis:

1. Early congenital syphilis
   A. Under 6 months of age:
      Aqueous procaine penicillin G, ten daily intramuscular doses totaling 100,000 to 200,000 units/kg.
   B. Six months to 2 years of age:
      As above, *or* benzathine penicillin G,

100,000 units/kg intramuscularly in one single dose.

2. Late congenital syphilis
   A. Ages 2 to 11 years, or weighing less than 70 pounds:
      Same as for 6 months to 2 years.
   B. Twelve years or older, but weighing more than 70 pounds:
      Same treatment as for adult-acquired syphilis, with comparable time and progression of infection.

SAUER NOTES: On Syphilis

1. Any patient treated for gonorrhea should have a serologic test for syphilis (STS) 4 to 6 weeks later.

2. Persons with HIV infection acquired through sexual contact or intravenous drug abuse should be tested for syphilis.

3. Seventy-five percent of the persons who acquire syphilis suffer no serious manifestations of the disease.

4. Syphilis does not cause vesicular or bullous skin lesions, except in infants with congenital infection.

Primary Stage

1. *Syphilis should be ruled in or out in the diagnosis of any penile or vulvar sores.*

2. Multiple primary chancres are moderately common.

Secondary Stage

1. The rash of secondary syphilis, except for the rare follicular form, does not itch.

2. Secondary syphilis should be ruled in or out in any patient with a generalized, nonpruritic rash. A high index of suspicion is necessary.

Latent Stage

The diagnosis of "latent syphilis" cannot be made for a particular patient unless cerebrospinal fluid tests have been done and are negative for syphilis.

Tertiary Stage

1. Tertiary syphilis should be considered in any patient with a chronic granuloma of the skin, particularly if it has an annular or circular configuration.

2. Invasion of the central nervous system occurs in the primary and the secondary stages of the disease. A cerebrospinal fluid test is indicated during these stages.

3. If the cerebrospinal fluid tests for syphilis are negative in a patient who has had syphilis for 4 years, central nervous system syphilis usually will not occur, and future spinal punctures are not necessary.

4. Twenty percent of patients with late asymptomatic neurosyphilis have a negative STS.

Congenital Syphilis

An STS should be done on every pregnant woman to prevent congenital syphilis of the newborn.

Serology

1. The serologic test for syphilis may be negative in the early days of the primary chancre. The STS is always positive in the secondary stage; an exception to this rule is in patients with AIDS.

2. A quantitative STS should be done on all syphilitic patients to evaluate the response to treatment or the development of relapse or reinfection.

3. The finding of a low-titer STS in a patient not previously treated for syphilis calls for a careful evaluation to rule out a *biologic false-positive reaction.*

LYME DISEASE

Originally described as Lyme arthritis, Lyme disease is caused by a spirochete that is transmitted by several species of *Ixodes* tick. The disease has been reported from 32 states and on every continent except Antarctica. Clinical manifestations include erythema chronicum migrans (ECM) skin lesions, flu-like symptoms, and possible neurologic, cardiac, and rheumatologic involvement.

PRIMARY LESION. The erythematous circular rash appears at the site of the tick bite and enlarges with central clearing, but multiple ECM eruptions can occur. The rash typically develops from 2 to 30 days after the bite. The bite area can become necrotic.

SECONDARY LESION. Multiple ECM eruptions can develop.

DISTRIBUTION. Usually ECM begins at the site of the tick bite.

SEASON. The disease occurs from late May through early fall.

COURSE. In untreated patients the ECM lesions may last only 10 to 14 days, they may persist for months, or they may come and go over a year's time. The bite papule and ECM fade rapidly after therapy is begun.

SUBJECTIVE COMPLAINTS. Flulike symptoms, with fever, chills, myalgia, and headache, appear with the rash. Later other organs may be affected.

ETIOLOGY. The spirochete *Borrelia burgdorferi* is transmitted by *Ixodes* ticks and possibly by the hard-bodied ticks. The white-tailed deer and white-footed mouse are preferred hosts of the tick.

DIAGNOSIS. High index of suspicion, history of tick bite (patient is not always aware of bite), previous "ringworm-type" rash, and, later, positive Lyme disease antibody titer are required.

Differential Diagnosis

Systemically many diseases can be considered with fever, myalgia, cardiac, joint, or neurologic manifestations.

Cutaneously the ECM rash can resemble an allergic reaction or tinea.

Treatment

Early in the disease, the antibiotic of choice is tetracycline, 500 mg, q.i.d. for 10 to 20 days.

BIBLIOGRAPHY

Syphilis

Arnold HL: Penicillin and early syphilis. JAMA 251:2011, 1984

Baum EW et al: Secondary syphilis, still the great imitator. JAMA 249:3069, 1983

Centers for Disease Control: Sexually transmitted diseases (STD) treatment guidelines. J Am Acad Dermatol 14:707, 1986

Centers for Disease Control: Syphilis and congenital syphilis—United States, 1985–1988. Arch Dermatol 124:1485, 1988

Centers for Disease Control: Recommendations for diagnosing and treating syphilis in HIV-infected patients. Arch Dermatol 125:15, 1989

Rudolph AH, Duncan WC, Kettler AH: Treponemal infections. J Am Acad Dermatol 18:1121, 1988

Sexually Transmitted Diseases (STD) Bulletin. Monthly. F & M Projects, 152 Madison Avenue, New York, NY 10016

Lyme Disease

Krafchik B: Lyme disease. Int J Dermatol 28:71, 1989

Kurgansky D, Burnett JW: *Borrelia burgdorferi* infections. Cutis 43:407, 1989

Mertz LE, Wobig GH, Duffy J et al: Ticks, spirochetes and new diagnostic tests for Lyme disease. Mayo Clin Proc 60:402, 1985

somewhat effective in preventing or decreasing the frequency of recurrence.

The difficult management problem with recurrent genital herpes simplex is that women and men are frightened of the disease and of the effect of herpes on a newborn. This serious problem of infecting the newborn is rare but has received a lot of lay publicity. Reassure the woman, and the man, that this is a rare complication of herpes simplex. If the mother, after careful examination, does not have the infection at the time of birth, the chance of infection of the infant is almost nonexistent. If the mother has herpes lesions before delivery, she can have cesarean section delivery and should the newborn get herpes simplex, therapy with acyclovir is beneficial; however, this is a serious problem.

KAPOSI'S VARICELLIFORM ERUPTION

Kaposi's varicelliform eruption (see Plate 52) is an uncommon but severe complication in children who have atopic eczema. It results from self-inoculation by scratching, due to the virus of either herpes simplex (eczema herpeticum) or vaccinia. In the former type, a history of exposure to fever blisters may or may not be obtained. The vaccinia form (eczema vaccinatum) should be nonexistent now. With either type, the child is acutely ill, has a high fever, and has generalized, umbilicated, chickenpox-like skin lesions.

Acyclovir administered intravenously has proved beneficial in halting the progression of the disease and in promoting faster healing.

Supportive therapy consists of antibiotics systemically, intravenous infusions, and a calamine-like shake lotion, locally.

HERPESVIRUS INFECTION IN IMMUNOCOMPROMISED PATIENTS

Severe, ulcerative life-threatening HSV infections can develop in immunocompromised children and adults who have undergone organ transplantation, have lymphomas or advanced metastatic carcinoma, have AIDS, or are receiving systemic corticosteroid or antimetabolite therapy.

Intravenous acyclovir therapy is helpful in controlling the viral proliferation.

ZOSTER
(Plates 50, 54, and 89)

Shingles is a common viral disease characterized by the appearance of several groups of vesicles distributed along a cutaneous nerve segment. Zoster and chickenpox are believed to be caused by the same virus. Susceptible children who are exposed to cases of zoster often develop chickenpox. Less commonly, older persons exposed to chickenpox may get zoster.

PRIMARY LESIONS. Multiple groups of vesicles or crusted lesions appear.

SECONDARY LESIONS. Bacterial infection with pustules occurs, rarely progressing to hemorrhagic gangrenous ulcers and scarring.

DISTRIBUTION. Unilateral eruption follows a nerve distribution, frequently in the thoracic region, the face, the neck, and less frequently the lumbosacral area and elsewhere. Eye involvement can be serious. Bilateral involvement of the body is rare but not fatal, contrary to the old wives' tale.

COURSE. New crops of vesicles can appear for 3 to 5 days. The vesicles then dry up and form crusts, which take 3 weeks, on the average, to disappear. The general health is seldom affected, except for low-grade fever and malaise. Recurrences are rare. The *post-herpetic pain* can persist for months in aged patients.

SUBJECTIVE COMPLAINTS. Pain of a neuritic type can precede the eruption and, if in the abdominal area, can lead to erroneous diagnoses and surgical procedures. The common simple pain of young persons with shingles is readily treated and soon disappears. On the other hand, the severe, true *post-herpetic pain* of older patients can be very serious. In order to evaluate critically the therapeutic response to the many agents said to relieve this severe pain, *a nerve distribution pain should not be labeled as the true post-herpetic type unless it has been present for over 30 days.* If this strict criterion is adhered to, many newly proclaimed treatments for such pain will be found to be of limited value.

ster is caused by a virus simi-
t causes chickenpox. Trauma
lay a role in development of
ingles. "Nervousness" plays

Severe cases of herpes zoster can develop in immunocompromised patients (see Chap. 18).

CONTAGIOUSNESS. The interrelationship between shingles and chickenpox has been referred to previously.

LABORATORY FINDINGS. Isolation and identification of the virus is not an office procedure.

Differential Diagnosis

Of the neuritic-type pain that precedes the skin lesions: appendicitis, ureteral colic, sciatica, migraine, and so on.

Of the eruption: herpes simplex (see single group of vesicles, recurrence history, refer to preceding section); blistered burn from hot application for neuritic pain (very commonly the patient really has shingles and erroneously attributes the blisters to the hot application for the preceding herpetic pain).

Treatment

CASE 1

A 40-year-old woman presents with multiple grouped vesicles on right cheek and forehead, causing moderately severe pain.

1. Reassure the patient that shingles, except in the elderly, is not a serious disease, and advise her not to believe what her well-meaning friends will tell her about the disease.
2. Supply the name of an ophthalmologist to consult, to rule in or out eye complications.
3. Hydrocortisone 1% lotion q.s.   60.0
   Sig: Apply locally to skin b.i.d.
4. Analgesic tablets   #50
   Sig: 1 to 2 tablets q.i.d. as needed for pain
5. Acyclovir (Zovirax) capsules, 200 mg #35
   Sig: 5 capsules a day in divided doses.
   I do not believe that this therapy is indicated for every case of zoster, but it is prescribed quite frequently.

CASE 2

A 70-year-old man presented with extensive zoster on the right side of the the buttocks and down the thigh.

1. The above therapy and admonitions apply also.
2. Prednisone, 10 mg   #50
   Sig: 1 tablet q.i.d. for 6 days, then 2 tablets every morning.
   (There is evidence that early systemic corticosteroid therapy is beneficial and can decrease the post-herpetic pain problem.)
3. Acyclovir (Zovirax) capsules, 200 mg #50
   Sig: 5 capsules a day in divided doses for 6 days, then 1 capsule t.i.d.

CASE 3

A 70-year-old man presented with *severe post-herpetic pain* of 5 weeks' duration.

1. Reassure the patient that the majority of patients who have post-herpetic pain lose it gradually, day by day, week by week. It is extremely rare for the pain to remain persistent, but, when this does happen, it can be disabling. Be optimistic, however. The following treatment can alleviate the neuritis.
2. Capsaicin (Zostrix) cream, 45 g
   Sig: apply three to four times a day locally. This treatment is of benefit for some patients.
3. Prednisone tablets, 10 mg   #40
   Sig: 2 tablets every morning for 6 days; then decrease dose slowly as symptoms subside.
4. Sedative capsule   #10
   Sig: 1 capsule h.s. for sleep.
5. For resistant cases, consult larger texts for additional therapy or refer the patient to a pain clinic.

CASE 4

A 28-year-old man with AIDS has an extensive case of zoster on the right chest wall and also disseminated lesions.

Hospitalization is necessary for supportive therapy and for intravenous acyclovir therapy (see Chap. 18).

CHICKENPOX

Chickenpox is a common viral disease of childhood that is characterized by the development of tense vesicles, first on the trunk and then spreading, to a milder extent, to the face and the extremities. New crops of vesicles appear for 3 to 5 days, and healing of the individual lesions occurs in a week. The disease occurs 10 to 14 days after exposure to another child with chickenpox or to an adult with zoster. The clear vesicle becomes a pustule and then a crusted lesion before dropping off. Itching is more prominent during the healing stage.

Treatment

1. Usually nothing indicated, or
2. Menthol   0.25%
   Nonalcoholic white shake lotion (p. 38) or
   hydrocortisone, 1% lotion q.s.   120.0
   Sig: Apply locally t.i.d. for itching.
3. Benadryl hydrochloride elixir   60.0
   Sig: 1 teaspoon t.i.d. for moderately severe itching.

SMALLPOX

Smallpox is an apparently eradicated viral disease. For historical interest here are some facts about smallpox and vaccination.

Smallpox is characterized by the development, after an incubation period of 1 to 3 weeks, of prodromal symptoms of high fever, chills, and various aches. After 3 to 4 days a rash develops, with lowering of the fever. The individual lesions are most extensive on the face and the extremities; they come out as a single shower and progress from papule to vesicle, and, in 5 to 10 days, to pustule. With the occurrence of the pustule the fever goes up again, with a high white blood cell count. Hemorrhagic lesions usually indicate a severe form of the disease.

Alastrim is a mild form of smallpox resulting from a less virulent strain of the virus.

Varioloid is a mild form of smallpox that occurs in vaccinated persons. However, this strain of virus is very virulent, and when transmitted to a nonvaccinated person often causes a fulminating disease.

Severe systemic complications of smallpox include pneumonia, secondary bacterial skin infection, and encephalitis.

Treatment

Prophylactic treatment consists of vaccination. The best technique is by multiple puncture.

VACCINIA

Vaccinia is produced by the inoculation of the vaccinia virus into the skin of a person who has no immunity.

The *primary vaccination reaction* follows this timetable (the multiple puncture technique should be used): A red papule on a red base develops on the fourth day, becomes vesicular in 3 more days and pustular in 2 to 3 more days, and then gradually dries to form a crust, which drops off within 3 to 4 weeks after the vaccination. A mild systemic reaction may occur during the pustular stage. The vaccination site should be kept dry and uncovered.

Generalized vaccinia is rare but can occur from autoinoculation, by scratching, in atopic eczema patients (see *eczema vaccinatum*, p. 185). A biologic false-positive serologic test for syphilis develops in approximately 20% of vaccinated persons. The test becomes negative within 2 to 4 months.

A *vaccinoid reaction* develops in a partially immune person. A pustule with some surrounding redness occurs within 1 week.

An *immune reaction* consists of a papule that develops in 2 days, which may or may not persist for 1 week.

An *absent reaction* indicates that the vaccine was inactivated by the procedure (*e.g.*, alcohol used in cleaning the site) or that the vaccine was impotent.

A successful vaccination offers protection from smallpox within 3 weeks, and this immunity lasts for approximately 7 years or longer.

COWPOX

Jenner used the cowpox virus to vaccinate humans against smallpox. For that reason, the vaccinia virus and the cowpox virus have been believed to be the same. Evidence now exists that proves these viruses to be different, presumably as a result of a change in the vaccinia virus through years of passage. The term *cowpox* is now reserved for the viral disease of cows that occurs in Europe. Humans can get the disease from infected teats and udders. A solitary nodule appears, usually on the hand, which eventually suppurates and then heals in 4 to 8 weeks.

WARTS (VERRUCAE)
(Plates 49, 51, 54, and 75)

Warts, or verrucae, are very common small tumors of the skin. It is doubtful if any human escapes this viral infection. Warts have been played with for centuries, and cures have been attributed to burying a dead black cat in the graveyard at midnight and other such feats. The interesting fact is that these examples of psychotherapy do work. Physicians attempt the same type of therapy under more professional guise and are pleased, but not surprised, when such therapy is effective. Children, fortunately, are most amenable to this suggestion therapy. On the other hand, however, every physician is also familiar with the stubborn wart that has been literally blasted from its mooring in the skin but keeps recurring.

The human papillomavirus (HPV) is a DNA virus. To date, 42 types of HPV have been identified by immunocytologic and molecular biologic techniques. Several of the types can cause clinically similar warts.

The various *clinical* types of warts relate to the appearance of the growth and to its location. The treatment varies somewhat for each clinical type of wart and will be discussed separately for each type.

Common Wart
(Plate 51)

The appearance is a papillary growth, slightly raised above the skin surface, varying from pinhead size to large clusters of pea-sized tumors. These warts are seen most commonly on the hands. Rarely, they have to be differentiated from *seborrheic keratoses* (flatter, darker, velvety tumors of older adults; see Chap. 33) and *pigmented verrucous nevi* (projections are not dry and rough to touch; longer duration; biopsy may be indicated; see Chap. 33).

Treatment

1. Suggestion therapy can be attempted, particularly with children. One form of such therapy consists of the application by the physician of a colored solution, such as podophyllum in alcohol, 25% solution. This has the added benefit of being a cell-destroying chemical.

2. Single small (under 6 mm) warts in adults or older children are removed best by electrosurgery. The recurrence rate is minimal, and one treatment usually suffices. The technique is to cleanse the area, anesthetize the site with 1% procaine or other local anesthetic, destroy the tumor with any form of electrosurgery (see Chap. 6), snip off or curette out the dead tissue, and desiccate the base. Recurrences can be attributed to failure to remove the dead tissue and to destroy the lesion adequately to its full depth. No dressing should be applied. The site will heal in 5 to 14 days with only minimal bacterial infection and scar formation. Warts around the nails have a high recurrence rate, and cure usually requires removal of part of the overlying nail.

3. If available, liquid nitrogen therapy is quite simple, effective, but moderately painful (see Chap. 6). The important admonition here is *freeze lightly* and not deeply.

SAUER NOTES:

1. A successful method of removing one or several warts, even in children, is the light application of liquid nitrogen to the wart followed by electrosurgery while the wart is thawing.

2. It is amazing how much electrosurgery some patients can tolerate before you need to stop the electrosurgery. In those moments of toleration, many warts can be cured, or the procedure can be repeated every 3 weeks as necessary.

---

4. Salicylic acid   10%
   Flexible collodion q.s.   30.0
   Sig: Apply to warts cautiously every night for 5 to 7 nights. If irritation occurs, stop

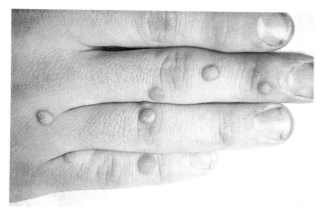

(A) Common warts on hand

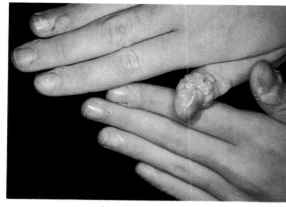

(B) Common and periungual warts

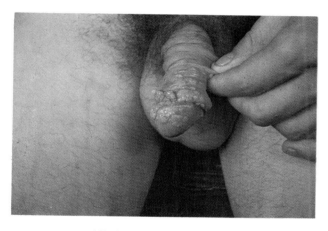

(C) Moist warts on penis

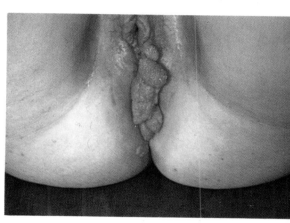

(D) Moist warts on female genital area

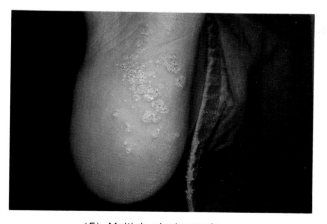

(E) Multiple plantar warts

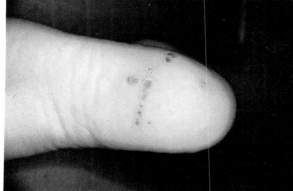

(F) Plantar warts that recurred in surgical excision site

Plate 51. **Warts.** (*Reed & Carnrick Pharmaceuticals*)

the application for three to four nights and resume again as necessary. The dead tissue can be removed with scissors.

Several prescription and proprietary medications of this therapy are available, such as Duoplant (27% salicylic acid), Duofilm (16.7% salicylic acid), Occlusal, and Compound W. Trans-plantar contains 21% salicylic acid in a dermal patch delivery system.

This type of treatment is applicable for the patient with 20 or more warts on one hand, or for larger warts to avoid scarring. The purpose is to remove as many warts as possible in this manner over a period of several weeks. Any remaining warts can be removed by electrosurgery or liquid nitrogen.

5. Another form of treatment for multiple warts or for warts in children is as follows:

A mild corticosteroid cream   15.0

Sig: Apply a very small quantity to each wart at night. Then cover the wart with Saran Wrap, Actiderm, or Blenderm Tape and leave the occlusive dressing on all night or for 24 hours. Repeat nightly.

This treatment has the advantage of being painless and quite effective. Salicylic acid (2% to 4%) can be added to the cream for further benefit.

6. Vitamin A, 50,000 units   #50

Sig: 1 tablet a day for no longer than 3 months.

For the resistant case in an adult, and for the patient who says, "Doctor, aren't there any pills I can take for these warts," vitamin A is safe and warts have disappeared after such a course of treatment.

Filiform Warts

Filiform warts have long, finger-like projections from the skin and most commonly appear on the eyelids, the face, and the neck. They are to be differentiated from *cutaneous horns* (which are seen in elderly patients with actinic keratosis or squamous cell carcinoma at the base and have a hard keratin horn; see Chap. 33), and from *pedunculated fibromas* (which occur on the neck and the axillae of middle-aged men and women; see Chap. 33).

Treatment

1. Without anesthesia, snip off the wart with a small scissors and apply trichloroacetic acid solution (saturated) cautiously to the base. This is a fast and effective method, especially for children.
2. Electrosurgery can be performed as described previously for common warts.
3. Light application of liquid nitrogen is effective.

An annoying variant of this type of wart is the case with multiple small *filiform warts of the beard area*. Low-intensity electrosurgery without anesthesia is well tolerated and effective for these warts. However, in order to achieve a permanent cure, the patient should be seen every 3 to 4 weeks for as long a period as necessary to remove the young warts that are in the process of enlarging. The physician's job is to keep ahead of these warts and eliminate the reinfection that occurs from shaving.

Flat Warts
(Plate 49)

These small, flat tumors are often barely visible but can occur in clusters of 10 to 30 or more. They are commonly seen on the forehead and the dorsum of the hand and should be differentiated from small *seborrheic keratoses* or *nonpigmented nevi*. On women's legs, they are spread by shaving.

Flat warts can also occur on the penis and cervix. Acetic acid 3% to 5%, or vinegar solution, applied for 5 to 15 minutes to the area, with the use of a hand lens or colposcope, aids visualization. The flat warts appear whitish. Warts of HPV types 16 and 18 are believed to be related to the development of cervical cancer.

Bowenoid papulosis on the anogenital area and penis can clinically resemble flat warts. Histologically the flat papules exhibit changes of squamous cell carcinoma *in situ*. The course is usually benign. HPV have been found in these lesions.

Treatment

1. For flat warts on the face, cautiously use liquid nitrogen or light electrosurgery. *Use*

care not to scar. Retin A Gel (0.01%) locally once a day removes some flat warts. Suggestion therapy is effective for these warts in children.

2. For hand or leg flat warts, light electrosurgery is effective and tolerated quite well.
3. For genital flat warts, saturated solution of trichloroacetic acid, applied by the physician with great care, is beneficial. Light liquid nitrogen, electrosurgery, or both are effective. This is a tender area and local anesthesia is often necessary. Laser therapy is promoted by some.

Some cases in adults can exhaust your therapeutic modalities, only to have the warts disappear with time.

Moist Warts (Condylomata Acuminata)
(Plates 51 and 54)

Moist warts are quite characteristic, single or multiple, soft, nonhorny masses that appear in the anogenital areas and, less commonly, between the toes and at the corners of the mouth. They are not always of a venereal nature. However, moist warts in the anal orifice of a child can be a sign of sexual abuse.

Genitoanal warts are predominantly induced by human papillomavirus types 6, 11, 16, and 18.

Treatment

1. Podophyllum resin in alcohol (25% solution). Apply once to the warts, cautiously. Second or third treatments are usually necessary at weekly intervals. To prevent excessive irritation, the site should be bathed within 3 to 6 hours after the application.
2. Occasionally liquid nitrogen or electrosurgery with local anesthesia is necessary.
3. Interferon alfa-2b (Intron A) is available for injection into the warts—*many* injections are needed.

Plantar Warts
(Plate 51)

(This is the layman's "planter's warts," which I am sure they believe are related to "Planter's Peanuts.") As the name signifies, this wart occurs on the sole of the foot, is flat,

extends deep into the thick skin, and, *on superficial trimming reveals small pinpoint-sized bleeding points.* Varying degrees of disability can be produced from the pressure type of pain. Single or multiple lesions can be present. The name *mosaic wart* is applied when the warts have coalesced into larger patches. One of the most vexing problems in dermatology is the patient with half of the sole of a foot covered with these warts.

Plantar warts are to be differentiated from a *callus* (no bleeding points visible on superficial trimming) and from *scar tissue from a previous treatment* (no bleeding points seen).

SAUER NOTE:

Never treat a plantar lesion as a wart until you have proved your diagnosis by trimming to reveal the bleeding points of the wart. Too many punctate keratoses and calluses are mistaken for plantar warts.

Treatment

It would be impossible to list all of the forms of therapy that have proved to be curative for plantar warts or any other warts, but here are some favorite forms of therapy. I wager that if you start with number 1 and proceed to number 6, either the warts will have left, or your patient will have gone to another physician.

1. Electrosurgery. This is the simplest and most successful form of therapy for a single small (under 6 mm) plantar wart. The procedure is the same as for common warts except that the downgrowth of the plantar wart is greater. Local anesthesia is usually necessary, and the injection is painful. Healing takes from 3 to 4 weeks to be complete. Some bleeding is to be expected a few days after the surgery. Most patients do not complain of much pain during the healing stage.
2. Liquid nitrogen therapy. This can be applied in two ways. When applied for 10 to 15 seconds, a blister will form in 24 hours and deep peeling of the wart will ensue. This can be quite painful but is effective.

When applied lightly for 5 to 8 seconds,

the larger warts or multiple warts can be removed gradually on several visits with less pain and disability.

3. Trichloroacetic acid–tape technique. This is useful for children and cases with multiple or large plantar warts. The procedure is as follows: pare down the wart with a sharp knife, apply trichloroacetic acid solution (saturated) to the wart, then cover the area with plain tape. Leave the tape on for 5 to 7 days. Then remove the tape and curette out the dead wart tissue. Usually, more wart will remain, and the procedure is repeated until the wart is destroyed. This course of treatment may take several weeks. After the first two visits the site may become tender and secondarily infected. If the disability and the infection are severe, therapy should be stopped temporarily and hot soaks instituted.

4. Fluorinated corticosteroid–occlusive dressing therapy. Have the patient apply a small amount of corticosteroid cream to the wart or warts at night and cover with Saran Wrap, Handi-Wrap, Actiderm, or Blenderm Tape. Leave on for 12 to 24 to 48 hours and reapply. This form of treatment is painless.

5. Cantharidin (Verrusol or Cantharone) is applied by the physician to the pared wart. Use caution and do not get this vesicant on the surrounding normal skin. For a thick wart you can cover with adhesive tape and leave on for 12 to 24 hours. This treatment can cause pain and infection, but it is quite effective. The resulting blister can be trimmed off in 1 or 2 weeks and the medicine reapplied, if necessary.

6. X-ray therapy. This painless form of therapy can be used for single small warts. Only a dermatologist or a radiologist should administer this treatment. The cure rate is fairly high.

MOLLUSCUM CONTAGIOSUM
(Plate 52)

Molluscum contagiosum is an uncommon viral infection of the skin that is characterized by the occurrence, usually in children or sexually active young adults, of one or multiple small skin tumors. These growths occasionally develop in the scratched areas of patients with *atopic eczema*.

The causative agent is a large DNA-containing poxvirus.

PRIMARY LESION. An umbilicated, firm, waxy, skin-colored, raised papule, varying in diameter from 2 to 5 mm and, rarely, larger.

SECONDARY LESION. The skin is inflamed from bacterial infection.

DISTRIBUTION. Most commonly the papules appear on the trunk, face, arms, and genital area but can occur anywhere.

COURSE. Onset of lesions is insidious, owing to lack of symptoms. Trauma or infection of a lesion causes it to disappear. Recurrences are rare, if lesions are removed adequately.

CONTAGIOUSNESS. By direct contact or autoinoculation.

Differential Diagnosis

Warts: no umbilication, not waxy (see earlier in this chapter).
Keratoacanthoma: most commonly in older adults; larger lesion; rapid growth; biopsy findings characteristic (see Chap. 33).
Basal cell carcinoma: in older adults; slow growing; biopsy findings characteristic (see Chap. 33).

Treatment

A 6-year-old child presents with ten small molluscum papules on his arms and upper trunk.

1. Verrusol (contains cantharidin, salicylic acid, and podophyllin). A drop is applied with care by the physician on each lesion. A blister will form. This is very effective and painless therapy.

2. Curettement. Rapidly curette each lesion, apply pressure to stop bleeding, then apply bandage. A small amount of trichloroacetic acid (saturated solution) on the broken pointed end of a swab stick helps to stop prolonged bleeding. Two or three visits may be necessary to treat recurrent lesions and new ones that have popped up.

3. Electrosurgery. Done lightly and rapidly, this is another effective method, especially for adults. It is not necessary to destroy the entire lesion, as for a wart, but only to induce some trauma and mild infection.

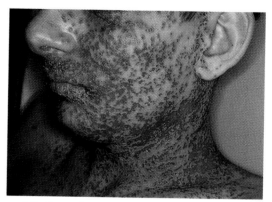

(A) Kaposi's varicelliform eruption: herpes simplex inoculated on atopic eczema

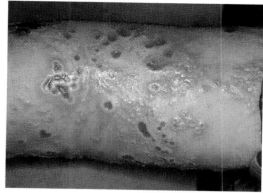

(B) Kaposi's varicelliform eruption: smallpox vaccination inoculated on atopic eczema, age 4

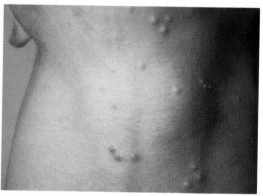

(C) Molluscum contagiosum on neck

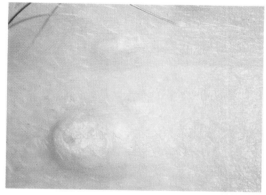

(D) Molluscum contagiosum close-up (*Drs. L. Calkins, A. Lemoine, and Hyde*)

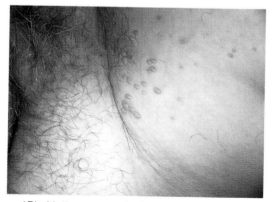

(E) Molluscum contagiosum of vulvar area

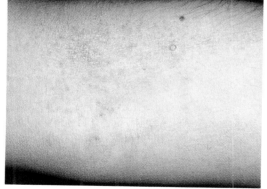

(F) Molluscum contagiosum with atopic eczema of cubital fossae

Plate 52. **Kaposi's varicelliform eruption and molluscum contagiosum.** (*Glaxo Dermatology*)

LYMPHOGRANULOMA VENEREUM

Lymphogranuloma venereum is an uncommon venereal disease characterized by a primary lesion on the genitals and secondary changes involving the draining lymph channels and glands.

The primary erosion or blister is rarely seen, especially on the female patient. Within 10 to 30 days after exposure, the inguinal nodes, particularly in the male patient, enlarge unilaterally. This inguinal mass may rupture if treatment is delayed. In the female patient the lymph drainage most commonly is toward the pelvic and the perirectal nodes, and their enlargement may be overlooked. Low-grade fever, malaise, and generalized lymphadenopathy frequently occur during the adenitis stage. Scarlatina-like rashes and erythema nodosum lesions also may develop. The later manifestations of lymphogranuloma venereum occur as the result of scarring of the lymph channels and fibrosis of the nodes. These changes result in rectal stricture, swelling of the penis or the vulva, and ulceration.

ETIOLOGY. Lymphogranuloma venerum is caused by the obligate intracellular parasite *Chlamydia trachomatis*, serotypes L_1, L_2, and L_3.

DIAGNOSIS. A complement fixation test (LGV-CFT) becomes positive 3 to 4 weeks after the onset of the disease in 80% to 90% of the patients.

Treatment

Tetracycline, 500 mg q.i.d., and minocycline, 100 mg b.i.d., are the drugs of choice. These are most effective in the early stages and should be continued for at least 3 weeks.

Fluctuant inguinal nodes should be aspirated to prevent rupture.

MEASLES (RUBEOLA)

Measles is a very common childhood disease. The characteristic points are as follows: the incubation period averages 14 days before the appearance of the rash. The prodromal stage appears around the 9th day after exposure and consists of fever, conjunctivitis, running nose, Koplik spots, and even a faint red rash. The Koplik spots measure from 1 to 3 mm in diameter, are bluish white on a red base, and occur bilaterally on the mucous membrane around the parotid duct and on the lower lip. With increasing fever and cough the "morbilliform" rash appears, first behind the ears and on the forehead, then spreads over face, neck, trunk, and extremities. The fever begins to fall as the rash comes out. The rash is a faint, reddish, patchy eruption, occasionally papular. Scaling occurs in the end stage.

Complications include secondary bacterial infection and encephalitis.

Differential Diagnosis

German measles: postauricular nodes; milder fever and rash; no Koplik spots (see following section).

Scarlet fever: circumoral pallor; rash brighter red and confluent (see Chap. 15).

Drug eruption: history of new drugs; usually no fever (see Chap. 9).

Infectious mononucleosis: rash similar; characteristic blood picture; high titer of heterophil antibodies.

Treatment

PROPHYLACTIC. Measles virus vaccine, live, attenuated, can be administered.

ACTIVE. Supportive therapy for the cough, bed rest, and protection from bright light are measures for the active disease. The antibiotics have eliminated most of the bacterial complications. Corticosteroids are of value for the rare but serious complication of encephalitis.

GERMAN MEASLES (RUBELLA)

While German measles is a benign disease of children, it is serious if it develops in a pregnant woman during the first trimester, since it causes anomalies in a low percentage of newborns.

The incubation period is around 18 days, and, as in measles, there may be a short prodromal stage of fever and malaise. The rash also resembles measles, since it occurs first on the face and then spreads. However, the redness is less intense and the rash disappears within 2 to 3 days. Enlargement of the cervi-

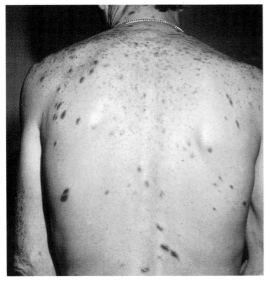

(A) Disseminated Kaposi's sarcoma: multiple red to brown papules and plaques distributed along the skin tension lines in a homosexual man with AIDS

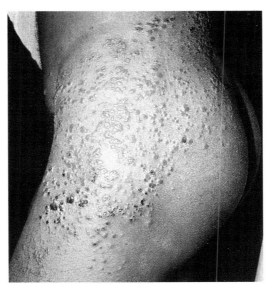

(B) Herpes zoster: umbilicated vesicles in a dermatomal distribution in a homosexual man with AIDS

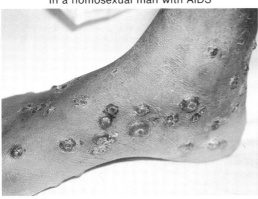

(C) Ecthymatous herpes varicella-zoster: crusted erosions and blisters on the foot of a patient with AIDS

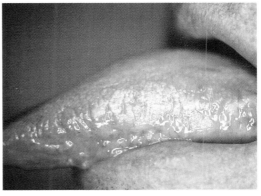

(D) Oral hairy leukoplakia: filamentous white papules on the sides of the tongue

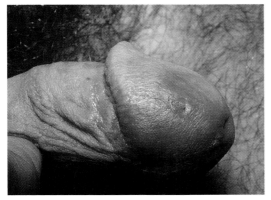

(E) Kaposi's sarcoma: an ill-defined purple plaque on the glans penis of a homosexual man with AIDS

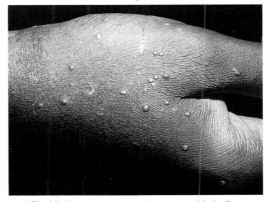

(F) Molluscum contagiosum: multiple firm white papules scattered over the dorsal hand and forearm in a Haitian man with AIDS

Plate 53. **Cutaneous diseases associated with HIV infection.** (*Drs. J. Rico and N. Prose*) (*Owen/Galderma*)

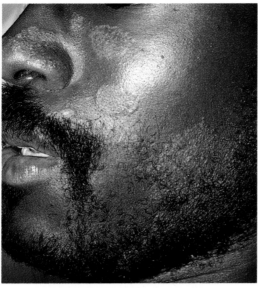

(A) Seborrheic dermatitis: annular scaling plaques on the nasolabial fold and cheeks

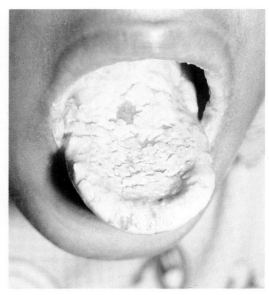

(B) Oral candidiasis: white plaques on the tongue of a child with AIDS

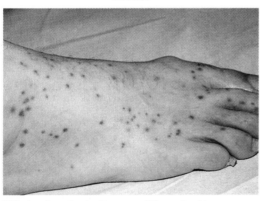

(C) Leukocytoclastic vasculitis: palpable purpura on the lower leg. This patient developed vasculitis after receiving trimethoprim-sulfamethoxazole

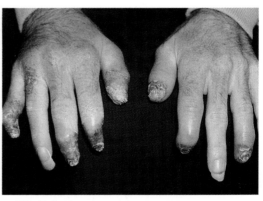

(D) Reiter's disease: psoriasiform dermatitis involving the distal fingers. Note the joint changes due to active arthritis

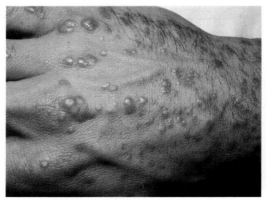

(E) Disseminated granuloma annulare: discrete annular pink papules on the dorsal hand

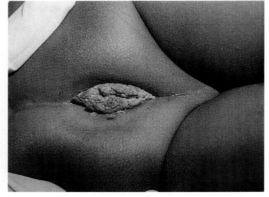

(F) Condyloma acuminata: fungating perianal warts in a child infected with HIV

Plate 54. **Cutaneous diseases associated with human immunodeficiency virus (HIV) infection.** (Drs. J. Rico and N. Prose)

petic gingivostomatitis can significantly impede adequate oral intake. *Herpes zoster* is not uncommon in children and adults with HIV infection. The occurrence of this cutaneous disease in a patient at risk for AIDS may identify those infected with HIV. Dissemination of both herpes simplex and herpes zoster to extracutaneous sites has been reported.

Molluscum contagiosum in patients with HIV infection often presents as disseminated disease or with large atypical lesions. Finally, *human papillomavirus* infection, particularly condylomata acuminata, may present as large, fungating lesions.

Fungal Infections

The most common mucocutaneous eruption in patients infected with HIV is oral *candidiasis* or thrush. A number of these patients may develop esophageal involvement with characteristic ulcerations visible on endoscopy or barium swallow. Candidiasis involving the diaper area is a significant problem in children with AIDS. Candidal paronychia has also been reported.

Cutaneous fungal infections may occur as extensive scaling papules and plaques or may involve atypical sites. In the adult population, *onychomycosis* is common. Cutaneous involvement of disseminated deep fungal infections including *cryptococcosis*, *histoplasmosis*, and *blastomycosis* have been reported in patients with AIDS.

Bacterial Diseases

Infants and children with AIDS are particularly at risk for bacterial infections; cutaneous bacterial diseases including *cellulitis* and *impetigo* are frequent. In adults, *acneiform eruptions* and extensive *folliculitis* have been reported.

Other Infections

Syphilis, like HIV infection, is a sexually transmitted disease that predominately affects young adults. In particular, patients with AIDS who are homosexual/bisexual or are intravenous drug users are at increased risk for syphilis. Patients coinfected with syphilis and HIV may be serologically (RPR, FTA) nega-tive despite active infection. Occasionally, they do not respond to standard antibiotic regimens and develop complications of syphilis. Those caring for patients with HIV infection or syphilis are urged to review the recommendations of the Centers for Disease Control for diagnosis and treatment.

Mycobacteria may involve the skin in patients with AIDS either as a primary cellulitis with *Mycobacterium avium-intracellulare*, or with secondary spread of *M. tuberculosis*, as in scrofula.

Infestations

"Atypical scabies" has been reported in both adults and children with AIDS. The rash tends to be highly pruritic, and patients present with widespread, keratotic papules similar clinically to Norwegian scabies.

Inflammatory Conditions

Seborrheic dermatitis is seen in up to 50% of the patients with HIV infection, in both those with AIDS and ARC. Clinically, seborrheic dermatitis in these patients tends to be more florid and less responsive to therapy than in the nonimmunocompromised host.

Psoriasis and *Reiter's disease* have been reported in 1% to 5% of patients with evidence of HIV infection. Psoriasis may flare in those with previously stable plaque-type disease or develop *de novo*. *Reiter's disease*, manifested by psoriasiform dermatitis, keratoderma blenorrhagica, seronegative spondyloarthropathy, urethritis, balanitis, uveitis, or conjunctivitis, is more common in patients with AIDS and is associated with the histocompatibility locus antigen HLA-B27. Therapy with zidovudine (azidothymidine [AZT]) appears to benefit some patients with severe AIDS-associated psoriasis. Conversely, the initiation of methotrexate for psoriasis and Reiter's disease in several patients with underlying HIV disease was associated with rapidly progressive immunodeficiency.

Atopic dermatitis has been reported to flare or to develop *de novo* in children and adults with HIV infection. *Drug eruptions* particularly due to trimethoprim-sulfamethoxazole, and other antibiotics, are common in patients with AIDS. Generalized *granuloma annulare* may be seen with widespread annular dermal papules.

Papular eruption of HIV infection was described by James and co-workers as multiple, 2- to 5-mm flesh-colored papules on the face, neck, and upper thorax that were often pruritic.

Neoplasms

B-cell lymphoma, which commonly involves the central nervous system in patients with AIDS, has been rarely reported to disseminate to skin. The lesions were described as small ulcerated papules or nodules.

Cutaneous malignancies, including metastatic basal cell carcinoma, squamous cell carcinoma, and malignant melanoma, have been reported in patients with HIV infection. With the advent of therapeutic agents to improve survival in patients with AIDS, we most likely will see an increased incidence of cutaneous malignancy.

Other Conditions

Vasculitis may occur as a manifestation of a drug eruption or may be idiopathic. Most commonly, vasculitis presents as palpable purpura on the extremities and there is histologic evidence of leukocytoclasis. The differential diagnosis includes septic emboli or other infections.

Patients with AIDS and chronic diarrhea or AIDS-wasting syndrome, particularly children, are at risk for *cutaneous manifestations of nutritional deficiencies.* Scurvy, acrodermatitis enteropathica, and cutaneous manifestations of vitamin B deficiency have been reported.

Other conditions involve the skin in patients infected with HIV. *Pruritus* may be one of the initial symptoms of HIV infection and is often incapacitating. Patients may present with excoriations, lesions of lichen simplex chronicus, prurigo nodularis, or minimal skin changes. *Xerosis,* which is not specific for HIV infection and can be seen in a variety of chronic illnesses, has been reported in up to 30% of patients with HIV infection. Finally, an evanescent *morbilliform rash* has been associated with acute seroconversion.

SKIN DISORDERS SPECIFIC FOR HIV INFECTION
(Plates 53 and 54)

There are several skin disorders seen in HIV-infected patients that appear to be restricted to this population (Table 18–2). The appearance of any of these lesions in an otherwise healthy patient should raise the suspicion of possible HIV infection. These include *disseminated Kaposi's sarcoma, disseminated cat-scratch disease, oral hairy leukoplakia, combined fungal-viral infections,* and *chronic varicella-zoster infection.*

Disseminated Kaposi's sarcoma was one of the initial manifestations of HIV infection; the first cases were reported in 1980, in previously healthy homosexual/bisexual men. Since then, Kaposi's sarcoma has remained a disease predominately seen in that subgroup of patients and has been infrequently reported in intravenous drug users, in those who acquire the disease through heterosexual contact, and in children. Disseminated Kaposi's sarcoma associated with AIDS differs from classic Kaposi's sarcoma in that the majority of patients present with multiple papules, plaques, or tumors involving the integument and mucosa. Visceral involvement occurs in 25% and may terminate in systemic hemorrhage. The lesions generally are asymptomatic. However, patients may complain of pruritus or pain, and large lesions may ulcerate. The treatment of isolated lesions by excision, cryotherapy, or local irradiation may offer palliation or cosmetic improvement. Recently, the administration of daily subcutaneous interferon alfa has been shown to induce remission and improve survival in some patients, particularly in those who are not profoundly immunosuppressed.

Kaposi's sarcoma is generally accepted to be a proliferation of endothelial cells. A host of other vascular lesions have also been re-

Table 18–2
Lesions Specific for AIDS

Disseminated Kaposi's sarcoma
Disseminated cat-scratch disease
Oral hairy leukoplakia
Combined infections
Ecthymatous varicella-zoster

ported in patients with HIV infection, particularly homosexual/bisexual men, and include telangiectasia, angiolipoma, and pyogenic granuloma. Some investigators have postulated that Kaposi's sarcoma and other vascular lesions in patients with AIDS are a consequence of stimulation by an endothelial growth factor produced by HIV-infected cells.

Disseminated cat-scratch disease has been noted to occur in patients with AIDS and ARC. This unique illness is characterized by the development of fever, chills, and weight loss and the evolution of numerous angiomatous nodules. The etiologic agent is the bacillus that causes cat-scratch disease. Treatment with oral erythromycin leads to the rapid resolution of both skin lesions and systemic symptoms.

Oral hairy leukoplakia is an asymptomatic benign process that presents as filamentous white papules on the lateral sides of the tongue. It is unique to patients with AIDS, ARC, or asymptomatic antibody-positive persons. Oral hairy leukoplakia is probably due to a mixed infection of Epstein-Barr virus and human papillomavirus. The lesions can be treated topically with tretinoin (Retin-A), and patients often improve after treatment with acyclovir.

Complex viral and fungal lesions involving the skin may be hyperkeratotic, vegetating, or ulcerative. Herpesvirus, papillomavirus, and fungal elements have been cultured or observed on biopsy.

Chronic ecthymatous varicella-zoster virus infection is a specific mucocutaneous infection that can occur in patients with AIDS with a previous history of varicella-zoster exposure. Patients may present either with dermatomal vesicles that subsequently ulcerate and disseminate or with frank ulcers. Children with HIV infection and varicella may also develop disseminated ecthymatous varicella-zoster infection. These lesions are often recalcitrant to therapy and may heal with scarring.

BIBLIOGRAPHY

Alessi E, Berti E, Cusini M et al: Oral hairy leukoplakia. J Am Acad Dermatol 22:79, 1990

Kaplan MH, Sadick N, McNutt NS et al: Dermatologic findings and manifestations of acquired immunodeficiency syndrome (AIDS). J Am Acad Dermatol 16:485, 1987

Leyden JJ: Infection in the immunocompromised host. Arch Dermatol 121:855, 1985

Penneys NS, Hicks B: Unusual cutaneous lesions associated with acquired immunodeficiency syndrome. J Am Acad Dermatol 13:845, 1985

Prose NS, Mendez H, Menikoff H et al: Pediatric human immunodeficiency virus and its cutaneous manifestations. Pediatr Dermatol 4:67, 1987

Weisman K, Petersen CS, Sondergaard J, Wantzin GL: Skin Signs in AIDS. Copenhagen, Munksgaard, 1988

19

Dermatologic Mycology

Fungi can be present as part of the normal flora of the skin or as abnormal inhabitants. Dermatologists are concerned with the abnormal inhabitants, or pathogenic fungi. However, so-called nonpathogenic fungi can proliferate and invade immunosuppressed persons.

Pathogenic fungi have a predilection for certain body areas; most commonly it is the skin, but the lungs, the brain, and other organs can be infected. Pathogenic fungi can invade the skin *superficially* and *deeply* and are thus divided into these two groups.

SUPERFICIAL FUNGAL INFECTIONS

The superficial fungi live on the dead horny layer of the skin and elaborate an enzyme that enables them to digest keratin, causing the superficial skin to scale and disintegrate, the nails to crumble, and the hairs to break off. The deeper reactions of vesicles, erythema, and infiltration are presumably due to the fungi liberating an exotoxin. Fungi are also capable of eliciting an allergic or id reaction.

It will be necessary to define a few mycologic terms before proceeding farther. When a skin scraping, a hair, or a culture growth is examined with the microscope in a wet preparation (see Chap. 2 and Fig. 2–3), the two structural elements of the fungi will be seen: the spores and the hyphae.

Spores are the reproducing bodies of the fungi. Sexual and asexual forms occur. Spores are rarely seen in skin scrapings.

Hyphae are threadlike, branching filaments that grow out from the fungus spore. The hyphae are the identifying filaments seen in skin scrapings in potassium hydroxide (KOH) solution.

Mycelia are matted clumps of hyphae that grow on culture plates.

Culture media vary greatly in content, but modifications of Sabouraud's dextrose agar are used to grow the superficial fungi (see Fig. 2–4). Sabouraud's agar and corn meal agar are both used to identify the deep fungi. Hyphae and spores grow on the media, and identification of the species of fungi is established by the gross appearance of the mycelia, the color of the substrate, and the microscopic appearance of the spores and the hyphae when a sample of the growth is placed on a slide. Some media show a color change when pathogenic fungi are isolated.

Classification

The latest classification divides the superficial fungi into three genera: *Microsporum,* *Epidermophyton,* and *Trichophyton.* Only two of these species invade the hair: *Microsporum* and *Trichophyton.* As seen in a KOH preparation, *Microsporum* causes an ecothrix infection of the hair shaft, whereas *Trichophyton* causes either an ectothrix or an endothrix infection. The ectothrix fungi cause the formation of an external spore sheath around the hair, whereas the endothrix fungi do not. The filaments of mycelia penetrate the hair in both types of infection.

The species of fungi is correlated with the

SAUER NOTES:

Since the discovery of the specific systemic antifungal agents griseofulvin and ketoconazole, many physicians have believed that (1) these agents are indicated for every fungus infection and (2) most skin diseases are due to a fungus, so they should treat the patient with the antifungal agent and make a diagnosis later. Both of these assumptions are erroneous.

1. Correct diagnosis of a fungal infection is necessary. Do not prescribe an oral antifungal drug for your patient if you are not sure of the diagnosis. Griseofulvin or ketoconazole are of no value in treating atopic eczema, contact dermatitis, psoriasis, pityriasis rosea, and so on.

2. Except for tinea of the scalp and nails, true fungal infections will be noticeably improved after only 2 to 3 weeks of oral antifungal therapy. If there is no improvement, the diagnosis of the dermatosis as a fungus disease is erroneous and the therapy should be stopped.

3. Treat with adequate dosage. Know (1) the correct daily dose for the particular type of fungal infection and (2) the correct duration of such dosage.

4. In general, oral griseofulvin or ketoconazole therapy should not be used to treat tinea of the feet and tinea of the toenails. The recurrence rate after completion of therapy is very high.

5. Do not treat candidal infections with oral griseofulvin. Very commonly, candidal intertrigo of the groin or candidal paronychias are erroneously treated with griseofulvin. Griseofulvin is of no value in these conditions. Since it is a penicillin-related drug, it usually aggravates the candidiasis.

6. Tinea versicolor does not respond to oral griseofulvin therapy.

7. So-called fungal infection of the ear does not respond to oral antifungal therapy. Most external ear diseases are not caused by a fungus (see External Otitis, Chap. 11).

8. Ketoconazole therapy can produce side-effects, including anaphylaxis, hepatotoxicity, and impotence. Consult the current literature on this subject, and monitor the patient carefully.

clinical diseases in Table 19–1. The organism causing tinea versicolor is not included in this table because it does not liberate a keratolytic enzyme.

Clinical Classifications

Superficial fungal infections of the skin affect various sites of the body. The clinical lesions, the species of fungi, and the therapy vary for these different sites. Therefore, fungal diseases of the skin are classified, for clinical purposes, according to the location of the infection. These clinical types are as follows:

Tinea of the feet (tinea pedis)
Tinea of the hands (tinea manus)
Tinea of the nails (onychomycosis)
Tinea of the groin (tinea cruris)
Tinea of the smooth skin (tinea corporis)
Tinea of the scalp (tinea capitis)
Tinea of the beard (tinea barbae)
Dermatophytid
Tinea versicolor (see Chap. 14).
Tinea of the external ear (see External Otitis, Chap. 11).

Tinea of the Feet
(Plates 55 and 56)

Tinea of the feet (athlete's foot, fungal infection of the feet, ringworm of the feet) is a very common skin infection. Many persons have the disease and are not even aware of it. The clinical appearance varies.

PRIMARY LESIONS. *Acute form:* blisters occur on the soles and the sides of feet or between the toes. *Chronic form:* lesions are dry and scaly.

SECONDARY LESIONS. Bacterial infection of the blisters is very common; maceration and fissures are also seen.

COURSE. Recurrent acute infections can lead to a chronic infection. If the toenails become infected, a cure is highly improbable, since this focus is very difficult to eradicate.

The species of fungus influences the response to therapy. Most vesicular, acute fungal infections are due to *T. mentagrophytes* and respond readily to correct treatment. The chronic scaly type of infection is usually due to *T. rubrum* and is exceedingly difficult, if not impossible, to cure.

(text continues on page 208)

Table 19–1
Relationship of Fungi to Body Areas

FUNGUS	FEET AND HANDS	NAILS	GROIN	SMOOTH SKIN	SCALP	BEARD
Microsporum species						
M. audouini	0	0	0	Uncommon	Uncommon	0
M. canis	0	0	0	Common	Uncommon	Rare
M. gypseum	0	0	0	Rare	Rare	0
Epidermophyton species						
E. floccosum	Mod. common	Rare	Common	Mod. common	0	0
Trichophyton species Endothrix species						
T. schoenleini	0	Rare	0	Rare	(Favus) rare	0
T. violaceum	0	Rare	0	0	Rare	Rare
T. tonsurans	0	Rare	0	Rare	Mod. common	0
Ectothrix species						
T. mentagrophytes	Common	Mod. common	Common	Rare	Rare	Mod. common
T. rubrum	Common	Common	Mod. common	Rare	0	Rare
T. verrucosum	0	0	0	Rare	Rare	Rare

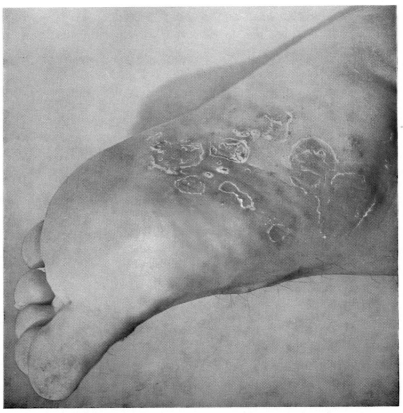

Plate 55. **Tinea of the foot.** This dry, scaly form of fungus infection is usually due to *T. rubrum*. (*Smith Kline & French Laboratories*)

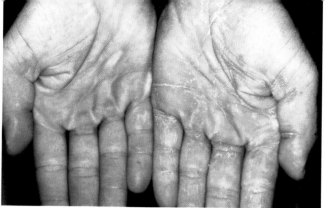

(A) Tinea of the left palm only, due to
T. mentagrophytes

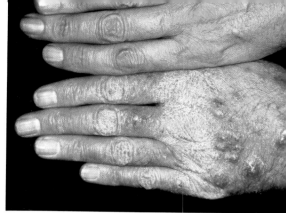

(B) Deep tinea of left hand, due to
T. mentagrophytes

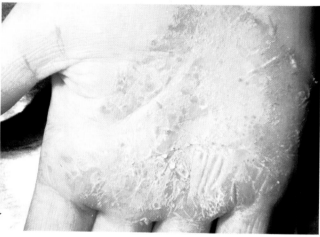

(C) Tinea of the palm, due to *T. rubrum*

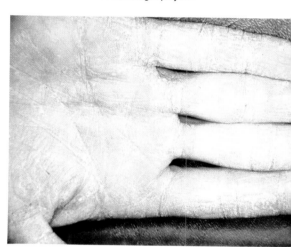

(D) Tinea of the palm, of dry, scaly type,
due to *T. rubrum*

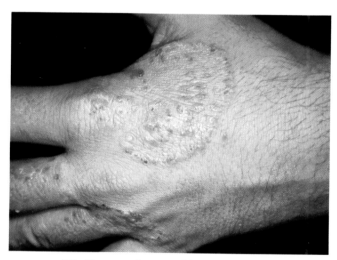

(E) Tinea on dorsum of hand, due to
T. mentagrophytes, in a diabetic, age 15

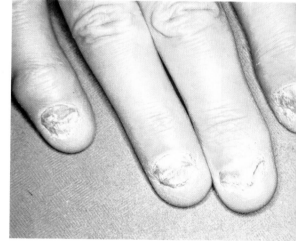

(F) Tinea of fingernails, due to *T. rubrum*

Plate 57. **Tinea of the hand and fingernails.** Tinea of the hand usually affects only one hand, but both feet. Thus, it is called "one hand, two foot syndrome." (*Duke Laboratories, Inc.*)

211

Once developed, the infected nail serves as a resistant focus for future skin infection.

PRIMARY LESIONS. Distal and lateral detachment of the nail occurs with subsequent thickening and deformity.

SECONDARY LESIONS. Bacterial infection can result from the pressure of shoes on the deformed nail and surrounding skin.

DISTRIBUTION. The infection usually begins in the fifth toenail and may remain there or spread to involve the other nails.

COURSE. *Tinea of the toenails can rarely be cured.* Aside from the deformity and an occasional mild flare-up of acute tinea, treatment is not necessary. Progression is slow, and spontaneous cures are rare.

Tinea of the fingernails can be cured, but the treatment usually takes months.

ETIOLOGY. This type of tinea is usually due to *T. rubrum* and, less importantly, to *T. mentagrophytes.*

LABORATORY FINDINGS. These organisms can be found in a KOH preparation of a scraping and occasionally can be grown on culture media. The material should be gathered from the debris under the nail plate.

Differential Diagnosis

(See also Chapter 26, *Diseases Affecting the Nails.*)

Nail injury: get history of injury, although tinea infection often starts in an injured nail; absence of fungi.
Psoriasis of fingernails: pitting, red areas under nail with resulting detachment; psoriasis elsewhere, usually; no fungi found (see Chap. 14).
Psoriasis of toenails: impossible to differentiate from tinea, since most psoriatic nails have some secondary fungal invasion.
Candidiasis of fingernails: common in housewives; paronychial involvement common; Candida found (see later in this chapter).
Green nails: This fingernail infection yields *Candida albicans* and *Pseudomonas aeruginosa* most commonly. Clinically, there is a distal detachment of the nail plate, with underlying greenish brown debris. For cure, complete débridement of the detached part of the nail is necessary, plus local antifungal therapy.

Treatment

TINEA OF FINGERNAILS

A young salesman presents with a fungal infection in three fingernails of 9 months' duration. The surrounding skin shows mild redness and scaling.

1. Griseofulvin therapy. This oral therapy is the treatment of choice.

    Griseofulvin ultrafine types (250–330 mg or equivalent) b.i.d. or t.i.d. is used for approximately 9 months. Therapy is stopped when there is no clinical evidence of infection (crumbling, thickening of nail plate, or subungual debris) and no cultural or KOH-ink mount evidence of fungi.
2. Ketoconazole therapy. If the patient and the physician are aware of the possibility of liver and other toxicity, then a 200-mg tablet once a day for 9 months might be curative. Monitor the patient closely.

TINEA OF TOENAILS

A 45-year-old woman presented with three infected toenails on the right foot and two on the left foot. These are causing mild pain when she wears certain tight-fitting shoes. Scaliness of soles of feet is also evident.

1. Griseofulvin or ketoconazole therapy. This oral therapy is *not* effective or indicated for tinea of the toenails. I have never seen a case that was cured. Apparently some dermatologists have cured cases after oral therapy was continued for several years or when oral therapy was combined with evulsion of the toenails. Nonetheless, I do not recommend it. The only time such therapy for toenails is prescribed, in my practice, is when the patient understands the problem but still wants to attempt a cure or a cosmetic improvement. At least 12 months of griseofulvin therapy is necessary. Women respond to this therapy better than men.
2. Antifungal solution, 15 ml.

    For the patient who wants to "do something," applications two to four times a day for months might help some mild cases. One can combine this therapy with débridement of the nails.
3. Débriding of thick nails by patient, dermatologist, or podiatrist offers obvious relief from discomfort. This can be accomplished by the use of nail clippers or filing or picking away with a broken piece of

glass, knife, or a motor-driven drill (see Chap. 37).

4. Surgical evulsion of the toenail is rarely curative. As stated previously, this surgical approach can be combined with oral griseofulvin therapy with probable enhancement of the end result.

Tinea of the Groin
(Fig. 19–2)

Tinea of the groin is a common, itching, annoying fungal infection appearing usually in men and often concurrently with tinea of the feet. Home remedies often result in a contact dermatitis that adds "fuel to the fire."

PRIMARY LESIONS. Bilateral, fan-shaped, red, scaly patches with a sharp, slightly raised border occur. Small vesicles may be seen in the active border.

SECONDARY LESIONS. Oozing, crusting, edema, and secondary bacterial infection are evident. In chronic cases lichenification may be marked.

DISTRIBUTION. The infection affects the crural fold, extending to involve scrotum, penis, thighs, perianal area, and buttocks.

COURSE. The type of fungus influences the course, but most acute cases respond rapidly to treatment. Other factors that affect the course and recurrences are obesity, hot weather, sweating, and chafing garments.

ETIOLOGY. Tinea of the groin is commonly due to the fungi of tinea of the feet, *T. rubrum,* and *T. mentagrophytes,* and also the fungus *E. floccosum.*

CONTAGIOUSNESS. This is minimal, even between husband and wife.

LABORATORY FINDINGS. The organism is found in KOH preparations of scrapings and can be grown on culture. Take material from the active border (see Chap. 2).

Differential Diagnosis

Candidiasis: no sharp border; fine scales, oozing, redness, satellite pustule-like lesions at edges; more common in obese females; *Candida* found (see later in this chapter and Plate 60).

Contact dermatitis: often coexistent but can be separate entity; new contactant history; no fungi found; no active border (see Chap. 9).

Prickly heat: pustular, papular; no active border, no fungi; may also be present with tinea (see Chap. 36).

Neurodermatitis: unilateral, usually; may have resulted from old chronic tinea; no fungi (see Chap. 11).

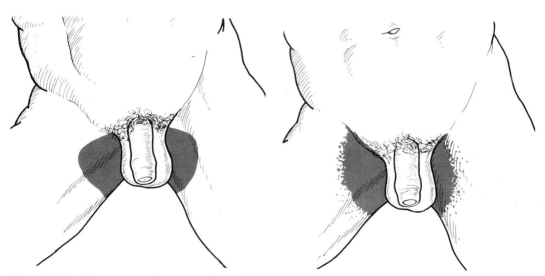

Figure 19–2. Dermograms for comparison of tinea of crural area and candidiasis of crural area. (*Left*) Tinea of crural area. Note sharp border of lesions. (See also Plate 58.) (*Right*) Candidiasis of crural area. Note indefinite border with satellite pustule-like lesions as edge. Candidiasis can also involve the scrotum. (See also Plate 61.)

Psoriasis: usually unilateral; may or may not have raised border; psoriasis elsewhere; no fungi (see Chap. 14).

Erythrasma: faint redness, fine scaling with no elevated border, also seen in axilla and webs of toes; reddish fluorescence under Wood's light; due to a diphtheroid organism called *Corynebacterium minutissimum* (see Chap. 15).

Treatment

1. Oozing, red dermatitis with sharp border occurs in crural area of young man.
   A. Since the infection usually comes from chronic tinea of the feet, to prevent recurrences advise the patient to dry the feet last and not the groin area last when taking a bath.
   B. Vinegar wet packs
      Sig: ½ cup of white vinegar to 1 quart of warm water. Wet the sheeting or thin toweling and apply to area for 15 minutes twice a day.
   C. Antifungal cream   15.0
      or Lotrisone cream   15.0
      Sig: b.i.d. locally.
      The Lotrisone cream contains a moderate-potency corticosteroid that can only be used for a short time (up to 6 weeks) in the groin or anal areas. Striae or atrophy could develop.

SAUER NOTE:

An effective therapy for tinea of the groin is:

Sulfur, ppt.	5%
Hydrocortisone	1%
Antifungal cream q.s.	15.0

Sig: Apply b.i.d. locally, and continue for 7 days after apparently clear (therapy-plus routine).

   D. Griseofulvin oral therapy
      Griseofulvin ultrafine types 250–330 mg
      Sig: 1 tab b.i.d. for 6 to 8 weeks for extensive case.
   E. Ketoconazole therapy is usually not indicated.

Tinea of the Smooth Skin
(Plates 58, 59, and 93E)

The familiar ringworm of the skin is most common in children because of their intimacy with animals and other children. The lay public believes that *most* skin conditions are "ringworm," and many physicians erroneously agree with them.

PRIMARY LESIONS. Round, oval, or semicircular scaly patches have a slightly raised border that commonly is vesicular. Rarely, deep, ulcerated, granulomatous lesions are due to superficial fungi.

SECONDARY LESIONS. Bacterial infection, particularly at the advancing border, is common in association with certain fungi, such as *M. canis* and *T. mentagrophytes.*

COURSE. Infection is short lived, if treated correctly. It seldom recurs unless treatment is inadequate.

ETIOLOGY. This disorder is most commonly due to *M. canis* from kittens and puppies and less commonly due to *E. floccosum* and *T. mentagrophytes* from groin and foot infections.

CONTAGIOUSNESS. The incidence is high.

LABORATORY FINDINGS. Same as for previously discussed fungal diseases.

Differential Diagnosis

Pityriasis rosea: history of herald patch; sudden shower of oval lesions; fungi not found (see Chap. 14).

Impetigo: vesicular, crusted; most commonly on face; no fungi found (see Chap. 15).

Contact dermatitis: no sharp border or central healing; may be coexistent with ringworm worsened by overtreatment (see Chap. 9).

Treatment

A child has several 2- to 4-cm sized scaly lesions on his arms of 1 week's duration. He has a new kitten that he holds and plays with.

1. Examine the scalp, preferably with a Wood's light, to rule out scalp infection.
2. Advise the mother regarding moderate isolation procedures in relation to the family and others.

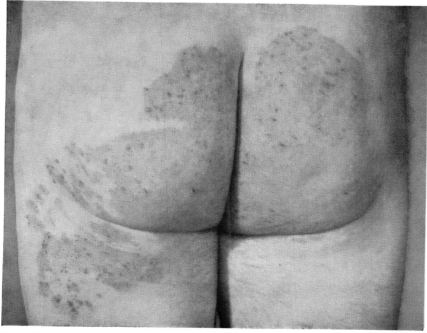

Plate 58. **Tinea of the smooth skin.** This infection on the buttocks had spread from the crural region. (*Smith Kline & French Laboratories*)

3. Antifungal salve q.s.   15.0
   Sig: Apply b.i.d. locally.
   (Antifungal bases that can be used are listed on p. 208 under Tinea of the Feet.)

SUBSEQUENT VISIT OF RESISTANT CASE OR A NEW WIDESPREAD CASE: GRISEOFULVIN ORAL THERAPY

Griseofulvin (ultrafine types) can be given in tablet or oral suspension form. The usual dose for children is 165 mg b.i.d., but the pharmaceutical company's product information sheet should be consulted. Therapy should be maintained for 3 to 6 weeks or until lesions are gone. Occasionally a higher dose is needed in deeper forms of infection.

Ketoconazole therapy is usually not necessary or indicated.

Tinea of the Scalp
(Plate 93)

Tinea of the scalp is the most common cause of patchy hair loss in children (Fig. 19–3). Endemic cases are with us always, but epidemics, usually due to the human type, were, until the discovery of griseofulvin, the real therapeutic problem. Griseofulvin orally

finds its greatest therapeutic usefulness and triumph in the management of tinea of the scalp. Before griseofulvin, children with the human type of scalp tinea had to be subjected to traumatic shampoos and salves for weeks or months, or they had to be epilated by x-ray. Often they were kept out of school for this entire period of therapy.

Ketoconazole systemic therapy is available for griseofulvin resistant cases, if these truly occur in tinea of the scalp.

Tinea capitis infections can be divided into two clinical types: (1) *noninflammatory* and (2) *inflammatory*. The treatment, the cause, and the course vary for these two types.

Noninflammatory Type

PRIMARY LESIONS. Grayish, scaly, round patches with broken-off hairs are seen, causing balding areas. The size of the areas varies.

SECONDARY LESIONS. Bacterial infection and id reactions are rare. A noninflammatory patch can become inflamed spontaneously or as the result of strong local treatment. Scarring almost never occurs. "Black dot" hairs are seen with *T. tonsurans* infection.

(text continues on page 218)

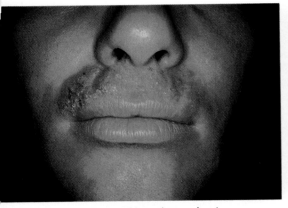

(A) Tinea of beard area due to
T. mentagrophytes

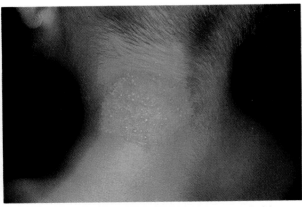

(B) Tinea of posterior neck area probably
due to *T. verrucosum*

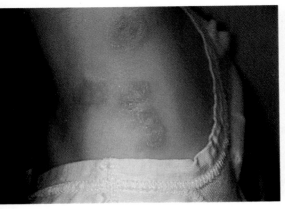

(C) Tinea of side of neck due to
T. mentagrophytes

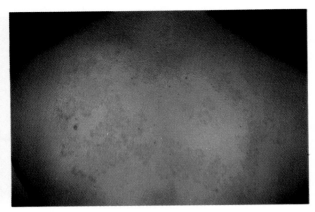

(D) Extensive tinea of back

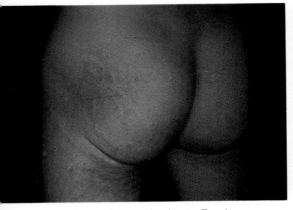

(E) Tinea of buttocks due to *T. rubrum*

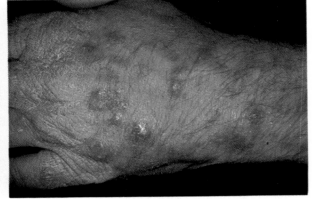

(F) Tinea profundus on dorsum of hand due to
T. mentagrophytes

Plate 59. **Tinea of smooth skin and of beard.** (*Ortho Pharmaceutical Corp.*)

(*A*) Due to *M. audouini.* Note absence of visible inflammation.

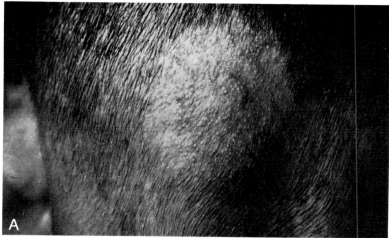

(*B*) Due to *T. tonsurans.* Wood's light examination revealed no fluorescence.

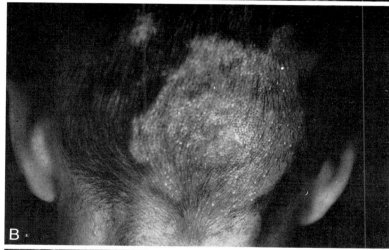

(*C*) Due to *T. mentagrophytes.* Note inflammation.

(*D*) Favus, due to *T. schoenleini,* of 11 years' duration

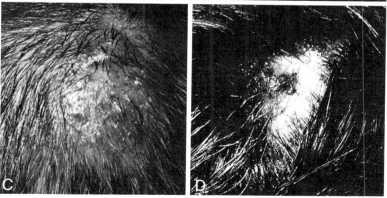

Figure 19–3   **Tinea of the scalp.** (See also Plate 93)

DISTRIBUTION. The infection is most common in the posterior scalp region. Body ringworm from the scalp lesions is common, particularly on the neck and the shoulders.

SAUER NOTES:

1. Examine the scalp in any child who has body ringworm.
2. *Perform hair KOH mounts, cultures, or Wood's light examination of suspicious scalp areas.*

COURSE. The incubation period in and on the hair is short, but clinical evidence of the infection cannot be expected less than 3 weeks after inoculation. Parents often do not notice the infection for another 3 weeks to several months, particularly in girls. Spontaneous cures are rare in 2 to 6 months but after that time occur with greater frequency. Some cases last for years, if untreated. Recurrence of the infection after the cure of a previous episode is rare but not impossible, since adequate immunity does not develop.

AGE-GROUP. Infection of the noninflammatory type is most common between the ages of 3 and 8 and is rare after the age of puberty. This adult resistance to infection is attributed in part to the higher content of fungistatic fatty acids in the sebum after puberty. This research laboratory finding had great therapeutic significance, and the direct outgrowth was the development of Desenex, Timofax, Salundek, and other fatty acid ointments and powders.

T. tonsurans infection is mainly seen in black urban preadolescent children. Spontaneous cures at puberty, particularly for girls, do not always occur.

ETIOLOGY. The noninflammatory type of scalp ringworm is caused most frequently by *T. tonsurans* and occasionally by *M. canis* and *M. audouini*. *M. audouini* and *T. tonsurans* are anthropophilic fungi (human-to-human passage only), whereas *M. canis* is a zoophilic fungus (animals are the original source, mainly kittens and puppies).

CONTAGIOUSNESS. The case can be a part of a large urban epidemic.

LABORATORY FINDINGS. *Wood's light examination of the scalp hairs* is an important diagnostic test, but hairs infected with *T. tonsurans* do not fluoresce. The Wood's light is a specially filtered ultraviolet light. The hairs infected with *M. audouini* and *M. canis* fluoresce with a bright yellowish green color (see Plate 93). *The bright fluorescence of fungus-infected hairs is not to be confused with the white or dull yellow color emitted by lint particles or sulfur-laden scales.* An inexpensive but excellent Wood's light is described in Chapter 37.

Microscopic examination of the infected hairs in 20% KOH solution shows an ectothrix arrangement of the spores when due to the *Microsporum* species and endothrix spores when due to *T. tonsurans*. Culture is necessary for species identification (see Fig. 2–4). The cultural characteristics of the various fungi can be found in many larger dermatologic or mycologic texts and will not be presented here.

Prophylactic Treatment

1. Infected persons may attend school, provided that (a) the child wears a cotton stockinette cap at all times (no swapping allowed) and (b) a note must be presented from the physician every 3 weeks, stating that the child is under a physician's care. Infected children should be restricted from theaters, churches, and other public places. Consult your own health department for specific rulings.
2. Inspection of all susceptible schoolchildren with a Wood's light by school nurse every 4 weeks during an epidemic.
3. Wash hair after every haircut by a barber or beautician.
4. Provide parent and teacher education on methods of spread of disease, particularly during an epidemic.
5. Suggest provision for individual storage of clothing, particularly caps, in school and home.

Active Treatment

1. Griseofulvin oral therapy. The ultrafine types of griseofulvin (Fulvicin U/F, Fulvicin P/G, Gris-Peg, Grifulvin V, and Grisactin) can be administered in tablet form or liquid suspension (not all brands available

in liquid form). The usual dose for a child aged 4 to 8 is 250 mg b.i.d., but some require a larger dose. The duration of therapy is usually 6 to 8 weeks. Both dose and duration have to be individualized and based on clinical, Wood's light, or culture response.

2. Ketoconazole oral therapy. This type of therapy is usually not indicated or necessary. For children aged 2 to 12 the minimum dosage is 3.3 mg/kg/day.

3. Manual epilation of hairs. Near the end of therapy, the remaining infected and fluorescent hairs can be plucked out, or the involved area can be shaved closely. This will eliminate the infected distal end of the growing hair.

Inflammatory Type

PRIMARY LESIONS. Pustular, scaly, round patches with broken-off hairs are found, resulting in bald areas.

SECONDARY LESIONS. Bacterial-like infection is common. When the secondary reaction is marked, the area becomes swollen and tender. This inflammation is called a *kerion.* Minimal scarring sometimes remains.

DISTRIBUTION. Any scalp area is involved. Concurrent body ringworm infection is common.

COURSE. Duration is much shorter than the noninflammatory type of infection. Spontaneous cures will result after 2 to 4 months in many cases, even if untreated, except for the *T. tonsurans* type.

ETIOLOGY. The inflammatory type of scalp ringworm is most commonly caused by *T. tonsurans* and *M. canis* and rarely by *M. audouini,* *M. gypseum,* *T. mentagrophytes,* and *T. verrucosum.* Except for *T. tonsurans* and *M. audouini* the species are zoophilic, that is, passed from infected animals or soil.

CONTAGIOUSNESS. The incidence is high in children and farmers. It is mainly endemic, except for cases due to *M. audouini.*

LABORATORY FINDINGS. Microscopic examination of the infected hairs in 20% KOH solution shows an ectothrix arrangement of the spores, but *T. tonsurans* shows endothrix spores. The hairs infected with *M. canis* and *M. audouini* fluoresce with a bright yellowish green color under the Wood's light.

DIFFERENTIAL DIAGNOSIS (see Table 19–2).

Prophylactic Treatment

This is the same as for noninflammatory cases.

Active Treatment

1. Griseofulvin oral therapy (as under noninflammatory type).

2. Local therapy. For some mild cases of the inflammatory type, or where drug expense is a factor, local therapy can be used with good results.

Bactroban Ointment   15.0

Sig: Apply locally b.i.d. The scalp and the hair should be shampooed nightly.

Table 19–2
Differential Diagnosis of Scalp Dermatoses

DERMATOSIS	WOOD'S LIGHT	SCALES	REDNESS	HAIR LOSS	REMARKS
Tinea capitis	±	Dry or crusted	Uncommon	Yes	Back of scalp, child
Alopecia areata (Chap. 16)	−	None	No	Yes	Exclamation point hairs at edges
Seborrheic dermatitis (Chap. 13)	−	Greasy	Yes	No	Diffuse scaling
Psoriasis (Chap. 14)	−	Thick and dry	Yes	No	Look at elbows, knees, and nails
Trichotillomania (Chap. 27)	−	None	No	Yes	Psychoneurotic child
Pyoderma (Chap. 15) (with or without lice)	−	Crusted	Yes	Occasional	Poor hygiene

3. If kerion is severe, with or without griseofulvin therapy:
   A. Burow's solution wet packs.
      Sig: 1 Domeboro packet to 1 pint of warm water. Apply soaked cloths for 15 minutes twice a day.
   B. Antibiotic therapy orally helps to eliminate secondary bacterial infection.

Tinea of the Beard
(Plate 59)

Fungal infection is a rare cause of dermatitis in the beard area. Farmers occasionally contract it from infected cattle. Any presumed bacterial infection of the beard that does not respond readily to proper treatment should be examined for fungi.

PRIMARY LESIONS. Follicular, pustular, or sharp-bordered ringworm-type lesions or deep, boggy, inflammatory masses are seen.

SECONDARY LESIONS. Bacterial infection is common. Scarring is unusual.

ETIOLOGY (see Table 19–1).

Differential Diagnosis

Bacterial folliculitis: acute onset, rapid spread; no definite border; responds rather rapidly to local therapy; no fungi found on examination of hairs or culture (see Chap. 15).

Treatment

A farmer presents with a quarter-sized, boggy, inflammatory, pustular mass on his chin of 3 weeks' duration.

1. Have veterinarian inspect cattle, if farmer is not aware of source of infection.
2. Burow's solution wet packs
   Sig: 1 Domeboro packet to 1 pint of hot water. Apply wet cloths to area for 15 minutes t.i.d.
3. Antifungal cream, q.s.   15.0
   Sig: Apply locally b.i.d.
4. Griseofulvin oral therapy. The usual dose of griseofulvin, ultrafine type, for an adult is 250 to 330 mg b.i.d. for 6 to 8 weeks or longer, depending on clinical response or negative Sabouraud's culture.

5. Ketoconazole therapy. Therapy with this agent is rarely indicated.

Dermatophytid

During an acute episode of any fungal infection, an id eruption can develop over the body. This is a manifestation of an allergic reaction to the fungal infection. The most common id reaction occurs on the hands during an acute tinea infection on the feet. To assume a diagnosis of an id reaction, the following criteria should be followed: (1) the primary focus should be acutely infected with fungi, not chronically infected; (2) the id lesions must not contain fungi; and (3) the id eruption should disappear or wane following adequate treatment of the acute focus.

PRIMARY LESIONS. Vesicular eruption of the hands (primary lesion on the feet) and papulofollicular eruption on body (primary lesion commonly is scalp kerion) are found; pityriasis rosea–like id eruptions and others are seen less commonly.

SECONDARY LESIONS. Excoriation and infection occur, when itching is severe, which is unusual.

Treatment

1. Treat the primary focus of infection.
2. For a vesicular id reaction on the *hands:*
   A. Burow's solution soaks
      Sig: 1 Domeboro packet to 1 quart of cool water. Soak hands for 15 minutes b.i.d.
3. For an id reaction on the *body* that is moderately pruritic:
   A. Aveeno oatmeal bath
      Sig: 1 packet of Aveeno to 6 to 8 inches of cool water in a tub, once daily.
   B. Hydrocortisone 1% lotion   120.0
      Sig: Apply locally b.i.d.
      Menthol 0.25%, phenol 0.5%, or camphor 2% could be added to this lotion.
4. For a severely itching, *generalized* id eruption:
   A. Prednisone, 10 mg, or related corticosteroid tablets   #30
      Sig: 1 tablet q.i.d. for 2 days, then 2 tablets every morning for 7 days (or longer if necessary).

DEEP FUNGAL INFECTIONS

Those fungi that invade the skin deeply and go into living tissue are also capable of involving other organs. Only the skin manifestations of these deeply invading fungi will be discussed here.

The following diseases are included in this group of deep fungal infections (other, rarer, deep mycotic diseases will be found in the Dictionary-Index and in Chapter 36, *Geographic Skin Diseases*):

Candidiasis
Sporotrichosis
North American blastomycosis

Systemic fungus infections that were extremely rare are now being seen more frequently in those patients who are immunocompromised, such as patients on chemotherapy, organ transplant cases, and those with the acquired immunodeficiency syndrome.

Candidiasis
(Plates 60 through 62)

Candidiasis (moniliasis) is a fungal infection caused by *Candida albicans* that produces lesions in the mouth, the vagina, the skin, the nails, the lungs, or the gastrointestinal tract or occasionally a septicemia. The latter condition is seen in patients who are on long-term, high-dose antibiotic therapy and in those who are immunosuppressed. Since *C. albicans* exists commonly as a harmless skin inhabitant, the laboratory findings of this organism is not adequate proof of its pathogenicity and etiologic role. *Candida* commonly seed preexisting disease conditions. Concern here is with the *cutaneous* and the *mucocutaneous* candidal diseases. The following classification will be helpful.

I. **Cutaneous Candidiasis**
   A. *Localized Diseases*
      1. Candidal paronychia (see Plate 75). This common candidal infection is characterized by development of painful, red swellings of the skin around the nail plate. In chronic infections the nail becomes secondarily thickened and hardened. Candidal paronychia is commonly seen in housewives and those persons whose occupations predispose to frequent immersion of the hands in water.

      This nail involvement is to be differentiated from *superficial tinea of the nails* (the candidal infection does not cause the nail to lose its luster or to become crumbly, and debris does not accumulate beneath the nail) and from *bacterial paronychia* (this is more acute in onset and throbs with pain).

      2. Candidal intertrigo (see Fig. 19–2 and Plates 60 and 62). This moderately common condition is characterized by well-defined, red, eroded patches, with scaly, pustular or pustulovesicular diffuse borders. The most common sites are axillae, inframammary areas, umbilicus, genital area, anal area, and webs of toes and fingers. Obesity, diabetes, and systemic antibiotics predispose to the development of this intertriginous type.

      It is to be differentiated from *superficial tinea infections*, which are not as red and eroded, and from *seborrheic dermatitis*.
   B. *Generalized Cutaneous Candidiasis.* (see Plate 89) This rare infection involves the smooth skin, mucocutaneous orifices, and intertriginous areas. It follows in the wake of general debility, as seen in immunosuppressed patients, and was very resistant to treatment prior to the discovery of ketoconazole.

II. **Mucous Membrane Candidiasis** (see Plate 60)
   A. *Oral Candidiasis* (*Thrush* and *Perlèche*). Thrush is characterized by creamy white flakes on a red, inflamed mucous membrane. The tongue may be smooth and atrophic, or the papillae may be hypertrophic, as in the condition labeled "hairy tongue." Therapy with Mycostatin Pastilles (lozenges) is effective. Perlèche is seen as cracks or fissures at the corners of the mouth, usually associated with

(text continues on page 224)

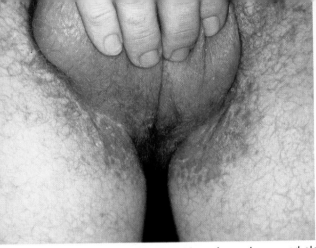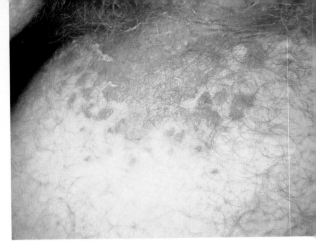

(*A* and *B*) Candidal intertrigo of crural area and close-up showing satellite lesions without the sharp border as seen in tinea cruris

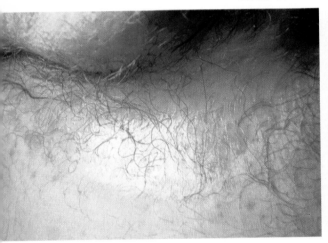

(*C*) Moist candidal intertrigo of crural area

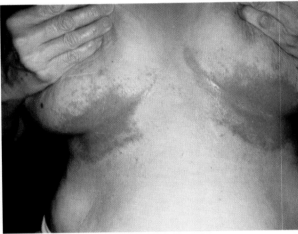

(*D*) Candidal intertrigo under breasts

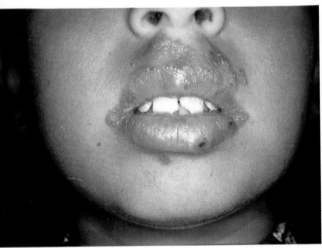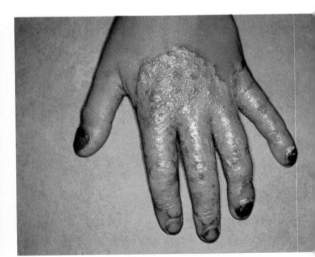

((*E* and *F*) Extensive candidiasis around the mouth and on dorsum of hand in child with Addison's disease

Plate 60. **Candidal infections.** (*See also* Plate 75, for candidal paronychia, and Plates 89 and 91, for infant candidal diseases.) (*Herbert Laboratories*)

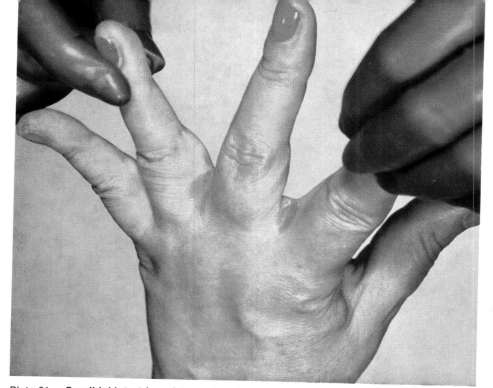

Plate 61. **Candidal intertrigo of the webs of the fingers.** (*Smith Kline & French Laboratories*)

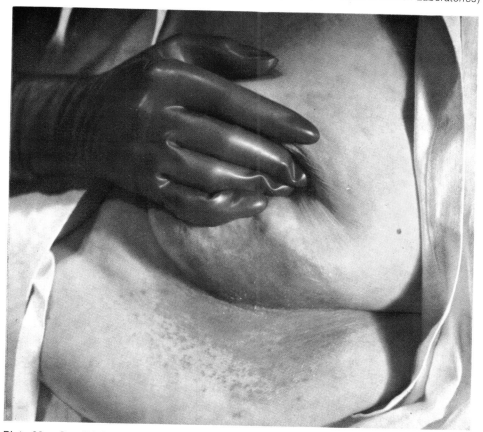

Plate 62. **Candidal intertrigo under the breast.** Note the lack of a definite border to the eruption, which distinguishes it from a tinea infection. (*Smith Kline & French Laboratories*)

candidal disease elsewhere, and a dietary deficiency. Thrush is seen commonly in immunosuppressed patients.

A noncandidal, clinically similar condition is commonly seen in *elderly persons with ill-fitting dentures* where the corners of the mouth override. Oral candidiasis is also to be differentiated from allergic conditions, such as those due to toothpaste or mouthwash.

B. *Candidal Vulvovaginitis.* The clinical picture is an oozing, red, sharply bordered skin infection surrounding an inflamed vagina that contains a buttermilk-like discharge. This type of candidal infection is frequently seen in pregnant women, diabetics, and those who have been on antibiotics systemically.

It is to be differentiated from an *allergic condition,* or from *trichomonal vaginitis.*

LABORATORY FINDINGS. Skin or mucous membrane scrapings placed in 20% KOH solution and examined with the high-power microscope lens will reveal small, oval, budding, thin-walled, yeastlike cells with occasional mycelia. Culture on Sabouraud's media will produce creamy dull-white colonies in 4 to 5 days. Further cultural studies on corn meal agar are necessary to identify the species as *C. albicans.*

Treatment

CASE 1

Candidal paronychia of two fingers is seen in a 37-year-old male bartender.

1. Advise patient concerning avoiding exposure of his hands to soap and water by wearing cotton gloves under rubber gloves, hiring a dishwasher, and so on.
2. Antifungal imidazole-type solution (Lotrimin or Mycelex Solution 1%)   15.0
   or Fungi-Nail   15.0
   Sig: Apply to base of nail q.i.d. (Continue treatment for several weeks.)
3. At night, apply:
   Lotrisone cream   15.0
   Sig: Apply locally h.s.

CASE 2

Candidal intertrigo of inframammary and crural region is seen in an elderly obese woman.

1. Advise the patient to wear pieces of cotton sheeting under breasts to keep the opposing tissues drier. Frequent bathing with through drying is helpful. Avoid use of an antibacterial soap.
2. Sulfur, ppt.   5%
   Hydrocortisone   1%
   Mycostatin cream, q.s.   30.0
   Sig: Apply locally t.i.d.
   (I prefer this compounded medication with Mycostatin cream as the base over the imidazole-type creams.)
3. Powder can be used over cream:
   Mycostatin Dusting Powder, q.s.   15.0
   Sig: Apply locally t.i.d.
4. Lotrisone cream   15.0
   Use b.i.d. for a short time only. It can cause atrophy and striae in intertriginous areas. *Limit the number of refills.*

CASE 3

Candidal vulvovaginitis is found in a woman who is 6 months' pregnant.

1. Mycostatin vaginal tablets, 100,000 units   #20
   Sig: Insert 1 tablet b.i.d. in vagina.
2. Monistat-Derm lotion, or
   Sulfur, ppt.   5%
   Hydrocortisone   1%
   Mycostatin cream, q.s.   30.0
   Sig: Apply locally b.i.d. to vulvar skin.

SAUER NOTES:

Do not treat a candidal infection with oral griseofulvin. This will intensify the candidal infection.

KETOCONAZOLE (Nizoral) THERAPY. In general this systemic therapy is rarely indicated for routine candidal infections. For chronic mucocutaneous candidiasis, ketoconazole can heal dramatically. For dosage information, study the package insert, or the bibliography. Monitor the patient carefully.

Sporotrichosis
(Plates 63 and 102)

Sporotrichosis is a granulomatous fungal infection of the skin and the subcutaneous tissues. Characteristically, a primary chancre

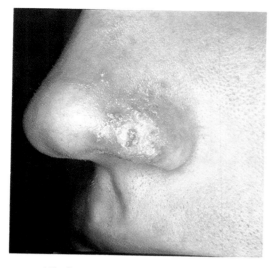

(A) Sporotrichotic primary lesion on the nose

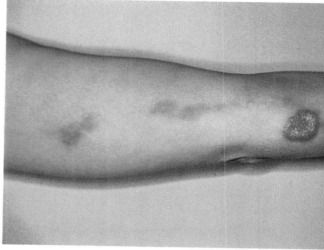

(B) Sporotrichotic chancre on arm with subcutaneous nodules

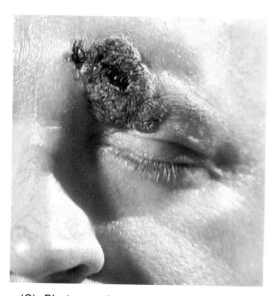

(C) Blastomycotic primary lesion of eyebrow

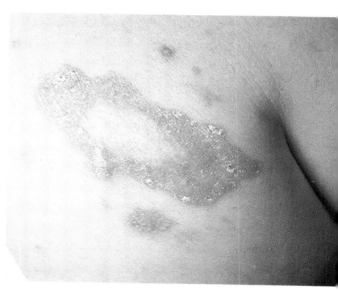

(D) Blastomycotic primary lesion on scapular area

Plate 63. **Deep fungus infections.** (*Stiefel Laboratories* [in part])

precedes more extensive skin involvement. Invasion of the internal viscera is rare (see Chap. 36).

PRIMARY LESION. A sporotrichotic chancre develops at the site of skin inoculation, which is commonly the hand and less commonly the face or the feet. The chancre begins as a painless, movable, subcutaneous nodule that eventually softens and breaks down to form an ulcer.

SECONDARY LESIONS. Within a few weeks subcutaneous nodules arise along the course of the draining lymphatics and form a chain of tumors that develop into ulcers. This is the classic clinical picture, of which there are variations.

COURSE. The development of the skin lesions is slow and rarely affects the general health.

ETIOLOGY. The causative agent is *Sporothrix schenckii*, a fungus that grows on wood and in the soil. It invades open wounds and is an occupational hazard of farmers, laborers, and miners.

LABORATORY FINDINGS. Cultures of the purulent material from unopened lesions readily grow on Sabouraud's media.

Differential Diagnosis

Consider any of the skin granulomas, such as *pyodermas, syphilis, tuberculosis, sarcoidosis,* and *leprosy.* An *ioderma* or *bromoderma* can cause a similar clinical picture.

Treatment

1. Saturated solution of potassium iodide, 60.0 ml
   Sig: On the first day, 10 drops t.i.d., p.c. added to milk or water; second day, 15 drops t.i.d.; third day, 20 drops t.i.d. and increase until 30 to 40 drops t.i.d. is given.

The initial doses may be smaller and the increase more gradual if one is concerned about tolerance. Watch for gastric irritation and ioderma. Continue this very specific treatment for 1 month after apparent cure.

2. Ketoconazole therapy.
   Ketoconazole (Nizoral), 200 mg
   Sig: 2 tablets a day for 8 weeks.
   Some cases are not helped. Monitor the patient closely as usual.

North American Blastomycosis
(Plate 63)

Two cutaneous forms of this disease are seen: (1) primary cutaneous blastomycosis and (2) secondary localized cutaneous blastomycosis.

Primary cutaneous blastomycosis occurs in laboratory workers and physicians following accidental inoculation. A primary chancre develops at the site of the inoculation, and the regional nodes enlarge. In a short time the primary lesion and nodes heal spontaneously, and the cure is complete.

The following discussion will be confined to the *secondary cutaneous form.* Systemic blastomycosis is rarer than the cutaneous forms but is seen occasionally in immunosuppressed patients.

PRIMARY LESION (secondary, localized, cutaneous form). The lesion begins as a papule that ulcerates and slowly spreads peripherally, with a warty, pustular, raised border. The face, the hands, and the feet are involved most commonly.

SECONDARY LESION. Central healing of the ulcer occurs gradually with resultant thick scar.

COURSE. A large lesion develops over several months. Therapy is moderately effective on a long-term basis. Relapses are common.

ETIOLOGY. The fungus *Blastomyces dermatitidis* is believed to invade the lungs primarily and the skin secondarily as a metastic lesion. High native immunity prevents the development of more than one skin lesion. This immunity is low in the rare systemic form of blastomycosis in which multiple lesions occur in the skin, the bones, and other organs. This fungal disease affects adult males most frequently.

LABORATORY FINDINGS. Collect the material for a 20% KOH solution mount from the pustules at the border of the lesion. Round, budding organisms can be found in this manner or in a culture mount. A chest roentgenogram is indicated in every case.

Differential Diagnosis

Consider any of the granuloma-producing diseases, such as *tuberculosis, syphilis, iodide or bromide drug eruption, pyoderma,* and *neoplasm.*

Treatment

1. Surgical excision and plastic repair of early lesions is quite effective.
2. Amphotericin B suppresses the chronic lesion more effectively than any other drug. It is administered by intravenous infusion, daily, in varying schedules, which are described in larger texts or reviews.
3. Ketoconazole therapy on a long-term basis is also beneficial. Higher than normal dosages for a longer period of time are necessary for immunosuppressed patients.

BIBLIOGRAPHY

Andre J, Achten G: Onychomycosis. Int J Dermatol 26:481, 1987

Conti-Diaz IA, Civila E, Asconegui F: Treatment of superficial and deep-seated mycoses with oral ketoconazole. Int J Dermatol 23:207, 1984

Herbert AA: Tinea capitis. Arch Dermatol 124:1554, 1988

Hudson CP, Callen JP: Systemic blastomycosis treated with ketoconzole. Arch Dermatol 120:536, 1984

Koneman EW, Roberts GD: Practical Laboratory Mycology, 3rd ed. Baltimore, Williams & Wilkins, 1985

Lambert DR, Siegle RJ, Camisa C: Griseofulvin and ketoconazole in the treatment of dermatophyte infections. Int J Dermatol 28:300, 1989

Lesher JL, Smith JG: Antifungal agents in dermatology. J Am Acad Dermatol 17:383, 1987

Matsumoto T, Ajello L: Current taxonomic concepts pertaining to the dermatophytes and related fungi. Int J Dermatol 26:491, 1987

Radentz WH: Opportunistic fungal infections in immunocompromised hosts. J Am Acad Dermatol 20:989, 1989

Terrell CL, Hermans PE: Antifungal agents used for deep-seated mycotic infections. Mayo Clin Proc 62:1116, 1987

Weitzman I: Saprophytic molds as agents of cutaneous and subcutaneous infection in the immunocompromised host. Arch Dermatol 122:1161, 1986

20

Granulomatous Dermatoses

When considered singularly these diseases are uncommon, but when all of the multitudinous granulomatous diseases are considered together, they form a group that is interesting, varied, and ubiquitous.

A granuloma is a focal chronic inflammatory response to tissue injury manifested by a histologic picture of an accumulation and proliferation of leukocytes, principally of the mononuclear type and its family of derivatives, the mononuclear phagocyte system. The immunologic components in granulomatous inflammation originate from cell-mediated or delayed hypersensitivity mechanisms controlled by thymus-dependent lymphocytes (T lymphocytes). Five groups of granulomatous inflammations have been promulgated (see Hirsh and Johnson in Bibliography):

Group 1 is the *epithelioid granulomas,* which include sarcoidosis, tuberculosis in certain forms, tuberculoid leprosy, tertiary syphilis, zirconium granuloma, beryllium granuloma, mercurial granuloma, and lichen nitidus.

Group 2, *histiocytic granulomas,* includes lepromatous leprosy, histoplasmosis, and leishmaniasis.

Group 3 is the group of *foreign-body granulomas,* including endogenous products (*e.g.,* hair, fat, keratin), minerals (*e.g.,* tattoos, silica, talc), plant and animal products (*e.g.,* cactus, suture, oil, insect parts), and synthetic agents such as synthetic hair.

Group 4 are the *necrobiotic/palisading granulomas,* such as granuloma annulare, necrobiosis lipoidica, rheumatoid nodule,

rheumatic fever nodule, cat-scratch disease, and lymphogranuloma venereum.

Group 5 is the *mixed inflammatory granulomas,* including many deep fungus infections such as blastomycosis and sporotrichosis, mycobacterial infections, granuloma inguinale, and chronic granulomatous disease.

Most of the above varied diseases are discussed with their appropriate etiologic classifications in the Dictionary-Index. Two of these granulomatous inflammations will be discussed in this chapter: *sarcoidosis,* which is an epithelioid granuloma in group 1, and *granuloma annulare,* which is in group 4 of necrobiotic/palisading granulomas.

SARCOIDOSIS
(Plate 64)

Sarcoidosis is an uncommon systemic granulomatous disease of unknown cause that affects skin, lungs, lymph nodes, liver, spleen, bones, and eyes. Any one of these organs or all of them may be involved with sarcoid granulomas. Lymphadenopathy is the most common single finding. Blacks are affected more often than whites. Only the skin manifestations of sarcoidosis will be discussed.

PRIMARY LESIONS. The superficial lesions consist of reddish papules, nodules, and plaques, which may be multiple or solitary and of varying size and configuration. Annular forms of skin sarcoidosis are common. These superficial lesions usually involve the face,

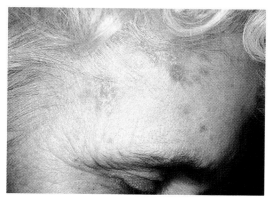

(A) Sarcoid of the forehead

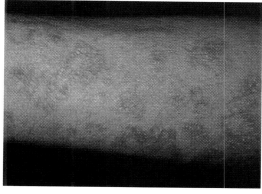

(B) Sarcoid on the forearm

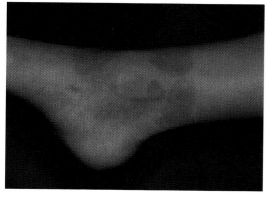

(C) Granuloma annulare on ankle
area

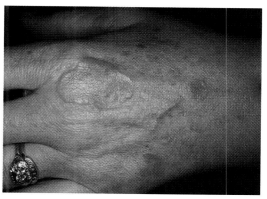

(D) Granuloma annulare on dorsum
of hand

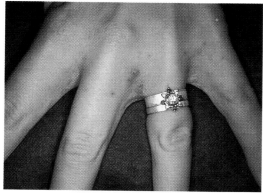

(E) Scabies on finger webs

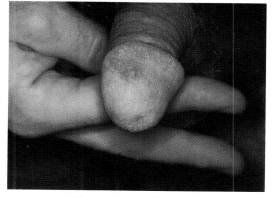

(F) Scabies on the penis

Plate 64. **Granulomas and scabies.** (*Hoechst-Roussel Pharmaceuticals Inc.*)

the shoulders, and the arms. Subcutaneous nodular forms and telangiectatic lesions are more rare.

SECONDARY LESIONS. Central healing can result in atrophy and scarring.

COURSE. Most cases of sarcoidosis run a chronic but benign course with remissions and exacerbations. Spontaneous "cure" is not unusual.

ETIOLOGY. The exact cause is unknown, but the clinicopathologic picture undoubtedly can be caused by several agents, including bacteria, fungi, and certain inorganic agents.

LABORATORY FINDINGS. The histopathology is quite characteristic and consists of epithelioid cells surrounded by Langhans' giant cells. No acid-fast bacilli are found, and caseation necrosis is absent. The tuberculin skin test is negative, but the Kveim test, using sarcoidal lymph node tissue, is positive after several weeks. The total blood serum protein is high and ranges from 7.5 to 10.0 g/dl, owing mainly to an increase in the globulin fraction.

Differential Diagnosis

Other granulomatous diseases: can be ruled out by biopsy and other appropriate studies.
Silica granulomas: histologically similar; a history of such injury can usually be obtained.

Treatment

Time appears to cure or cause remission of most cases of sarcoidosis, but corticosteroids and immunosuppressant drugs may be indicated for extensive cases.

GRANULOMA ANNULARE
(Plates 54 and 64)

Granuloma annulare is a moderately common skin problem. The usually encountered ring-shaped, red-bordered lesion is often mistaken for ringworm by the inexperienced (see Plate 60). Several clinical variations exist. The two most common are the *localized form* and the *generalized form.*

Females with granuloma annulare predominate over males in a ratio of 2.5 to 1. No ages are exempt, but the localized form is usually seen in patients in the first 3 decades of life and the generalized form in patients in the fourth to seventh decades.

PRIMARY LESIONS. In both the *localized form* and the *generalized form* the lesion is a red asymptomatic papule with no scaling. The papule may be solitary. Most frequently the lesion assumes a ring-shaped or arcuate configuration of papules that tends to enlarge centrifugally. Rarely are the rings over 5 cm in diameter. In the *localized form* of granuloma annulare the lesions appear mainly on the hands, arms, feet, and legs. In the *generalized form* there may be hundreds of the red or tan papular circinate lesions on the extremities and on the trunk.

SECONDARY LESIONS. On healing, the red color turns to brown before the lesions disappear.

COURSE. Both forms of granuloma annulare can resolve spontaneously after one to several years, but the generalized form is even more long lasting.

ETIOLOGY. The cause is unknown. An immune-complex vasculitis or a cell-mediated immunity has been proposed to be a factor in the disease, as has trauma.

LABORATORY FINDINGS. The histopathology is quite characteristic. The middle and upper dermis have focal areas of altered collagenous connective tissue surrounded by an infiltrate of histiocytic cells and lymphocytes. In some cases these cells infiltrate between the collagen bundles, giving a palisading effect. The term *necrobiosis* has been used to describe these changes. Some believe that the generalized form of granuloma annulare is associated with a higher incidence of diabetes mellitus.

Differential Diagnosis

Tinea corporis: usually itches and has a scaly red border; the fungus can be demonstrated with a potassium hydroxide scraping or Sabouraud culture (see Chap. 19).
Lichen planus, annular form: characterized by violaceous flat-topped papules with

Wickham's striae; mucous membrane lesions are usually seen (see Chap. 14).

Secondary syphilis: can be clinically similar but will have a positive serology (see Chap. 16).

Other granulomatous diseases: can usually be distinguished by biopsy.

There is a *subcutaneous form of granuloma annulare* that is difficult to separate histologically from the *rheumatoid nodule.*

Treatment

LOCALIZED FORM. Many cases respond to the application of a corticosteroid cream covered for 8 hours a day with an occlusive dressing such as Saran wrap. Intralesional corticosteroids (see p. 106) are very effective for a case with only a few lesions.

GENERALIZED FORM. Numerous remedies have been tried with anecdotal benefit.

BIBLIOGRAPHY

Buechner SA, Winkelmann RK, Banks PM: T-cell subsets in cutaneous sarcoidosis. Arch Dermatol 119:728, 1983

Hirsh BC, Johnson WC: Concepts of granulomatous inflammation. Int J Dermatol 23:90, 1984

Kerdel FA, Moschella SL: Sarcoidosis. J Am Acad Dermatol 11:1, 1984

Reyes-Flores O: Granulomas induced by living agents. Int J Dermatol 25:158, 1986

Steiner A, Pehamberger H, Wolff K: Sulfone treatment of granuloma annulare. J Am Acad Dermatol 13:1004, 1985

Veien NK, Stahl D, Brodthagen H: Cutaneous sarcoidosis in caucasians. J Am Acad Dermatol 16:534, 1987

21

Dermatologic Parasitology

Dermatologic parasitology is a very extensive subject and includes the dermatoses due to three main groups of organisms: protozoa, helminths, and arthropods.

The *protozoal dermatoses* are exemplified by the various forms of trypanosomiasis and leishmaniasis (see Chap. 36).

Helminthic dermatoses include those due to roundworms (ground itch, creeping eruption, filariasis, and other rare tropical diseases) and those due to flatworms (schistosomiasis, swimmer's itch, and others) (see Chap. 36).

Arthropod dermatoses are divided into those caused by two classes of organisms: the arachnids (spiders, scorpions, ticks, and mites) and the insects (lice, bugs, flies, moths, beetles, bees, and fleas). Lyme disease is caused by a spirochete that is transmitted by a tick and is discussed in Chapter 16.

In this chapter *scabies,* caused by a mite, and *pediculosis,* caused by lice, are discussed.

Flea bites, chigger bites, creeping eruption, swimmer's itch, and *tropical dermatoses* are discussed in Chapter 36, *Geographic Skin Diseases.*

SCABIES
(Plate 64)

Scabies is usually more prevalent in a populace ravaged by war, famine, or disease, when personal hygiene becomes relatively unimportant. However, there are unexplained cyclic epidemics of this parasitic infestation. In the 1970s and 1980s such a cycle plagued Americans. In normal times scabies is rarely seen except in schoolchildren, among the elderly in nursing care centers, or in poorer populations under crowded conditions. It can be a sexually transmitted disease.

SAUER NOTES:

1. Scabies should be ruled out in any generalized excoriated eruption.
2. Always ask if other members of the household itch.

PRIMARY LESIONS. A burrow caused by the female of the mite *Sarcoptes scabiei* (Fig. 21–1) measures approximately 2 mm in length and can be hidden by the secondary eruption. Small vesicles may overlie the burrows.

SECONDARY LESIONS. Excoriations of the burrows may be the only visible pathology. In severe, chronic cases, bacterial infection may be extensive and may take the form of impetigo, cellulitis, and furunculosis.

DISTRIBUTION. Most commonly the excoriations are seen on the lower abdomen and the back, with extension to the pubic and the axillary areas, the legs, the arms, and the webs of the fingers (uncommon).

SUBJECTIVE COMPLAINTS. Itching is intense, particularly at night, when the patient is warm and in bed and the mite is more ac-

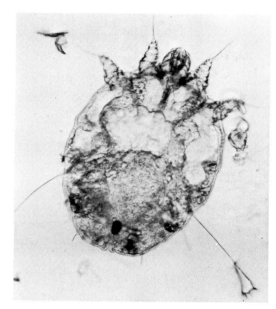

Figure 21–1. **The female of the mite Sarcoptes scabiei.** The small, oval, black body near the anal opening is a fecal pellet. Proximal to it is a vague, much larger, oval, pale-edged mass—an egg. (*Dr. H. Parlette*)

tive. However, many skin diseases itch worse at night, presumably due to a lower itch threshold when relaxation occurs.

COURSE. The mite can persist for months and years ("seven-year itch") in untreated, unclean persons.

CONTAGIOUSNESS. Other members of the household or intimate contacts may or may not have the disease, depending on cleanliness and the severity of the infestation.

LABORATORY FINDINGS. The female scabies mite, ova, and fecal pellets may be seen in curetted burrows examined under the low-power magnification of the microscope (see Fig. 21–1). Potassium hydroxide (20% solution) can be used to clear the tissue, as with fungus smears. Another method of collection is to scrape the burrow through immersion oil and then transfer the scrapings to the microscopic slides. Skill is necessary to uncover the mite by curetting or scraping.

Differential Diagnosis

Pyoderma: rule out concurrent parasitic infestation: positive history of high carbohy-

drate diet or diabetes mellitus; only mild itching (see Chap. 15).

Pediculosis pubis: lice and eggs on and around hairs; distribution different (see following section).

Winter itch: no burrows; seasonal incidence; elderly patient, usually; worse on legs and back (see Chap. 11).

Dermatitis herpetiformis: vesicles, urticaria; excoriated papules; eosinophilia; no burrows (see Chap. 22).

Neurotic excoriations: nervous person; patient admits picking at lesions; no burrows.

Parasitophobia: usually the patient brings to the office pieces of skin and debris; showing the patient the debris under a microscope helps to convince him of the absence of parasites. This is a difficult problem to manage.

Treatment

ADULTS AND OLDER CHILDREN

1. Inspect or question concerning itching in other members of the family or intimate contacts to rule out infestation in them. Any infested household members must be treated at the same time as the patient to prevent "ping-pong" infestation.
2. Instruct patient to bathe thoroughly, scrubbing the involved areas with a brush.
3. Lindane (Kwell or Scabene) lotion
   Sig: Apply to the entire body from the neck down.
4. After 24 hours bathe carefully and change to clean clothes and bedding.

SAUER NOTES:

1. I have the patient *repeat* the lotion application in 1 week, leaving it on again for 24 hours.
2. Tell the patient that the itching can persist for weeks.

---

5. Washing, dry cleaning, or ironing of clothes or bedding is sufficient to destroy the mite. Sterilization is unnecessary.
6. Itching may persist for a few days or even for 2 to 3 weeks in spite of the destruction of the mite. For this apply b.i.d.:

A. Crotamiton (Eurax) cream q.s.　　60.0
This cream has scabicidal power and antipruritic action combined.

B. Corticosteroid systemic therapy may be indicated for 10 to 14 days.

7. If itching persists after 4 weeks, reexamine the patient carefully. It takes a lot of reassurance to convince these itchy patients that they are not still infested with scabies.

NEWBORNS AND INFANTS

1. General instructions are as above.

2. Lindane lotion used in newborns and infants has caused convulsions.

3. Eurax cream　　　　　　　　　60.0
Sig: Apply b.i.d. locally to affected areas only, or

4. Sulfur, ppt.　　　　　　　　　5%
Water-washable cream base q.s.　　60.0
Sig: Apply b.i.d. to affected areas.

PEDICULOSIS

Lice infestation affects persons of all ages, but usually those in the lower-income strata are affected most often because of lack of cleanliness and infrequent changes of clothing. It is also seen as a sexually transmitted disease.

Three clinical entities are produced: (1) infestation of the hair by the head louse *Pediculus humanus capitis:* (2) infestation of the body by *P. humanus corporis,* and (3) infestation of the pubic area by the pubic louse *Phthirus pubis* (Fig. 21–2). Since lice bite the skin and live on the blood, it is impossible for them to live without human contact. The readily visible oval eggs or nits are attached to hairs or to clothing fibers by the female louse. After the eggs hatch, the newly born lice mature within 30 days. Then the female louse can live for another 30 days and deposit a few eggs daily.

PRIMARY LESIONS.　　The bite is not unusual but is seldom seen because of the secondary changes produced by the resulting intense itching. In the *scalp* and *pubic form* the nits are found on the hairs, but the lice are found only occasionally. In the *body form* the nits and the lice can be found after careful searching in the seams of the clothing.

SECONDARY LESIONS.　　In the *scalp form* the skin is red and excoriated, with such severe secondary bacterial infection, in some cases, that the hairs become matted together in a crusty, foul-smelling "cap." Regional lymphadenopathy is common. A morbilliform

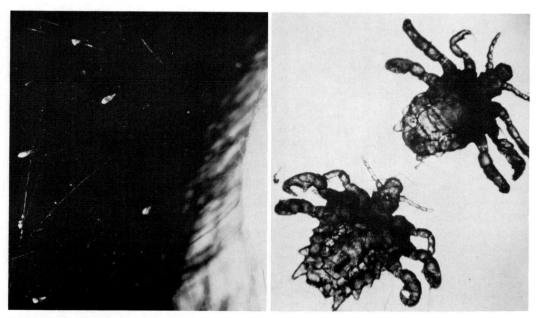

Figure 21–2.　　**Pediculosis.** (*Left*) Nits on scalp hair behind ear. (*Dr. L. Hyde*) (*Right*) Pubic louse or *Phthirus pubis* as seen with 7.5× lens of microscope. (*Dr. J. Boley*)

rash on the body, an id reaction, is seen in long-standing cases.

In the *body form* linear excoriations and secondary infection, seen mainly on the shoulders, the belt-line, and the buttocks, mask the primary bites.

In the *pubic form* the secondary excoriations are again dominant and produce some matting of the hairs. This louse can also infest body, axillary, and eyelash hairs. An unusual eruption on the abdomen, the thighs, and the arms, called *maculae cerulae,* because of the bluish gray, pea-sized macules, can occur in chronic cases of pubic pediculosis.

Differential Diagnosis

PEDICULOSIS CAPITIS
Bacterial infection of the scalp: responds rapidly to correct antibacterial therapy (see Chap. 15).

SAUER NOTE:

All cases of scalp pyoderma must be examined closely for a primary lice infestation.

Seborrheic dermatitis or dandruff: the scales of dandruff are readily detached from the hair, while oval nits are not so easily removed (see Chap. 13).
Hair casts: resemble nits but can be pulled off more easily; no eggs seen on microscopic examination.

PEDICULOSIS CORPORIS
Scabies: may be small burrows; distribution of lesions different; no lice in clothes (see beginning of this chapter).
Senile or winter itch: history helpful; dry skin, aggravated by bathing; will not find lice in clothes (see Chap. 11).

PEDICULOSIS PUBIS
Scabies: no nits; burrows in pubic area and elsewhere (see beginning of this chapter).
Pyoderma secondary to contact dermatitis, from condoms, contraceptive jellies, new underwear, douches: history important; acute onset, no nits (see Chap. 15).
Seborrheic dermatitis, when in eyebrows and eyelashes: no nits found (see Chap. 13).

Treatment

1. Pediculosis Capitis
   A. Shampoos or rinses:
      1) Permethrin (Nix) creme rinse   60.0
         Sig: Use as a rinse for 10 minutes after a shampoo. Only one application is necessary.
      2) Lindane (Kwell or Scabene) shampoo   60.0
         Sig: Shampoo and comb hair thoroughly. Leave on the hair for 4 minutes. Shampoo again in 3 days.
      3) Pyrethrins (RID, R&C)   60.0
         Sig: Apply to scalp for 10 minutes and rinse off. Apply again in 7 days (nonprescription).
   B. For secondary scalp infection:
      1) Trim hair as much as possible and agreeable with the patient.
      2) Shampoo hair once a day with an antiseborrhea-type shampoo.
      3) Bactroban or Polysporin ointment.   15.0
         Sig: Apply to scalp b.i.d.
   C. Change and clean bedding and headwear after 24 hours of treatment. Storage of headwear for 30 days will destroy the lice and the nits.
2. Pediculosis Corporis
   A. Calamine lotion, q.s.   120.0
      Sig: Apply locally b.i.d. for itching. (The lice and the nits are in the clothing.)
   B. Have the clothing laundered or dry cleaned. If this is impossible, dusting with 10% lindane powder will kill the parasites. Care should be taken to prevent reinfestation. Storage of clothing for 30 days will kill both nits and lice.
3. Pediculosis Pubis: Treatment is the same as for scalp form.

BIBLIOGRAPHY

Centers for Disease Control: Scabies in health-care facilities—Iowa. Arch Dermatol 124:837, 1988

Modly CE, Burnett JW: Tick-borne dermatologic diseases. Cutis 41:244, 1988

Orkin M, Maibach HI: Cutaneous Infestations and Insect Bites. New York, Marcel Dekker, 1985

Rasmussen JE: Lindane, a prudent approach. Arch Dermatol 123:1008, 1987

22

Bullous Dermatoses

To medical students and practitioners alike, the bullous skin diseases appear most dramatic. One of these diseases, pemphigus, is undoubtedly greatly responsible for the aura that surrounds the exhibition and the discussion of an unfortunate patient with a bullous disease. Happy would be the instructor who could behold such student interest when a case of acne or hand dermatitis is being presented.

In almost all cases of bullous diseases, it is necessary to examine a fresh tissue biopsy specimen for deposits of immune reactants, immunoglobulins, and complement components, at or near the basement membrane zone. Routine histologic examination of a formalin-fixed biopsy specimen is of course also usually indicated. (See Chap. 10, *Dermatologic Immunology*.)

Three bullous diseases are discussed in this chapter: pemphigus vulgaris, dermatitis herpetiformis, and erythema multiforme bullosum. However, other bullous skin diseases do occur, and in this introduction they will be differentiated from these three.

BULLOUS IMPETIGO. The name of *pemphigus neonatorum* has been attached to this pyodermic skin infection because of the resemblance of the large bullae in this disease to pemphigus. This term should be abandoned. Bullous impetigo is to be differentiated from the other bullous diseases by its occurrence in infants and children, rapid development of the individual bullae, presence of impetigo lesions in siblings, and rapid response to local antibiotic therapy (see Chaps. 15 and 34).

CONTACT DERMATITIS DUE TO POISON IVY OR SIMILAR PLANTS. Bullae and vesicles are seen in linear configuration. A history of pulling weeds or burning brush is usually obtained, and a past history of poison ivy or related dermatitis is common. The duration of disease is 10 to 14 days (see Chap. 9).

DRUG ERUPTION. Elicit drug history (particularly of sulfonamides and iodides). The eruption usually clears on discontinuing drugs. Bullae appear rapidly (see Chap. 9).

EPIDERMOLYSIS BULLOSA (see Plate 80). This rare, chronic, hereditary skin disease is manifested by the formation of bullae, usually on the hands and the feet, following trauma. The full clinical and immunologic spectra of these diseases have not been completely defined.

The *simple form,* of dominant inheritance, can begin in infancy or adulthood with the formation of tense, slightly itching bullae at the sites of pressure, which heal quickly without scarring. Forced marches or jogging can initiate this disease in patients who have the heredity factor. Such cases are usually treated erroneously as athlete's foot. The disease is worse in the summer or may be present only at this time.

The *dystrophic form,* of recessive inheritance, begins in infancy like the simple form, but as time elapses the bullae become hemorrhagic, heal slowly, and leave scars that can amputate digits; death can result from secondary infection. Mucous membrane lesions are more common in the dystrophic form than in the simple form. Treatment is supportive.

A lethal, nonscarring form is of recessive inheritance also but is usually fatal within a few months. (See Chap. 32.)

FAMILIAL BENIGN CHRONIC PEMPHIGUS (HAILEY-HAILEY DISEASE). This is a rare, hereditary bullous eruption that is most common on the neck and in the axillae. It can be distinguished from pemphigus by its chronicity and benign nature and by its histologic picture. (See Chap. 32.) Some consider this disease to be a bullous variety of *keratosis follicularis (Darier's disease)*.

PORPHYRIA. The congenital erythropoietic type and the chronic hepatic type (porphyria cutanea tarda) commonly have bullae on the sun-exposed areas of the body. See Dictionary-Index under *Porphyria* and also p. 296.

BULLOUS PEMPHIGOID (see Plate 98). This chronic bullous eruption most commonly occurring in elderly adults usually is not fatal. It is differentiated from *Pemphigus vulgaris* by the histologic presence of subepidermal bullae without acantholysis and quite specific immunofluorescent autoantibodies in the basement membrane zone; from *erythema multiforme* by its chronicity, absence of iris lesions and histology; and from *dermatitis herpetiformis* by the absence of response to sulfapyridine or dapsone therapy (some bullous pemphigoid cases do respond to this therapy) and by histology.

CICATRICIAL PEMPHIGOID (Fig. 22–1 and Plate 98). This disabling but nonfatal bullous eruption of the mucous membranes most commonly involves the eyes. As the result of scarring, which is characteristic of this disease and separates it from true pemphigus, the

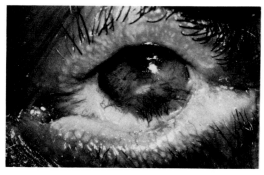

Figure 22–1. Pemphigoid, cicatricial type of eye. (*Drs. L. Calkins and A. Lemoine*)

eyesight is eventually lost. Over 50% of the cases have skin lesions. Histologically, the bullae are subepidermal and do not show acantholysis. There is quite a bit of immunologic similarity between this disease and bullous pemphigoid.

LINEAR IgA BULLOUS DISEASE. Most of the children and adults with this disease differ from classic dermatitis herpetiformis in the morphology and distribution of their lesions, have a poorer response to dapsone, and have linear IgA anti–basement membrane zone antibodies.

INCONTINENTIA PIGMENTI. The first stage of this rare disease of infants manifests itself with bullous lesions, primarily on the hands and feet. See Chap. 34 and Plates 90 and 91.

TOXIC EPIDERMAL NECROLYSIS. This rare disease is characterized by large bullae and a quite generalized Nikolsky sign, in which large sheets of epidermis become detached from the underlying skin. The mucous membranes are frequently involved. The patient is toxic. Adults are most commonly affected. In many instances it is difficult to separate this disease clinically from severe erythema multiforme–like disease (*Stevens-Johnson syndrome*). Drugs are usually the causative factor. Most commonly implicated are sulfonamides, anticonvulsants, and nonsteroidal anti-inflammatory drugs. There may be a genetic predisposition to this bullous drug reaction. Therapy is supportive, combined with systemic corticosteroids, but an appreciable number of cases are fatal.

STAPHYLOCOCCAL SCALDED SKIN SYNDROME. Clinically, this disorder is similar to toxic epidermal necrolysis but has been separated from this disease because of the finding that phage group 2 *Staphylococcus aureus* is the usual cause. In newborns, this formerly was known as *Ritter von Ritterschein's disease*. It also occurs in children. The prognosis is very favorable.

IMPETIGO HERPETIFORMIS. One of the rarest of skin diseases, this disease is characterized by groups of pustules mainly seen in the axillae and the groin, high fever, prostration, severe malaise, and, generally, a fatal outcome. It occurs most commonly in pregnant or postpartum women. It can be distinguished from *pemphigus vegetans* or *dermati-*

tis herpetiformis by the fact that these diseases do not produce such general, acute, toxic manifestations.

In spite of high medical student and general practitioner interest in the bullous skin conditions, the diagnosis and the management of the three main diseases, particularly pemphigus vulgaris and dermatitis herpetiformis, should be in the realm of the dermatologist. In this chapter the salient features of these diseases are presented, with therapy skimmed over lightly.

PEMPHIGUS VULGARIS
(Plates 1 F, 65, and 98)

Even though pemphigus vulgaris is rare, most physicians see several cases of this disease early in their careers. Patients with pemphigus usually have to be hospitalized at one time or another during the course of the disease, and, as a result, the hospital personnel and staff are exposed to this most miserable, odoriferous, debilitating skin disease. Prior to the advent of corticosteroid therapy, the disease was eventually fatal.

PRIMARY LESIONS. The early lesions of pemphigus are small vesicles or bullae on apparently normal skin. Redness of the base of the bullae is unusual. Without treatment, the bullae enlarge and spread, and new ones balloon up on different areas of the skin or the mucous membranes. Rupturing of the bullae leaves large eroded areas. The Nikolsky sign is positive; that is, a top layer of the skin adjacent to a bulla readily separates from the underlying skin after firm but gentle pressure.

SECONDARY LESIONS. Bacterial infection with crusting is marked and accounts, in part, for the characteristic mousy odor. Lesions that heal spontaneously or under therapy do not leave scars.

COURSE. When untreated, pemphigus vulgaris can be rapidly fatal or assume a slow lingering course, with debility, painful mouth and body erosions, systemic bacterial infection, and toxemia. Spontaneous temporary remissions do occur without therapy. The following clinical variations of pemphigus also exist:

Pemphigus vegetans is characterized by the development of large granulomatous masses in the intertriginous areas of the axillae and the groin. Secondary bacterial infection, while present in all cases of pemphigus, is most marked in this form. Pemphigus vegetans is to be differentiated from a granulomatous *ioderma* or *bromoderma* (see Chap. 9) and from *impetigo herpetiformis* (see beginning of this chapter).

Pemphigus foliaceus appears as a scaly, moist, generalized exfoliative dermatitis. The characteristic mousy odor of pemphigus is dominant in this variant, which is also remarkable for its chronicity. The response to corticosteroid therapy is less favorable in the foliaceus form than in the other types. (See also Chap. 36 for a Brazilian form.)

Pemphigus erythematosus clinically resembles a mixture of pemphigus vulgaris, seborrheic dermatitis, and lupus erythematosus. The distribution of the red, greasy, crusted, and eroded lesions is on the butterfly area of the face, the sternal area, the scalp, and occasionally in the mouth. The course is more chronic than for pemphigus vulgaris, and remissions are common.

Some dermatologists believe that pemphigus foliaceus and pemphigus erythematosus may be distinct diseases from pemphigus vulgaris and vegetans.

ETIOLOGY. The cause of pemphigus vulgaris is unknown, but autoimmunity is a factor.

LABORATORY FINDINGS. The histopathology of early cases is quite characteristic and serves to differentiate most cases of pemphigus vulgaris from dermatitis herpetiformis and the other bullous diseases. Acantholysis, or separation of intercellular contact between the keratinocytes, is characteristic. The bulla is intraepidermal. Cytologic smears (Tzanck test) for diagnosis of pemphigus vulgaris will reveal numerous rounded acantholytic epidermal cells with large nuclei in condensed cytoplasm. Antiepithelial autoantibodies against the intercellular substance are found by direct and indirect immunofluorescent tests. Fresh tissue biopsy specimens taken from noninvolved skin will best show immunoglobulins. Indirect tests are performed on serum.

niated mercury in white petrolatum can be prescribed for a very slow bleaching effect.

VITILIGO
(Plate 67)

CLINICAL LESIONS. Irregular areas of depigmented skin are occasionally seen with a hyperpigmented border.

DISTRIBUTION. Most commonly the lesions occur on the face and the dorsum of hands and feet, but they can occur on all body areas.

COURSE. The disease is slowly progressive, but remissions and changes are frequent. It is more obvious during the summer because of the tanning of adjacent normal skin.

ETIOLOGY. The cause is unknown. Heredity is a factor in some cases.

Differential Diagnosis

Rule out causes of *secondary hypopigmentation* (see end of this chapter; Fig. 24–1.)

Treatment

An attractive young woman with large depigmented patches on her face and dorsum of hands asks if something can be done for her "white spots." Her sister has a few lesions.

1. *Cosmetics.* The use of the following covering or staining preparations is recommended: pancake-type cosmetics, such as Covermark, by Lydia O'Leary; Vitadye (Elder); walnut juice stain; or potassium permanganate solution in appropriate dilution. Many patients with vitiligo become quite proficient in the application of these agents.
2. *Corticosteroid cream therapy.* This is effective for early mild cases of vitiligo, especially when one is mainly concerned with face and hand lesions. Betamethasone valerate cream 0.1% (Valisone cream) can be prescribed for use on the hands for 4 months or so and for use on the face for only 3 months. Do not use on the eyelids or as full-body therapy.
3. Suntanning should be avoided because this accentuates the normal pigmentation

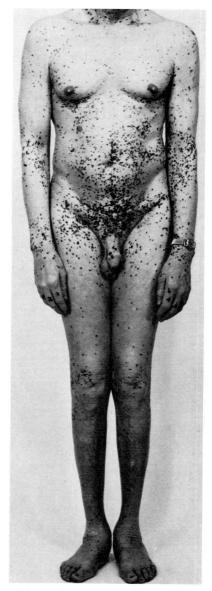

Figure 24–1. **Secondary hypopigmentation.** A marked example of loss of pigment that occurred in a black man following healing of an exfoliative dermatitis. Corticosteroids were used in the therapy.

and makes the nonpigmented vitiligo more noticeable.

If the patient desires a more specific treatment, the following can be suggested, with certain reservations:

4. *Psoralen derivatives.* For many years Egyptians along the Nile River chewed certain plants to cause the disappearance

of the white spots of vitiligo. Extraction of the chemicals from these plants revealed the psoralen derivatives to be the active agents, and one of these, 8-methoxypsoralen (8 MOP), was found to be the most effective. This chemical is available as Oxsoralen in 10-mg capsules and also as a topical liquid form. The oral form is to be ingested 2 hours before exposure to measured sun radiation. Consult the package insert. The results of the necessary long-term therapy with this routine have been so disappointing that I do not prescribe it any more.

Trisoralen is a synthetic psoralen in 5-mg tablets. The recommended dosage is 2 tablets taken 2 hours before measured sun exposure for a long-term course. Detailed instructions accompany the package. Some dermatologists believe this therapy to be more effective than Oxsoralen.

A short 2-week course of Oxsoralen capsules (20 mg/day) has been advocated for the purpose of acquiring a better and quicker *suntan*. The value of such a course has been questioned. The sun exposure must be gradual. *Oral psoralens plus self-administered UVA or UVB in "tanning booths" can produce severe burns, which may be fatal.*

5. *PUVA therapy.* The combination of oral psoralen therapy with UVA radiation has been somewhat successful in repigmenting vitiligo.

Classification of Pigmentary Disorders

I. **Melanin Hyperpigmentation or Melanoderma**
   A. Chloasma (melasma)
   B. Incontinentia pigmenti
   C. Secondary to skin diseases
      1. Chronic discoid lupus erythematosus
      2. Tinea versicolor
      3. Stasis dermatitis
      4. Many cases of dermatitis in blacks and other dark-skinned individuals (see Fig. 24–1)
      5. Scleroderma
      6. Porphyria cutanea tarda (see Plate 67)
   D. Secondary to external agents
      1. X-radiation
      2. Ultraviolet
      3. Sunlight
      4. Tars
      5. Photosensitizing chemicals, as in cosmetics, causing development of clinical entities labeled as Riehl's melanosis, poikiloderma of Civatte, berlock dermatitis (see Plate 67) and others.
   E. Secondary to internal disorders
      1. Addison's disease
      2. Chronic liver disease
      3. Pregnancy
      4. Hyperthyroidism
      5. Internal carcinoma causing malignant form of acanthosis nigricans
      6. Hormonal influence on benign acanthosis nigricans
      7. Intestinal polyposis causing mucous membrane pigmentation (Peutz-Jehger syndrome)
      8. Albright's syndrome
      9. Schilder's disease
      10. Fanconi's syndrome
   F. Secondary to drugs such as ACTH, estrogens, progesterone, melanocyte-stimulating hormone
II. **Nonmelanin Pigmentations**
   A. Argyria due to silver salt deposits
   B. Arsenical pigmentation due to ingestion of inorganic arsenic, as in Fowler's solution and Asiatic pills
   C. Pigmentation from heavy metals such as bismuth, gold, and mercury
   D. Tattoos
   E. Black dermographism, the common bluish black or green stain seen under watches and rings in certain persons from the deposit of the metallic particles reacting with chemicals already on the skin
   F. Hemosiderin granules in hemochromatosis or bronze diabetes
   G. Bile pigments from jaundice
   H. Yellow pigments following atabrine and chlorpromazine ingestion
   I. Carotene coloring in carotenemia
   J. Homogentisic acid polymer deposit in ochronosis

III. Hypopigmentation
  A. Albinism
  B. Vitiligo
  C. Leukoderma or acquired hypopigmentation
    1. Secondary to skin diseases such as tinea versicolor, chronic discoid lupus erythematosus localized scleroderma, psoriasis, secondary syphilis, pinta, and so on (see Fig. 24–1)
    2. Secondary to chemicals such as mercury compounds, monobenzyl ether of hydroquinone, and cortisone-type drugs given intralesionally, especially in blacks (see Plate 67)
    3. Secondary to internal diseases, such as hormonal diseases, and in Vogt-Koyanagi syndrome
    4. Associated with pigmented nevi (halo nevus or leukoderma acquisitum centrifugum)

BIBLIOGRAPHY

El Mofty AM, El Mofty M: Vitiligo. Int J Dermatol 19:237, 1980

Fulk CS: Primary disorders of hyperpigmentation. J Am Acad Dermatol 10:1, 1984

Hatchome N, Aiba S, Kato T et al: Possible functional impairment of Langerhans' cells in vitiliginous skin. Arch Dermatol 123:51, 1987

Kumari J: Vitiligo treated with topical clobetasol propionate. Arch Dermatol 120:631, 1984. Also summarizes betamethasone local therapy.

Taylor WOG: The albino fellowship. Int J Dermatol 21:84, 1982

25

Collagen Diseases

The diseases commonly included in this group are *lupus erythematosus, scleroderma,* and *dermatomyositis*. The skin manifestations are usually a dominant feature of these diseases, but in some cases, particularly systemic lupus erythematosus, skin lesions may be absent. Rheumatoid arthritis and periarteritis nodosa are often included in the collagen disease group but only occasionally are accompanied by skin lesions, usually of the erythema multiforme–like group (see Chaps. 10 and 12).

The onset of the collagen diseases is insidious, and the prognosis as to life is serious. It is not unusual to attach the label of "collagen disease" to a patient who has only minimal subjective and objective findings (malaise, weakness, vague joint and muscle pains, antibody and immunologic abnormalities, biologic false-positive serology, and high sedimentation rate) with the realization by the physician that months and years will have to elapse before a more exacting diagnosis of one of the above diseases can be made.

Considerable advances have been made in the laboratory testing directed toward differentiation of the several collagen diseases. The LE cell test was the first test developed, but it has been superceded by the antinuclear antibody (ANA) test, fluorescent ANA test, and many more complicated serologic and tissue tests (see Chap. 10).

If the ANA test is positive in a patient, then the fluorescent ANA test is usually indicated. The pattern of nuclear fluorescence, as well as the dilution of a serum at which fluorescence is lost, may provide important diagnostic and prognostic information.

For completeness and for a better understanding of these patterns, consult Table 10–3.

LUPUS ERYTHEMATOSUS
(Plates 68 and 69)

Systemic and discoid lupus erythematosus are clinically dissimilar but basically related diseases. The two diseases differ in regard to characteristic skin lesions, subjective complaints, other organ involvement, blood and tissue test findings, response to treatment, and eventual prognosis. However, rare cases of clinically classic discoid lupus erythematosus show laboratory evidence of the pathology seen with the systemic form of lupus erythematosus and can terminate as the disseminated disease. Certain early borderline cases are difficult to categorize, and some *subacute* forms may develop into the systemic disease. The variations of the systemic and the discoid forms of lupus erythematosus are shown in Table 25–1.

Discoid Lupus Erythematosus
(Plates 68, 69, and 98)

Differential Diagnosis

Systemic lupus erythematosus: see Table 25–1.

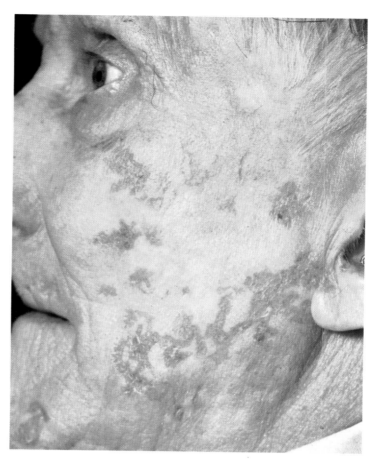

Plate 68. **Lupus erythematosus** (*Top*) Chronic discoid lupus erythematosus on the cheek of an elderly man. (*K.C.G.H., Truman Medical Center*)

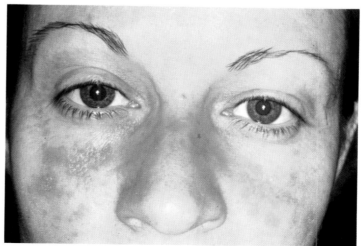

(*Bottom*) Systemic lupus erythematosus showing classic "butterfly" eruption. (*Drs. S. Wilson and W. Larson*) (*Smith Kline & French Laboratories*)

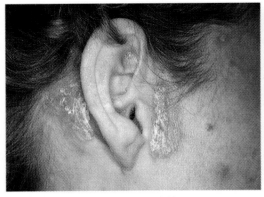

(A) Chronic discoid lupus
    erythematosus

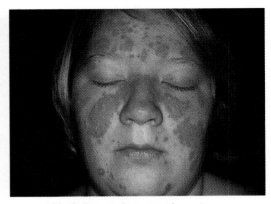

(B) Subacute lupus erythematosus

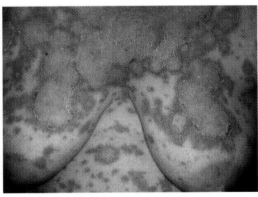

(C) Subacute lupus erythematosus

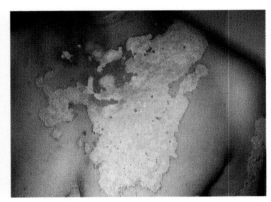

(D) Subacute lupus erythematosus

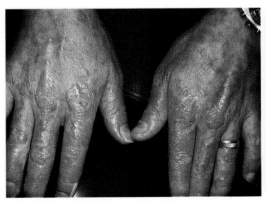

(E) Systemic lupus erythematosus
    of hands

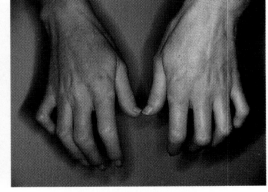

(F) Diffuse scleroderma of hands

Plate 69. **Lupus erythematosus and scleroderma.** (*Burroughs Wellcome Co.*)

Table 25–1
Comparison of Discoid with Systemic Lupus Erythematosus

	DISCOID	SYSTEMIC
Primary Lesions	Red, scaly, thickened, well-circumscribed patches with enlarged follicles and elevated border	Red, mildly scaly, diffuse, puffy lesions; purpura is also seen; bullae occur rarely.
Secondary Lesions	Atrophy, scarring, and pigmentary changes	No scarring; mild hyperpigmentation
Distribution	Face, mainly in "butterfly" area, but also on scalp, ears, arms, and chest; may not be symmetric	Face in "butterfly" area, arms, fingers, and legs; usually symmetric
Course	Very chronic, with gradual progression; slow healing under therapy; no effect on life	Acute onset with fever, rash, malaise, and joint pains. Most cases respond rather rapidly to corticosteroid and supportive therapy, but the prognosis for life is poor.
Season	Aggravated by intense sun exposure or radiation therapy	Same
Sex Incidence	Almost twice as common in females	Same
Systemic Pathology	None obvious	Nephritis, arthritis, epilepsy, pancarditis, hepatitis, and so on
Laboratory Findings	Biopsy characteristic in classic case. ANA and related tests are negative, as are other laboratory tests	Biopsy is useful, especially fresh tissue immunofluorescent studies. Leukopenia, anemia, albuminuria, increased sedimentation rate, positive ANA test, and biologic false-positive serologic test for syphilis are found.

Subacute cutaneous lupus erythematosus (see Plate 69): recurrent erythematous, scaly, annular, nonscarring, photosensitive lesions in a widespread pattern. Sixty percent of patients have antibodies to the Ro (SS-A) antigen, and about 75% have human leukocyte antigen HLA-DR3 phenotype.

Actinic dermatitis: many cases are grossly and histologically similar to systemic or discoid lupus erythematosus but get history of presence only in summer; faster response to antimalarial drugs and locally applied sunscreening agents.

Seborrheic dermatitis: lesions greasy, red, scaly, associated with scalp dandruff; occurs in eyebrows and scalp without hair loss; rapid response to antiseborrheic local therapy (see Chap. 13).

Any cutaneous granulomas: such as sarcoidosis (see Chap. 20), secondary and tertiary syphilis (see Chap. 16), and lupus vulgaris (see Chap. 15).

Cases with scarring alopecia (see Fig. 27–1) are to be differentiated from *alopecia cicatrisata* (see Chap. 27), *old tinea capitis of endothrix type* (see Chap. 19), *lichen planus* (see Chap. 14), and *folliculitis decalvans* (see Chap. 27).

Treatment

A young woman presents with two red, scaly, dime-sized lesions on her right cheek of 3 months' duration.

1. Laboratory workup should include a complete blood cell count, urinalysis, serology, ANA and related tests, sedimentation rate, and, usually, a biopsy. The tests should be normal, but the biopsy of fixed tissue and fresh tissue is rather characteristic of discoid lupus.

2. Fluorinated corticosteroid cream   15.0
   Sig: Apply b.i.d. locally to lesions.
   Do not use fluorinated corticosteroids creams on the face for long periods of time because atrophy and telangiectasia can develop.

3. Sunscreen cream with a sun protective factor (SPF) of 15 or more.

Sig: Apply to face as sunscreen for protection, reapplying frequently.

Chloroquine and related antimalarial-type drugs are very effective for this disease. However, because of an irreversible retinitis that has developed in a few patients on long-term therapy, this therapy is not advised, except when used by a physician very knowledgeable of the effects of these drugs.

Systemic Lupus Erythematosus
(Plates 68 and 69 and Fig. 25–1)

Differential Diagnosis

Discoid lupus erythematosus: see Table 25–1.

Subacute cutaneous lupus erythematosus: see preceding section under Differential Diagnosis.

Actinic dermatitis: skin lesions similar in appearance; usually only in summer; no altered laboratory studies; more rapid response to antimalarial drugs.

Seborrheic dermatitis: associated with scalp dandruff; responds to local antiseborrhea therapy (see Chap. 13).

Contact dermatitis: due to cosmetics, paint sprays, vegetation, hand creams; acute onset with no systemic symptoms; history helpful (see Chap. 9).

Dermatomyositis: muscle soreness and weakness (see at end of this chapter).

Drug eruption due to apresoline, hydralazine, and procainamide: can simulate systemic lupus; take history.

Mixed connective tissue disease: This is a distinct clinical syndrome sharing features of systemic lupus erythematosus, progressive systemic sclerosis, and polymyositis. A high titer of particulate fluorescent antinuclear antibody is significant.

Treatment

A young woman presents with diffuse red, puffy eruption on cheeks, nose, forehead, and at base of fingernails, of 1 week's duration. She complains of malaise, fever, joint pains, headache, and ankle edema that has become progressively worse in the past 3 weeks.

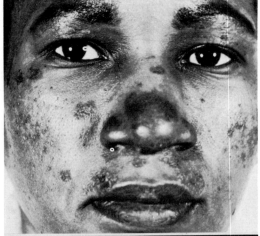
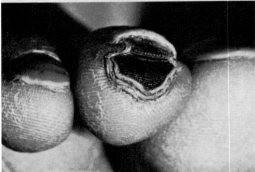

Figure 25–1. **Systemic lupus erythematosus.** (*Top*) Scaly, dark red lesions in a black woman. (*K.U.M.C.*) (*Bottom*) Gangrene of toe due to Raynaud's phenomenon in fatal case. (*Dr. R. Jordan*)

The patient should have a complete diagnostic workup and should be treated with corticosteroids, immunosuppressive agents, and any other supportive therapy, as indicated for the organs involved.

Remember that photosensitizing drugs, such as some diuretics and sulfonamide therapy, are contraindicated. Preferably, patients with systemic lupus should be primarily under the care of an internist, with assistance from the other specialties as needed.

SCLERODERMA
(Plates 69 and 70)

As in lupus erythematosus, there are two forms of scleroderma that are clinically unrelated, except for some common histopathologic changes in the skin. *Localized sclero-*

didal infection), *palmar erythema, spider hemangiomas,* and *pedunculated fibromas.* The following dermatoses are usually better, or disappear, during pregnancy: *psoriasis, acne* (can be worse), *alopecia areata,* and, possibly, *systemic scleroderma.*

MENOPAUSE STATE. Common physiologic changes in the skin of women during menopause include hot flashes, increased perspiration, increased hair growth on the face, and varying degrees of scalp hair loss. Other skin conditions associated with the menopause are *chloasma, pedunculated fibromas, localized neurodermatitis, vulvar pruritus, keratoderma climactericum* (palmar psoriasis), and *rosacea.*

GERIATRIC STATE (See Chap. 35, *Geriatric Dermatology*). The diffuse atrophy of the skin that occurs in the aged person is partially responsible for the dryness that results in *senile pruritus* and *winter itch.* Other changes include excessive wrinkling and hyperpigmentation of the skin. Specific dermatoses noted with increased frequency are *seborrheic* and *actinic keratoses, basal cell* and *squamous cell carcinomas, senile purpura, pedunculated fibromas,* and *capillary senile hemangiomas.*

RHEUMATIC FEVER. Nonspecific changes of increased sweating result in *prickly heat;* also *petechiae, urticaria, erythema nodosum, erythema multiforme,* and *rheumatic nodules* are seen.

POLYARTERITIS NODOSA. Polyarteritic nodules are specific, while purpura, erythema, and gangrene are nonspecific.

ENDANGITIS OBLITERANS (Buerger's Disease). This disease is characterized by superficial migrating thrombophlebitis, pallor or cyanosis, gangrene, and ulceration.

ULCERATIVE COLITIS. A characteristic ulcerative disease of the skin called *pyoderma gangrenosum* (see Plate 71) is associated quite frequently with ulcerative colitis, but the skin lesions can occur without this association. The ulcers are deep and foul smelling, spread rapidly, and characteristically have undermined edges with necrotic holes.

FRÖHLICH'S SYNDROME. This syndrome is due to hypopituitarism in the male. Feminine-type smooth skin and scant hair growth,

particularly in pubic and axillary regions, well-developed scalp hair, obesity, and small, thin fingernails are found.

ACROMEGALY. This disorder is caused by hyperpituitarism and excess growth-stimulating hormone. Skin changes due to overgrowth of the skeletal system, coarsened skin, deepened lines, increased sweating and oiliness, acne, increasing number of nevi, hyperpigmentation, and hypertrichosis occur.

CUSHING'S SYNDROME. Basophil adenoma of the pituitary gland is causative. Purplish atrophic striae, hyperpigmentation, hypertrichosis (in females and preadolescent males), and increased incidence of pyodermas are evident.

HYPERTHYROIDISM. The skin is moist and warm and has an evanescent erythema. There is hyperpigmentation (hypopigmentation, rarely), *seborrhea, acne, toxic alopecia,* and *nail atrophy. Localized myxedema* of the pretibial areas of the legs can develop and appears to be related to exophthalmos.

HYPOTHYROIDISM. The skin in generalized myxedema is cool, dry, scaly, thickened, and hyperpigmented. *Toxic alopecia,* with hair that is dull, dry, and coarse, and increased incidence of *pyodermas* are found.

ADDISON'S DISEASE. The most important dermatosis is hyperpigmentation (Plate 72), which is first seen on areas of friction, pressure, and irritation. Sweating is increased, and the axillary and pubic hair is shed.

DIABETES MELLITUS (Plate 73). Due to the increased amount of carbohydrate in the skin of patients with diabetes, skin infections occur with much higher frequency than in nondiabetic persons. These infections include *boils, carbuncles, ulcers, gangrene, candidiasis, tinea of the feet and the groin* (with or without secondary bacterial infection), and *infectious eczematoid dermatitis.* Other dermatoses seen are *pruritus, xanthoma diabeticorum,* and *necrobiosis lipoidica diabeticorum.*

LIPIDOSES. This complex group of metabolic diseases causes varying skin lesions, depending somewhat on the basic metabolic fault. The most common skin lesions are *xanthomas,* which are characterized by yellowish plaques or nodules readily seen on the skin

(*text continues on page 262*)

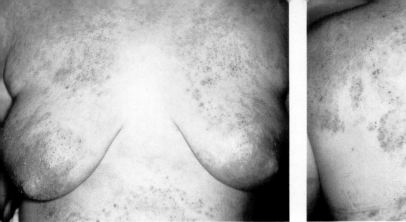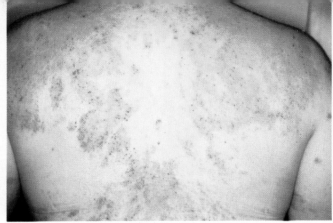

(*A* and *B*) Herpes gestationis associated with pregnancy (two different patients)

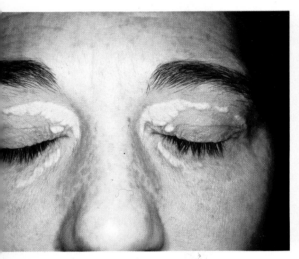

(*C*) Xanthelasma

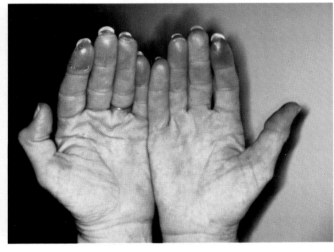

(*D*) Raynaud's disease with gangrene

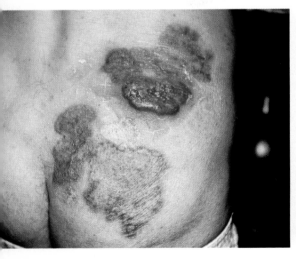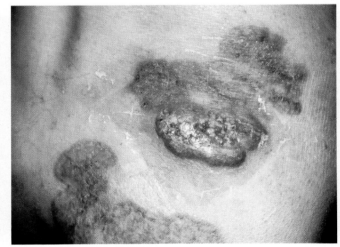

(*E*) Pyoderma gangrenosum of hip and (*F*) close-up showing both active and scarred, healed areas (this case was not associated with ulcerative colitis)

Plate 71. **Dermatoses due to internal disease.** (*Schering Corp.*)

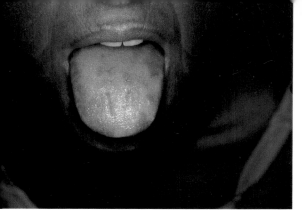

(A) Addison's disease, with hyperpigmentation of skin and tongue, in white woman

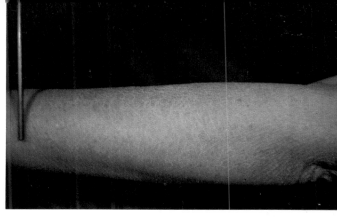

(B) Hypothyroidism, with "year-round dry skin"

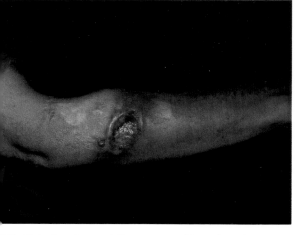

(C) Delusional excoriation on arm, "have to get the hairs out"

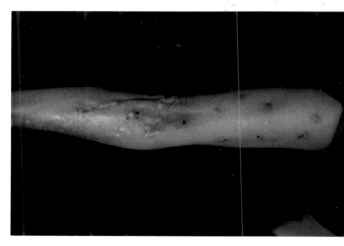

(D) Neurotic excoriations on the arm in a 47-year-old woman

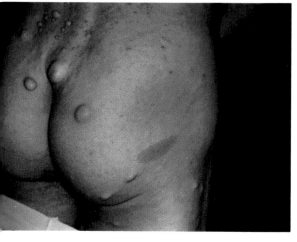

(E) Neurofibromatosis with café-au-lait lesion on buttocks

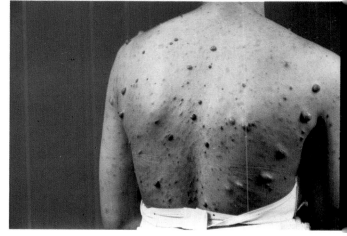

(F) Neurofibromatosis on the back (K.U.M.C.)

Plate 72. **Dermatoses due to internal disease** (Continued). (Reed & Carnrick)

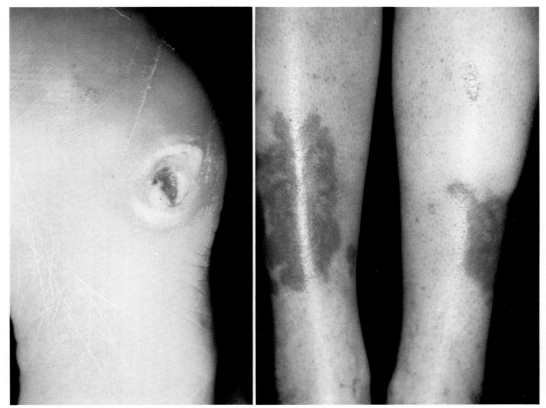

Plate 73. **Skin manifestations of diabetes mellitus.** (*Left*) Mal perforans of sole of foot of 3 years' duration. (*Right*) Necrobiosis lipoidica diabeticorum on anterior tibial area of legs. (*Dermik Laboratories, Inc. and Smith Kline & French Laboratories*)

surface. Xanthomatous lesions are either due to primary *hyperlipidemia*, or are the secondary result of a primary disease such as *alcoholism, diabetes mellitus, hypothyroidism*, and, less commonly, *obstructive jaundice, nephrotic syndrome*, and *dysproteinemia*.

The diagnosis of a patient with a xanthoma would begin with tests for fasting plasma cholesterol and triglycerides. These tests should uncover 95% of the patients with hyperlipidemia. If these tests are abnormal, then plasma turbidity studies and plasma lipoprotein electrophoresis should be performed. On the basis of abnormal lipoprotein patterns, five types of familial hyperlipidemia can be recognized.

Clinically there are five general types of xanthomas. They are tendinous xanthomas, planar xanthomas (most common form is *xanthelasma* or *xanthelasma palpebrarum*), tuberous xanthomas, eruptive xanthomas, and xanthoma disseminatum. These can usually be correlated with specific lipoproteins.

For secondary hyperlipidemia, therapy would be aimed at the primary disease. For familial hyperlipidemia, diet therapy and drug therapy must be considered, based on the type of disease.

Xanthoma-like deposits in the skin occur in several other diseases, namely the *histiocytosis* group of diseases, which are *Schüller-Christian syndrome, Letterer-Siwe disease*, and *eosinophilic granuloma*. Vesicular lesions can be seen in cases of Schüller-Christian syndrome, and a seborrheic-dermatitis–like picture is evident in Letterer-Siwe disease (see Fig. 34–3).

Extracellular lipid accumulations occur in *lipoid proteinosis, extracellular cholesterosis*, and *necrobiosis lipoidica diabeticorum*. Skin lesions of the latter occur mostly in women, on the anterior tibial area of the leg, and are characterized by sharply circumscribed, yellowish plaques with a bluish border. Diabetes is present in the majority of patients. Disturbances of phospholipid metabolism include *Niemann-Pick disease* and *Gaucher's disease*. Patients with both disorders develop a yellowish discoloration of the skin.

VITAMIN DEFICIENCIES. Dermatoses due to lack of vitamins are rare in the United States. However, a common question asked by many patients is, "Doctor, don't you think my trouble is due to lack of vitamins?" The answer in 99% of the cases is "No!"

Vitamin A. *Phrynoderma* is the name for generalized dry hyperkeratoses of the skin due to chronic and significant lack of vitamin A. Clinically, the texture of the skin resembles the surface of a nutmeg grater. Eye changes are often present, including night blindness and dryness of the eyeball.

Large doses of vitamin A (25,000 to 50,000 units t.i.d.) are used in the treatment of patients with *Darier's disease, pityriasis rubra pilaris, comedone acne,* and *xerosis* (dry skin). The value of this therapy has not been proved. Vitamin A therapy in high doses should be for only 4 to 6 months at a time, with cessation of therapy for 6 to 8 weeks before resuming it again.

Hypervitaminosis A, due to excessively high and persistent intake of vitamin A in drug or food form, causes hair loss, dry skin, irritability, weight loss, and enlargement of the liver and the spleen.

Isotretinoin (Accutane) is a vitamin A acid preparation that is beneficial for severe cystic acne and a few other rarer conditions.

Etretinate (Tegison), another synthetic derivative of vitamin A, is useful for pustular and exfoliative psoriasis. *Both Accutane and Tegison have severe side-effects, including fetal abnormalities. They should never be prescribed unless the physician and patient thoroughly understand the potential dangers of these vitamin A derivatives.*

Vitamin B Group. Clinically, a patient with a true vitamin B deficiency is deficient in all of the vitamins of this group. Thus the classic diseases of this group, *beriberi* and *pellagra,* have overlapping clinical signs and symptoms.

Vitamin B₁ (Thiamine). This deficiency is clinically manifested by *beriberi*. The cutaneous lesions consist of edema and redness of the soles of the feet.

Vitamin B₂ (Riboflavin). A deficiency of this vitamin has been linked with red fissures at the corners of the mouth and glossitis. This can occur in marked vitamin B₂ deficiency, but most cases with these clinical lesions are due to *contact dermatitis* or *malocclusion* of the lips from faulty dentures.

Nicotinic Acid. This deficiency leads to *pellagra,* but other vitamins of the B group are contributory. The skin lesions are a prominent part of pellagra and include redness of the exposed areas of hands, face, neck, and feet, which can go on to a fissured, scaling, infected dermatitis. Local trauma may spread the disease to other areas of the body. The disease is worse in the summer and heals with hyperpigmentation and mild scarring. Gastrointestinal and neurologic complications are serious.

The B group vitamins are administered with benefit to patients who have *rosacea*. Vitamin B₁₂ in doses of 1000 µg subcutaneously is questionably effective for cases of severe *seborrheic dermatitis.*

Vitamin C (Ascorbic Acid). *Scurvy* is now a rare disease, and the skin lesions are not specific. They include a follicular papular eruption, petechias, and purpura.

Vitamin D. No skin lesions have been attributed to lack of this vitamin. Vitamin D and vitamin D₂ (calciferol) have been used in the treatment of *lupus vulgaris.*

Vitamin E. It has been reported that vitamin E is effective in treating *pseudoxanthoma elasticum* and *epidermolysis bullosa* (Ayres and Mihan).

Vitamin K. Hypoprothrombinemia with purpura from various causes responds to vitamin K therapy.

Vitamin P (Hesperidin). Vitamin P appears to be beneficial for *chronic purpuric eruptions* of the Schamberg variety.

INTERNAL CANCER (Plate 74). Skin lesions may develop from internal malignancies either by metastatic spread or by the occurrence of nonspecific eruptions. The most interesting of the *nonspecific dermatoses* is the rare entity *acanthosis nigricans.* The presence of the velvety, papillary, pigmented hypertrophies

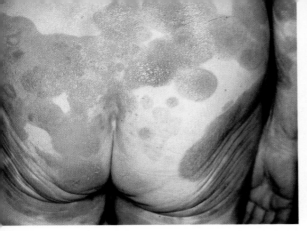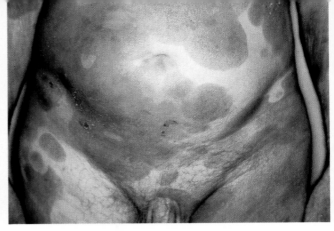

(A) Mycosis fungoides in plaque stage of buttocks and *(B)* abdomen of 79-year-old man

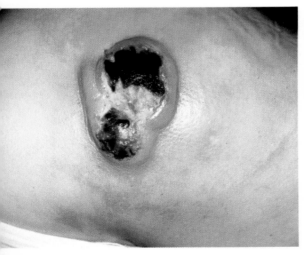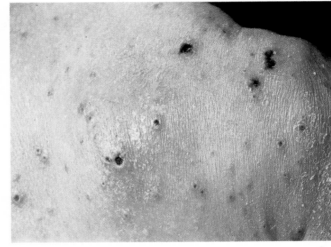

(C) Mycosis fungoides in tumor stage on thigh

(D) Nonspecific pyoderma with lymphocytic leukemia

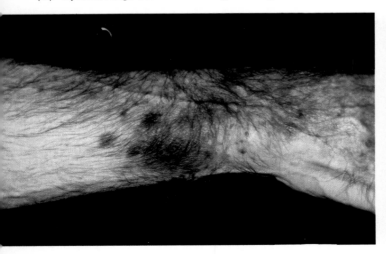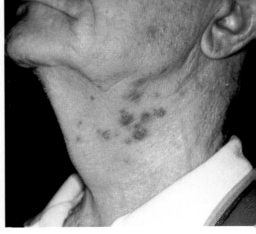

(E) Purpura of arm and *(F)* folliculitis of neck in same patient with myelogenous leukemia

Plate 74. **Dermatoses associated with lymphomas.** *(Syntex Laboratories, Inc.)*

of this disease in the axillae, the groin, and other moist areas of an adult will indicate an internal cancer, usually of the abdominal viscera, in over 50% of cases. A *benign form of acanthosis nigricans* exists in children and becomes most manifest at the age of puberty. This benign form is not associated with cancer.

A *dermatitis herpetiformis–like eruption* with vesicles and intense pruritus is seen occasionally in patients with an internal malignancy or lymphoma.

Purpuric lesions and pyodermas also occur as nonspecific changes in patients with malignancies (see Plate 74).

Specific skin lesions showing the malignancy or lymphoma on biopsy occur in *mycosis fungoides, leukemia, lymphomas,* and *metastatic skin lesions* from internal malignancies.

NEUROSES AND PSYCHOSES. A common belief among many members of the medical profession is that the majority of skin diseases are due to "nerves" or are a neurotic manifestation. This old idea is undoubtedly based on the familiar sight of the scratching skin patient; he just looks "nervous," and it makes one nervous and itchy merely to look at him. It is hard to know which came first for most patients, the itching or the nervousness. In my practice I tend to deemphasize the nervous element but not ignore it. My answer to patients and physicians who question the role of nerves in a particular case is to say that they play a definite role in many skin eruptions, but rarely are "nerves" the precipitating cause of a dermatosis. If a patient has an emotional problem and also has an itching dermatitis, a flare-up of the problem will intensify his itch, as it would aggravate another patient's duodenal ulcer or migraine headache.

Therapy for patients with skin disease, where "nerves" are believed to play a dominant part, can well be handled by the calm, receptive, attentive, interested general physician. Simple local therapy prescribed with the confidence of a competent physician will often establish in the patient the necessary faith that will cure his complaint. Occasionally, these patients will not respond to such therapy, and a rare case might benefit from special psychiatric care.

The following list will divide the psychocutaneous diseases into those believed to be (1) related to psychoses, (2) related to neuroses, and (3) of questionable psychic relationship.

Dermatoses Related to Psychoses

Factitial dermatitis: the patient denies that he is producing the skin disease. This is not to be confused with *neurotic excoriations.*

Skin lesions due to compulsive movements: an example is the chronic biting of an arm in a feeble-minded patient.

Delusions: of parasitism, cancer, syphilis, and so on (see Plate 72); various "proofs" are often presented by the patient to substantiate his or her existing belief.

Dysmorphic syndrome: patients have symptoms of cutaneous pain, burning, or other dysesthesias or, alternatively, have concerns about the structure and function of the skin or body contour. This is also called *cutaneous nondisease.* Symptoms most commonly involve the face, scalp, and genitals (vulvodynia). This is a serious psychotic problem. Haloperidol (Haldol) in a low dosage of 1 to 2 mg twice daily can be helpful (Koblenzer 1985).

Trichotillomania in adults: this is a rare cause of hair loss.

Dermatoses Related to Neuroses

Neurotic excoriations (see Plate 72): the patient admits picking or scratching the lesions.

Phobias: the patient fears contraction of a disease (*e.g.,* syphilophobia, acarophobia, cancerophobia, bacteriophobia).

Trichotillomania of children: this is not as serious as it is in adults. The physician's index of suspicion must be high to diagnose this disease (see Chap. 27).

Localized neurodermatitis (see Plate 16): the primary cause can be an insect bite, contact dermatitis due to a permanent wave, psoriasis, stasis dermatitis, or many other conditions that can initiate the scratching habit. The habit then outlives the disease, and the neurodermatitis cycle develops.

Dermatoses of Questionable Psychic Cause

Hyperhidrosis of palms and soles
Dyshidrosis
Alopecia areata
Lichen planus
Chronic urticaria
Rosacea

Atopic eczema
Psoriasis
Aphthous stomatitis
Primary pruritus, local or generalized

INTERNAL MANIFESTATIONS OF SKIN DISEASE

My purpose in this section is to list some of the internal phenomena that occur with certain diseases that primarily involve the skin. The collagen diseases belong in this group, particularly *lupus erythematosus* and *scleroderma*, and have been discussed earlier in this book (see Chap. 25).

ROSACEA. Eye lesions, such as keratitis, conjunctivitis, and blepharitis, are seen rather commonly.

ATOPIC ECZEMA. This is one manifestation of a triad of atopic conditions, the other two being bronchial asthma and hay fever. Eye cataracts are seen with severe forms of atopic eczema but only rarely. Blood eosinophilia is common.

PSORIASIS. This chronic papulosquamous eruption is associated with arthritis in a small number of cases. The psoriasis usually exists as one of the more severe forms of the disease, such as the exfoliative type, and frequently precedes the development of the arthritis. Most observers believe that the joint lesions are a form of rheumatoid arthritis.

URTICARIA PIGMENTOSA OR MASTOCYTO-SIS (see Plate 92). This rare maculopapular disease, mainly of children, is characterized by urtication of the lesions, following scratching. The skin lesions are composed of mast cells, and mast cell infiltrates are found in bone, liver, lymph nodes, and the thymus. The childhood form usually disappears spontaneously after a few years. The form in adults can last for years and eventuate in a lymphoma.

PSEUDOXANTHOMA ELASTICUM. This rare but characteristic skin disease of yellowish papules or plaques, mainly of the body folds, is a degeneration of the elastic tissue. Systemically, angioid streaks of the retina are seen in 25% of cases and result in a slowly progressive loss of visual acuity. Other systemic manifestations, undoubtedly due to the degeneration of elastic tissue in the arteries, include mental changes, intermittent claudication, absence of peripheral pulses, and intestinal hemorrhage.

INCONTINENTIA PIGMENTI (see Plates 90 and 91). This disease is a good example of the widening of clinical horizons. The pathology noted in the first early cases was a whorled hyperpigmentation of skin found in infants. Histologically, melanin was seen in the corium. This suggested that the epidermis was incontinent. It was later learned that when cases were seen at birth or soon after, the earliest stages of the disease were vesicular and bullous lesions and, then, lichenoid and warty lesions. The whorled hyperpigmentation was the third stage.

There is a familial or hereditary tendency in a few cases. Systemically, developmental defects have been found in an appreciable number of cases; these include faulty dentition, bone deformities, epilepsy, and mental deficiency.

NEUROFIBROMATOSIS (see Plates 72 and 92). Also known as von Recklinghausen's disease, this hereditary condition classically consists of pigmented patches (café-au-lait spots), pedunculated skin tumors, and nerve tumors. All of these lesions may not be present in a single case. Since internal nerves can be the site of the neurofibromas, deafness, paralysis, sensory disturbances, and epilepsy may be associated with them. Malignant degeneration of the tumors is not unusual.

BIBLIOGRAPHY

Barthelemy H, Chouvet B, Cambazard F: Skin and mucosal manifestations in vitamin deficiency. J Am Acad Dermatol 15:1263, 1986

Bishop ER: Monosymptomatic hypochondriacal syndromes in dermatology. J Am Acad Dermatol 9:152, 1983

Boulton AJM, Cutfield RG, Abouganem D et al: Necrobiosis lipoidica diabeticorum. J Am Acad Dermatol 18:530, 1988

Braverman IM: Skin Signs of Systemic Disease, 2nd ed. Philadelphia, WB Saunders, 1981

Callen JP, Jorizzo JL: Dermatologic signs of internal disease. Philadelphia, WB Saunders, 1988

Cruz PD, East C, Bergstresser PR: Dermal, subcutaneous, and tendon xanthomas. J Am Acad Dermatol 19:95, 1988

DiBacco RS, DeLeo VA: Mastocytosis and the mast cell. J Am Acad Dermatol 7:709, 1982

Feingold KR, Elias PM: Endocrine-skin interactions. J Am Acad Dermatol 19:1, 1988

Gould WM, Gragg TH: A dermatology–psychiatry liaison clinic. J Am Acad Dermatol 9:73, 1983

Harris BA, Sherertz EF, Flowers FP: Improvement of chronic neurotic excorations with oral doxepin therapy. Int J Dermatol 26:541, 1987

Hoeg JM, Gregg RE, Brewer HB: An approach to the management of hyperlipoproteinemia. JAMA 255:512, 1986

Kashihara-Sawami M, Horiguchi Y, Ikai K et al: Letterer-Siwe disease. J Am Acad Dermatol 18:559, 1988

Koblenzer CS: Psychosomatic concepts in dermatology. Arch Dermatol 119:501, 1983

Koblenzer CS: The dysmorphic syndrome. Arch Dermatol 121:780, 1985

Lookingbill DP, Spangler N, Sexton FM: Skin involvement as the presenting sign of internal carcinoma. J Am Acad Dermatol 22:19, 1990

Miller SJ: Nutritional deficiency and the skin. J Am Acad Dermatol 21:1, 1989

Parish LC, Fine E: Alcoholism and skin disease. Int J Dermatol 24:300, 1985

Parker F: Xanthomas and hyperlipidemias. J Am Acad Dermatol 13:1, 1985

Schwalgerle SM, Bergfeld WF, Senitzer D et al: Pyoderma gangrenosum: A review. J Am Acad Dermatol 18:559, 1988

Winton GB: Skin diseases aggravated by pregnancy. J Am Acad Dermatol 20:1, 1989

Wong C-K: Cutaneous amyloidoses. Int J Dermatol 26:273, 1987

27

Diseases Affecting the Hair

Thelda Kestenbaum, M.D.* and
Gordon C. Sauer, M.D.

The hair on an individual's scalp and body is a personal mark. Care of the scalp hair receives more attention, from both men and women, than care of any other part of the human anatomy. Thus, it is easy to understand the psychological problems caused by a disease of the hair. Unfortunately, however, two of the most common diseases of the hair, hereditary hair loss of the scalp and excessive hair growth on the face, cannot be prevented, contrary to magazine and newspaper advertisements.

Cosmetic aspects of hair and scalp care are covered in Chapter 8.

GRAY HAIR

Graying of the hair is a normal process of aging and develops earlier in whites than in blacks by about a decade. By age 50 years, half of whites are 50% gray. Premature graying may indicate underlying diseases such as pernicious anemia. Patchy gray hair may develop in areas of the scalp affected by *alopecia areata*. A frontal white patch of hair may be inherited as an autosomal dominant trait (*piebaldism*). Persons who are said to have "turned gray overnight" have probably had a diffuse form of alopecia areata in which the dark hairs were lost preferentially to gray hairs.

Elimination of gray hair is considered desirable by millions of persons, and there are a myriad of products on the market to help one achieve this goal. Hair dyes color on a temporary or permanent basis. The most common chemical that causes a hair dye contact dermatitis is paraphenylenediamine, which is on a standard tray of patch test substances in a dermatologist's office and should be tested for in a suspected case so as to avoid repeated episodes.

HIRSUTISM AND HYPERTRICHOSIS

Hirsutism is the excessive growth of terminal hair in a male sexual growth pattern. *Hypertrichosis* is the excessive growth of hair that is not in a male sexual growth pattern. Drugs can induce hirsutism or hypertrichosis.

Hirsutism

Hirsutism in women is often difficult to judge because there are major ethnic and racial variations. Women from Scandinavia and

* Assistant Professor of Medicine, Division of Dermatology, University of Kansas Medical Center, Kansas City, Kansas.

Asia are much less likely to have hirsutism than women from the Mediterranean regions.

Androgen excess and drug-induced hirsutism must be ruled out. Tests for dehydroepiandrosterone sulfate (DHEA-S), testosterone, follicle-stimulating hormone–luteinizing hormone (FSH/LH) ratio, and prolactin will help rule out endocrinologic causes. Androstenedione, cortisol, sex hormone binding proteins, and 17-hydroxyprogesterone levels may also be obtained, depending on clinical suspicion.

Among the diseases one needs to rule out in hirsutism are polycystic ovary disease, adrenal hyperplasia, Cushing's syndrome, adrenal tumors, ovarian tumors, and pituitary tumors.

The majority of women presenting with hirsutism will have no hormonal abnormalities or else minor ones and are placed in the familial or idiopathic group. As hormonal assays become more sophisticated, it is being appreciated that many patients in this group have subtle androgen "abnormalities." Do not let a familial history of hirsutism lull you into thinking a patient has "familial hirsutism." Remember that the congenital adrenal hyperplasias (21-hydroxylase defect and 11β hydroxylase defect) are inherited.

Treatment

Spironolactone (Aldactone) may be helpful in cases of idiopathic and familial hirsutism by interfering with androgen biosynthesis and by blocking the action of androgens at the receptor level.

Hypertrichosis

Hypertrichosis may be congenital or acquired. *Congenital* generalized types are very rare and have been described as being inherited and occurring sporadically. Some of the "dog-faced" or "monkey-faced" persons in circus sideshows probably had this condition. Fetal alcohol syndrome and fetal hydantoin syndrome may lead to congenital hypertrichosis. A host of rare syndromes may have congenital hypertrichosis as a feature. Congenital localized hypertrichosis has been noted on the margin of the pinna in infants of diabetic mothers. Localized congenital hypertrichosis over the base of the spine may be a marker of underlying spinal abnormalities.

Acquired hypertrichosis may be generalized or localized also. Acquired hypertrichosis lanuginosa ("malignant down") is a rare but striking cutaneous manifestation of internal malignancy. Fairly generalized hypertrichosis may occur in patients with diverse diseases such as porphyrias, dermatomyositis, anorexia nervosa, mercury intoxication, and head injuries. Drugs can induce hypertrichosis (Table 27–1). Localized acquired hypertrichosis may occur over areas of inflammatory dermatoses such as venous stasis or areas occluded by a plaster cast or may be a feature of a benign nevus.

Treatment

Treatment of hypertrichosis may include shaving, depilatories, bleaching, plucking, waxing (really a sort of plucking), and electrolysis. Electrolysis is the only permanent method of hair removal and usually requires more than one treatment to each hair follicle that one wishes to ablate. It should be done by someone trained in the technique. Inquiry should be made whether the operator uses sterile needles to deliver the electrical current to the hair follicle to prevent any possibility of accidental transmission of blood-borne disease.

Shaving, contrary to popular belief, does not increase the amount of hair that regrows. Chemical depilatories and bleaching agents are available over the counter and frequently prove effective but may be irritating to the skin of some persons. Waxing and plucking have the advantage of removing the unwanted hair for longer periods without re-treatment than does shaving. Plucking, waxing, and electrolysis may cause a folliculitis. Electrolysis also can cause scarring and is expensive.

Table 27–1
Drugs That Can Cause Hirsutism and Hypertrichosis

Hirsutism	Hypertrichosis
Androgens	Corticosteroids
Danazol	Diazoxide
	Minoxidil
	Penicillamine
	Phenytoin
	Psoralens
	Streptomycin

HAIR LOSS (ALOPECIA)

Alopecia of the scalp is of considerable concern to both men and women. It is helpful in differentiating among the many causes of alopecia to examine the hair and scalp and observe whether the hair loss is diffuse or patchy and whether the scalp appears scarred (Fig. 27–1). A careful history and physical examination of the hair and scalp is most important. Nonscarring hair loss is more common than scarring hair loss (Table 27–2).

Nonscarring Alopecia

Diffuse Nonscarring Alopecia

Among the more common causes of nonscarring hair loss are androgenetic hair loss, telogen effluvium, alopecia areata, trichotillomania, trauma, and tinea. An appropriate history and laboratory testing are necessary (Table 27–3).

One must exclude syphilis, thyroid disease, iron deficiency, drug-induced (Table 27–4) and toxin-induced (thallium, boric acid, heavy metal) causes, or systemic lupus erythematosus as etiologies. When acne and hirsutism or other reasons make one suspect an androgen excess, appropriate hormonal studies should be done. Careful questioning about current or recent illness, past medical history, weight loss, recent childbirth in women, drug ingestion, hair dressing procedures, and family history of baldness is important.

ANDROGENETIC HAIR LOSS. Androgenetic hair loss (also called pattern baldness, hereditary baldness, androgenic baldness,

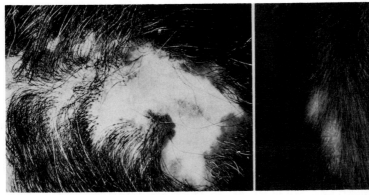

Chronic discoid lupus erythematosus
in a black patient

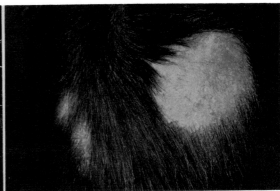

Tinea of the scalp

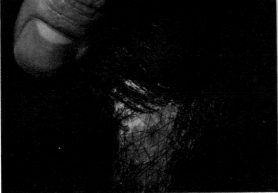

Alopecia cicatrisata

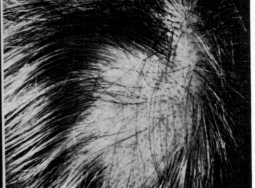

Traumatic alopecia

Figure 27–1. Hair loss due to various causes. The case of traumatic alopecia was caused by the accidental catching of the scalp hair in a rotary massaging instrument used on the patient's back.

Table 27–2
Characteristics of Nonscarring and Scarring Hair Loss

NONSCARRING HAIR LOSS	SCARRING HAIR LOSS
Diffuse	Tinea
Androgenetic (male pattern hair loss, female pattern hair loss)	Severe bacterial infection
Telogen effluvium (secondary to systemic disease, post partum, weight loss)	Hair loss associated with other skin disease (discoid lupus erythematosus, scleroderma, lichen planus)
Drugs and toxins	Trauma (chemical burns, radiation overdosage)
Endocrinopathy (hypothyroidism, hyperthyroidism)	Idiopathic (pseudopelade of Brocq or alopecia cicatrisata)
Hair loss associated with skin disease (systemic lupus erythematosus, exfoliative dermatitis)	Congenital (aplasia cutis, epidermal nevi)
Congenital syndromes (many associated with hair shaft defects—rare)	
Patchy	
Alopecia areata	
Traumatic (traction) alopecia	
Trichotillomania	
Tinea	
Secondary syphilis	

male pattern hair loss, and female pattern hair loss) is diagnosed by most lay persons, and they do not consult a physician. It is defined as an alopecia induced by androgens in those genetically predisposed, and it occurs in both men and women. The fact that it is probably the most common cause of nonscarring diffuse hair loss in women is underappreciated by both patients and physicians. Of course a workup to exclude other causes of diffuse hair loss should be done (see Table 27–3). In women with this problem the thinning is usually on the crown and its onset is usually in young adulthood. Telogen effluvium may be a feature of it.

TELOGEN EFFLUVIUM. Telogen effluvium is the shedding of an excessive number of hairs that are in the telogen (resting) phase. Normally about 13% of the scalp hairs are in telogen phase, 83% are in anagen (growth) phase, and the remainder are in catagen phase. It is normal to shed up to 100 hairs per day from the scalp. Various events such as childbirth, high fever, rapid and marked weight loss, drugs, and virtually any major bodily insult may increase the ratio of telogen to anagen hairs. Within 2 or 3 months after the triggering event, the patient notes an increase in hair shedding. It is reversible.

Postpartum alopecia deserves special mention as a type of telogen effluvium because a good history can often obviate doing an extensive workup when this is the suspected cause. In women with diffuse nonscarring hair loss it may account for almost 10% of the patients.

To estimate whether an excessive number of hairs are in a resting phase, grasp and lightly pull eight to ten closely grouped hairs; normally none to two hairs are pulled out. A more accurate method is to put pieces of a rubber tube around a straight forceps and pull about fifty hairs out by the roots. The hair bulbs are examined to determine whether there is a normal telogen-anagen ratio. An increase in number of telogen hair bulbs may be seen in androgenetic alopecia and sometimes in alopecia areata, so an abnormally high telogen-anagen ratio does not entirely rule out these other entities.

Treatment

ANDROGENETIC HAIR LOSS
1. Topical minoxidil (Rogaine) (60-ml bottle) may be helpful for this problem. It has been studied in men more than in women. Younger men (<40 years of age) with mild

Table 27–3
Laboratory Studies to Evaluate Nonscarring Alopecia

Baseline

Complete blood cell count

Ferritin

VDRL

Thyroxine, thyroid-stimulating hormone (consider thyroid antibodies)

Microscopic examination of hair

Fungal culture

Other

Scalp biopsy

ANA

Hormones (*e.g.,* dehydroepiandrosterone sulfate, testosterone, androstenedione)

Borate and thallium levels

Heavy metal screen

to moderate hair loss of less than 10 years' duration respond the best. It takes 12 months to see maximal response, and it is expensive. One milliliter is applied twice daily to the scalp with one of several different applicator types in the package. Slightly less than half of men using it will obtain significant improvement. The use of the drug must be maintained indefinitely to maintain the new hair growth.

Table 27–4
Some Drugs That Can Cause Alopecia

Chemotherapeutic drugs

Anticoagulants (heparin, coumadin)

Testosterone

Anabolic steroids (*e.g.,* danazol)

β-Blockers

Corticosteroids

Anticonvulsants (phenytoin, valproic acid, trimethadione)

Cholesterol-lowering drugs

Vitamin A

Oral contraceptives

Progesterone

Quinacrine

Captopril

Colchicine

Gold

Retinoids

Amphetamines

2. The surgical procedures of hair transplantation and scalp reduction are possible therapeutic modalities.

TELOGEN EFFLUVIUM

Treatment consists of pointing out the causative factor and reassuring the patient that he or she will not become bald. Usually the hair loss will slowly cease, and the normal hair pattern will be reestablished. Tell the patient that regrowth will take at least 6 months.

Nonscarring Patchy Alopecia

Alopecia areata (Fig. 27–2) is said to account for between 1% and 3% of patient visits to the offices of dermatologists. It is a nonscarring, usually patchy, but sometimes diffuse hair loss of unclear cause. Many cases are familial, and it is believed that this may well have an autoimmune etiology. It is seen more commonly in patients with atopic dermatitis, autoimmune thyroid disease, vitiligo, and Down's syndrome.

Usually this disease presents as an asymptomatic, totally bald area. Exclamation-mark hairs are often noted at the margin of the bald spot or spots. These are broken-off hairs that are thicker distally and thinner proximally near the scalp like the top part of an exclamation mark (!) and are considered pathognomonic of alopecia areata.

Typically the scalp is involved, but any hair-bearing area of the body may be affected, such as the eyelashes, eyebrows, and beard.

In the majority of cases in adults, in which only one or a few bald spots appear, regrowth occurs in 6 to 12 months, and reassurance is all that is needed. Factors that bode a bad prognosis are young age at onset and extensive early hair loss. When all the scalp hair is lost the term *alopecia totalis* is used; and if all body hair is lost, the term *alopecia universalis* is used. These latter two severe forms of alopecia areata have a bad prognosis and are fortunately rare.

Trichotillomania (Fig. 27–3 and Plate 93) is a self-inflicted hair pulling disorder that may affect up to 8 million Americans and is seen more commonly in females than in males. It seems to be linked with tics and habit disorders and is classified as a disturbance of impulse control (although it may be an obsessive-compulsive disorder). Trichotillomania usually begins in childhood and is a persistent problem. Certainly in children suf-

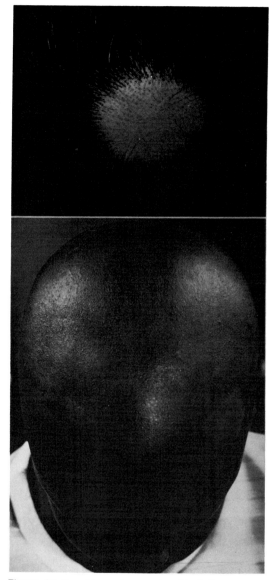

Figure 27–2. Alopecia areata. (*Top*) Single area on vertix of scalp. Exclamation point hairs are barely visible. (*Bottom*) Total alopecia of 4-year-old black girl.

fering from this condition some attempt at evaluating the child's home situation is in order to see if the emotional well-being of the child can be improved.

Traumatic alopecia (see Fig. 27–1) from cosmetic treatments to the hair may result in a patchy, nonscarring hair loss that is frequently especially marked around the periphery of the scalp. Frequent use of hair permanents, hair straighteners, and hair dyes can lead to

patchy hair loss marked by broken off hairs. Tight ponytails and tight braiding (especially "corn-row" braiding) may lead to hair loss that is usually nonscarring but in some persons can cause scarring. Inquiry about hair care is always necessary in evaluating patients with alopecia.

Tinea capitis (see Fig. 27–1 and Plate 93) is more commonly seen in children than in adults and can cause a patchy hair loss characterized by broken off hairs and scaling of the scalp. Currently in the United States the most common fungal organism causing this condition (*T. tonsurans*) does not cause fluorescence with a Wood's light. Usually tinea causes a nonscarring hair loss. A severely inflammatory tinea can result in scarring. A KOH slide and fungal culture establish this diagnosis. Therapy with oral griseofulvin, or possibly ketoconazole, is effective.

Secondary syphilis may cause a patchy, nonscarring hair loss or, less frequently, a diffuse, nonscarring hair loss. A serum VDRL test would be diagnostic.

Treatment

Topical corticosteroids and topical anthralin may be helpful and are fairly safe treatments for alopecia areata. Intralesional corticosteroids and PUVA have been used. Generally the adverse effects of systemic corticosteroids do not usually warrant their use. Appropriate referrals for hairpieces and informing the patient of the existence of the National Alopecia Areata Foundation for educational information and local support group information are often helpful in this frequently very stress-producing disorder that lacks an effective treatment.

Clomipramine, which is available on special protocol only, has been reported effective for some patients with trichotillomania.

Scarring (Cicatricial) Alopecia

Of the skin disorders that can lead to a scarring hair loss one should include discoid lupus erythematosus, scleroderma, lichen planus, tinea, and metastatic carcinoma. A skin biopsy and a fungal culture are indicated to help establish the diagnosis in cases of scarring alopecia.

Folliculitis decalvans is a chronic folliculitis of unclear cause. It is characterized by

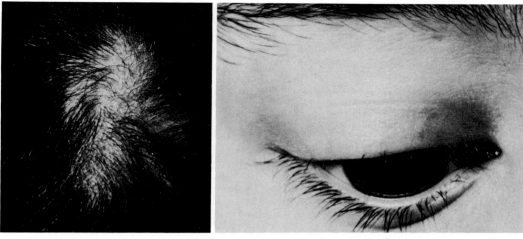

Figure 27–3.   **Trichotillomania.** (*Left*) On the scalp of a 9-year-old boy. (*Right*) Of the eyelashes of a 10-year-old girl.

recurrent, progressive pustules that gradually extend and destroy the hair follicle. Bacterial cultures may reveal *Staphylococcus aureus* but usually reveal nonpathogenic organisms. Fungal cultures should be done to exclude a scarring type of tinea capitis. Favus of the scalp caused by *Trichophyton schoenleini* may mimic this disease. Therapy with oral antibiotics is occasionally effective.

Pseudopelade of Brocq (alopecia cicatrisata) is a scarring alopecia of unknown cause (see Fig. 27–1). It probably represents an end stage of a skin disease such as lichen planus. There is no effective treatment.

MISCELLANEOUS DISORDERS AFFECTING THE HAIR

TRICHORRHEXIS NODOSA.   This is probably the most common hair shaft abnormality and is usually caused from traumatic hairdressing procedures. Clinically one sees circumferential tiny white specks on the hair shaft. When viewed under the microscope these areas prove to be transverse fractures resembling the bristles of two brooms interlocked in appearance. These fracture points often lead to breaking off of the hairs and the complaint that the hair does not grow as long as it used to. There may be inherited causes of trichorrhexis nodosa, but these are much more rare. Clinically these fracture points on the hair shaft may be confused with nits of head lice or hair casts.

TRICHOSTASIS SPINULOSA.   This is a common condition in adults that clinically resembles comedones ("blackheads") and occurs on the face or upper body. Retention of multiple vellus hairs (up to 50) is the cause of this problem. It may be treated with topical tretinoin (Retin-A) or waxing.

UNCOMBABLE HAIR SYNDROME ("Spunglass hair").   This interesting hair shaft abnormality is characterized by hair shafts that are triangular on cross section. On electron microscopy a longitudinal depression occurs. Clinically, onset is around 3 years of age when the hair seems totally wild and unamenable to combing and brushing. The hair is usually a silvery blond color. Although usually generalized, it can be localized. Eyebrows and eyelashes are normal. Spontaneous improvement may occur during childhood.

ACQUIRED PROGRESSIVE KINKING OF THE HAIR.   This odd and rare entity arises during the teens or early adult years. Gradually and progressively in a white person the hair becomes kinky, dry, and more unmanageable. It is unassociated with internal disease. Unlike uncombable hair, the hair shaft in this disorder is not triangular but is elliptical or irregular with partial twists at irregular intervals. The duration of anagen (growth phase) is said to be reduced. Oral retinoids may induce a clinically similar problem.

Interestingly, a seemingly converse clinical picture has been described in black patients with the acquired immunodeficiency syndrome who develop softer, silkier hair that replaces the previously kinky hair. In addition, the color is said to become ashen and the hair is sparse.

GREEN HAIR. The deposition of copper on the hair, from tap water used to wash the hair (or from swimming pool water), may cause a greenish hue in blond hair. Pretreating the hair with some types of conditioners may help prevent the discoloration. Shampooing with an edetic acid– or penicillamine-containing mixture may reduce the green color.

TWISTED HAIRS (PILI TORTI), BEADED HAIR (MONILETHRIX), RINGED HAIR (PILI ANNULATI). These three conditions may be different clinical manifestations of altered hair growth from hereditary and congenital causes. The terms are self-defining.

FRAGILITY OF THE HAIR SHAFT (FRAGILITAS CRINIUM). Longitudinal splitting and fraying of the hair shaft reflects structural weakness of the hair. The most common form is terminal splitting of the hair shaft seen in women who have allowed their hair to grow very long. This fragile hair can be associated

with trichorrhexis nodosa, monilethrix, and ringed hair.

LOOSE ANAGEN SYNDROME. In this disorder of children, usually blond girls aged 2 to 5 years, the loosely anchored hairs are in anagen stage and do not grow in length. It may be familial.

INGROWN HAIR (PILI INCARNATI). This common condition, seen particularly in blacks, is usually associated with *pseudofolliculitis* of the beard. Allowing a beard to grow or less frequent and less close shaving can be beneficial in eliminating ingrown hairs.

BIBLIOGRAPHY

Baden HP: Diseases of the Hair and Nails. Boca Raton, FL, CRC Press, 1986

Barrett S: Commercial hair analysis: Science or scam? JAMA 254:1041, 1985

Leonidas JR: Hair alteration in black patients with the acquired immunodeficiency syndrome. Cutis 39:537, 1987

Mitchell AJ, Krull EA (eds): Hair disorders. Dermatol Clin 5(3), 1987

Person JR: Green hair: Treatment with a penicillamine shampoo. Arch Dermatol 121:717, 1985

Pitts RL: Serum elevation of dehydroepiandrosterone sulfate associated with male pattern baldness in young men. J Am Acad Dermatol 16:571, 1987

Price VH, Gummer CL: Loose anagen syndrome. J Am Acad Dermatol 20:249, 1989

Rook A, Dawber R: Diseases of the Hair and Scalp. Boston, Blackwell Scientific Publications, 1982

Stern RS: Topical minoxidil. Arch Dermatol 123:62, 1987

Stroud JD: Diagnosis and management of the hair loss patient. Cutis 40:272, 1987

Swedo SE et al: A double-blind comparison of clomipramine and desipramine in the treatment of trichotillomania (hair pulling). N Engl J Med 321:497, 1989

SAUER NOTES:

1. Shaving the hair does not increase its growth.
2. Frequent shampooing does not damage normal scalp hair.
3. Dandruff, unless it becomes severely secondarily infected, does not cause hair loss.
4. Excessive brushing of the hair can cause hair breakage and hair loss.
5. Hair length is genetically predetermined by the duration of the anagen phase.

28

Diseases Affecting the Nails

Thelda Kestenbaum, M.D.* and
Gordon C. Sauer, M.D.

The most common nail dystrophies are caused by fungal infection, psoriasis, trauma, or impaired circulation. Nail diseases may be divided into (1) primary nail diseases, (2) nail dystrophies associated with cutaneous disease, and (3) nail dystrophies that reflect internal disease. There is considerable overlap between some of these categories.

Growth of fingernails is approximately 0.1 mm per day. Nails grow more rapidly on the middle fingernail than they do on the thumb or fifth finger. Toenails grow at one half or one third the fingernail rate. Diseases such as psoriasis or nail biting hasten nail growth. Old age and decreased circulation may slow nail growth.

Nail anatomy is discussed on page 6. The nail matrix is responsible primarily for the nail plate. Calcium only accounts for a small percent of the nail plate by weight, contrary to the notion of many persons.

PRIMARY NAIL DISEASES

Only the most *common* primary nail diseases are included in this chapter. The terminology for the *rare* primary conditions is very

complex and is defined at the end of this chapter.

Contact Reactions
(Plate 75)

Changes in the nails, mainly the fingernails, from cosmetic applications are related to the constant attempts by manufacturers to discover a nail polish or covering that will adhere to and become a part of the nail for the life of the person, or at least for the duration of a certain fad. Several years ago such a cosmetic panacea was discovered in the form of a base coat, but the nail rebelled, with the development of thickening and loosening of the nail plate. The use of artificial nails and a press-on type of covering results in splitting of the distal ends of the nail.

The usual culprits for contact dermatitis in nail cosmetics are methacrylates in sculptured nails and cyanoacrylates in nail glues. These reactions usually cause *onycholysis* (lifting up of the nail plate from the nail bed distally) and *paronychial infection,* which can be quite painful and disfiguring.

These nail-bed reactions are not related to, and should be differentiated from, the allergic sensitivity manifested by some women to chemicals in the nail polish. The fingernails, interestingly enough, do not react to this allergy, but the sensitivity shows up on the eyelids and the neck as a *contact dermatitis* (see

---

* Assistant Professor of Medicine, Division of Dermatology, University of Kansas Medical Center, Kansas City, Kansas.

276

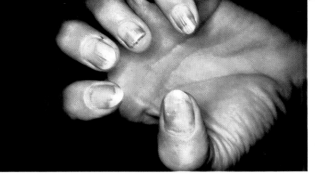

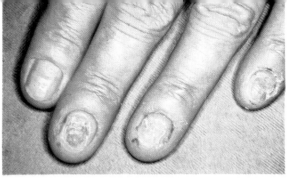

(A) Onycholysis contact reaction to nail hardener

(B) Onychotillomania or picking of nail plate

(C) Traumatic, habit-tic injury to plate

(D) Tinea due to *T. rubrum*

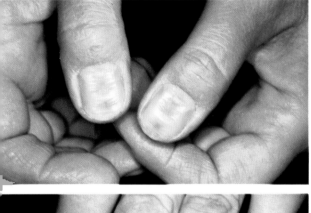

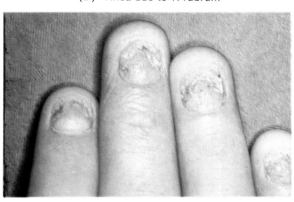

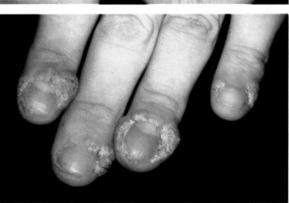

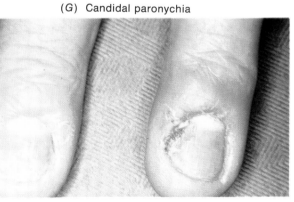

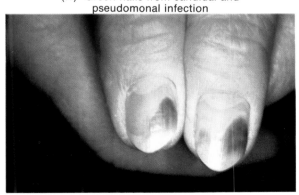

(E) Periungual warts in lymphoma patient

(F) Photosensitivity onycholysis from demeclocycline

(G) Candidal paronychia

(H) Green nails from candidal and
pseudomonal infection

Plate 75. **Nail disorders.** (*Westwood Pharmaceuticals*)

Chap. 9). The most common sensitizer in nail polish is toluene-sulfonamide formaldehyde resin.

Overuse of liquid cuticle removers may cause an irritant rather than an allergic contact dermatitis. These products usually contain sodium or potassium hydroxide.

Nail Biting (Onychophagia)

This common "nervous" habit of some children and fewer adults is very difficult to stop. Often the less attention that is paid to this tic the better, with the resulting cessation of the biting. Nail biting actually hastens the growth of nails. It is a good way to spread warts. The local application of distasteful chemicals to the nails seldom stops the biting.

Infections

Primary nail infections can occur from several causes.

Bacterial and candidal infections (see Plate 75) can cause paronychial reactions. *Candidal infections* are chronic and cause inflammation and swelling of the proximal and lateral nail folds. These infections are very resistant to therapy (see Chap. 19). *Bacterial paronychias* are more acute, are painful, and often require surgical drainage of the pus.

Green nails (see Plate 75) is a unique and distinctive infection from which *Candida albicans* and *Pseudomonas aeruginosa* can be cultured. Complete débridement of the detached part of the nail is necessary for a cure.

Ingrown Nails

The mechanism of this disorder is the growth of the lateral edge of the nail plate, usually of the big toe, into the adjacent skin groove. Tight-fitting shoes and improper nail trimming initiate the process. The result is a foreign-body type of reaction with pain, redness, swelling, and infection.

Prophylactic management is simple: the toenail, especially the big toenail, never should be trimmed in a semilunar manner but should be trimmed straight across, so that the corner lies above the skin groove.

Active treatment of an acute process consists of hot soaks and local application of an antiseptic tincture. After the pain has lessened, the placement of a pledget of cotton gently under the nail may be sufficient to raise the pointed corner up above the skin surface. More resistant cases are treated by removing the overlying skin by excision and suture, or by removing the lateral section of the nail back to the nail base, with or without destruction of the base by electrosurgery.

Hang Nails

Some patients are prone to develop small cutaneous tags from the lateral and posterior skin folds. Accidental or intentional pulling on these skin flaps tears into the deeper skin, with resultant bleeding and a painful raw area that is susceptible to bacterial infection. This can be prevented by removal of the hang nail with scissors.

Treatment of the infection, which may develop into a *bacterial paronychia*, is with hot soaks, local application of antiseptic tinctures or ointments, avoidance of covering dressings, and, in severe cases, use of systemic antibiotics.

Leukonychia

The common "white spots" of the nail plate have been responsible for many interesting homespun etiologic labels. Medically speaking, we cannot do much better regarding the cause. (I've always thought they followed the telling of white lies.) The histogenesis is also not known, but current theories propose that the white spots are due to tiny air bubbles in the nail or to the presence of incompletely keratinized cells, probably the result of minor injury. No treatment is indicated.

Hereditary leukonychia is very rare and involves all the fingernails and toenails (Plate 76).

Fragile or Brittle Nails

The distal splitting or peeling of the fingernail plate is a common complaint of women. In most instances the cause cannot be determined, but some cases are due to the "perma-

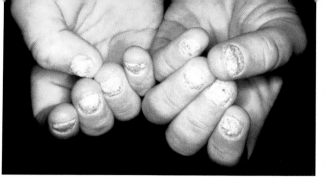
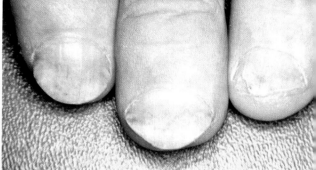

(*A* and *B*) Psoriasis of nails showing crumbling, pitting, and distal detachment of plates

(*C* and *D*) Lichen planus showing pterygium and plate atrophy on close-up of fingernails

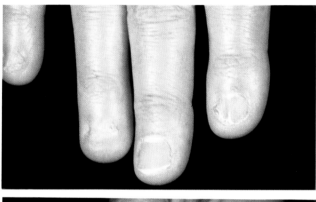
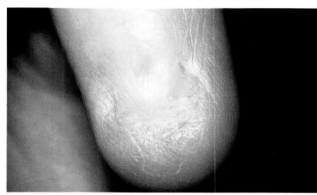

(*E*) Darier's disease of nails

(*F*) Medial canaliform dystrophy

(*G*) Beau's lines due to hyperpigmentation in black patient following x-irradiation

(*H*) Hereditary leukonychia totalis and partial onycholysis

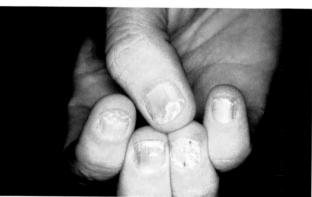
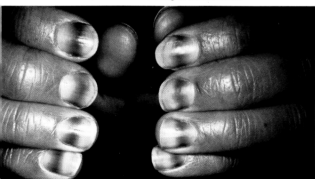

Plate 76. **Nail disorders.** (*Continued*).

nent" type of nail polishes or the solvents used in removing the polish. Other factors include poor peripheral circulation, iron deficiency, or gout.

Treatment is usually quite unsatisfactory. There is no question about the fact that the use of strong detergents, fingernail polish, and polish removers weakens the adhesion between the cell layers in the nail plate. Avoidance of these practices will, in 5 to 6 months, result in less or no splitting. Gently buffing the nail plate will physically remove some of the rough edges.

Onychorrhexis

Onychorrhexis is an excessive longitudinal striation of the nail plate and is seen commonly as a person ages. Persons with rheumatoid arthritis or decreased peripheral circulation, as well as skin diseases such as psoriasis, alopecia areata, lichen planus, or Darier's disease, may also develop this nail dystrophy.

Melanonychia

A longitudinal hyperpigmented band is most common in blacks but also seen in Asians. A solitary longitudinal streak in a white patient is cause for worry because, although it may just be caused by a nevus involving the nail matrix, it may also be caused by melanoma. A nail biopsy is frequently necessary to rule out this possibility.

Many drugs, especially the chemotherapeutic agents, can cause longitudinal nail hyperpigmentation.

NAIL DISEASE SECONDARY TO OTHER DERMATOSES

The nail, as one of the skin appendages, is susceptible to diseases of the skin adjacent to the nail or to dermatoses on distant areas. It is important to remember that a dermatitis of the skin can be made to heal rather rapidly, but that any concurrent nail involvement will take approximately 3 months to grow out with the nail. The "scar" remains on the nail much longer than on the skin.

Tinea of the Nails (Onychomycosis)
(Plate 75)

Disturbance of nail growth due to fungi is a commonly observed nail problem. The nail involvement occurs secondary to a primary foot and hand tinea. A major percentage of the male population have one or more thickened toenails, which almost invariably are caused by fungi. Females have onychomycosis of the toenails less frequently, and both sexes have fingernail involvement only rarely. Tinea of the nails is discussed in detail in Chapter 19.

Warts
(Plate 75)

Verrucae can occur anywhere on the body, but one of the most difficult warts to treat is the type that grows around the nail and under the nail plate. Nail biting can spread the wart virus. If a periungual wart is large and extends rather far under the nail, a deformed nail may result from the removal. The patient should be told about this possibility in advance. The management of these problem warts is discussed in Chapter 17.

Squamous cell carcinoma may be the diagnosis of a "recalcitrant wart." It has been associated with human papillomavirus 16. *Periungual fibromas* and *osteochrondromas* may mimic periungual warts. An especially painful "wart" may in fact be a *glomus tumor*.

Eczematous Eruptions of the Fingers

The eczematous skin eruptions include *contact dermatitis, atopic eczema*, and *nummular eczema*. The nail becomes involved when these dermatoses affect the adjacent skin. When the skin dermatitis heals, the nail will heal also, but, as stated previously, the mark of the dermatitis on the nail will take 3 months to disappear completely.

An unusual reaction of the nail is the development of a *highly polished nail surface* in some patients with severely itching *atopic eczema*. This is due to the habit of some atopic persons of constantly rubbing the skin with the flat nail surface instead of scratching with the distal end of the nail.

Psoriasis
(Plate 76)

An astute clinician can occasionally diagnose psoriasis by merely examining the nails. Often the only sign of psoriasis will be the nail changes for which the patient seeks medical advice. Psoriasis can cause any and all of the dystrophic changes of the nails. The most common changes are small pinpoint pits, with or without distal detachment of the nail. A proximal red halo frequently is present around the distal detachment. In severe psoriatic nail involvement there is complete disintegration of the plate surface, with massive subungual proliferation. Even these severe changes are usually asymptomatic.

Treatment of psoriasis of the nails is very unsatisfactory. If psoriasis is present on other areas and responds to therapy, the nails may also clear. Cordran tape applied over the nails is moderately effective.

Lichen Planus
(Plate 76)

Lichen planus is a papulosquamous disease that may cause a pterygium or winglike deformity of the nail, longitudinal ridging, thinning of the nail plate, thickening of the nail plate, or onycholysis, among other nail changes. As with psoriasis of the nails, treatment is not very effective.

Twenty Nail Dystrophy

A lackluster appearance with longitudinal striations, roughness, and some pitting may be seen in all twenty nails, usually in children. This may improve spontaneously over some years. Although this problem was described as a primary nail disease, many authors believe these are nail changes of psoriasis, lichen planus, or alopecia areata that are seen without other manifestations of the disorder.

Other Dermatoses
(Plate 76)

Nonspecific nail changes can occur along with *alopecia areata, Darier's disease, epidermolysis bullosa, ichthyosis, pityriasis rubra pilaris,* and other dermatoses.

NAIL DISEASE SECONDARY TO INTERNAL DISEASE

Changes in the nails can reflect internal disease. The great majority of these changes are nonspecific.

Beau's Lines
(Plate 76)

Beau's lines, or transverse furrows of the nails, may develop with any of a large group of cutaneous and systemic disturbances. The latter include many of the acute infectious febrile diseases, such as malaria, syphilis, and pulmonary tuberculosis, and coronary disease, pregnancy, collagen diseases, and emotional shock.

Beau's lines are due to a temporary growth disturbance in the nail plate. An analogy is the alteration in the annual growth rings of trees when affected by drought, fire, or pestilence. The width of Beau's lines varies directly with the duration of the internal disease. As stated before, the "scar" of this nail alteration will, for the fingernail, take approximately 3 months to grow out. Many are the awesome, astute, detective-like, laity-impressing deductions made by the clever physician when these lines are noted. A proper and impressive Sherlock Holmes–like statement on finding Beau's lines approximately half-way down all of the fingernails is, "I see that you had a rather severe illness about 6 weeks ago."

Hippocratic Nails

Clubbed nails and fingers are classically associated with chronic lung and heart disorders (Fig. 28–1). These changes apparently are due to the prolonged anoxemia that is present. Equally common is a congenital and hereditary form of hippocratic nails seen in healthy persons.

Koilonychia (Spoon Nails)

Koilonychia is a concavity of the nail plate classically associated with iron deficiency

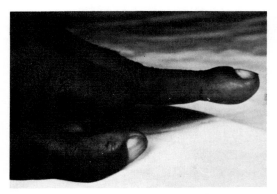

Figure 28–1. **Hippocratic or clubbed nails and fingers in black male with cardiovascular syphilis.**

anemia, but it may be seen in about half of the patients with hemochromatosis. Thyroid disease (hyperthyroidism and hypothyroidism) and polycythemia also may be associated. Probably most cases are not associated with internal diseases.

Koilonychia may be seen as part of some other skin diseases such as lichen planus, psoriasis, or syphilis. There is an autosomal dominant variety. It is common in infants on finger and toenails. Injury to the nail can produce this nail dystrophy.

Terry's Nails

Over 30 years ago Terry noticed that cirrhotic patients frequently had a whitish opacity to all but the distal several millimeters of nail plate of all the nails. It is not specific for hepatic disease and has been described in up to a fourth of hospitalized patients in general.

Mees' Lines

The appearance of transverse white bands in the nail plate and growing out with it classically has been associated with arsenic intoxication, but almost any severe illness can cause it. This is really a kind of generalized horizontal leukonychia occurring in all nails simultaneously.

Muehrcke's Lines

Double white horizontal lines in the nail bed can be seen in patients with chronic, severe hypoalbuminemia and therefore do not grow out with the nail plate as do Mees' lines. Any disease causing low albumin levels may give rise to this.

Syphilis

Of the three forms of syphilis, secondary syphilis is most likely to involve the nail. Fragile nails, onycholysis, onychorrhexis, koilonychia, pitting, onychomadesis, and hypertrophic nails (onychauxis) may result. Ripple, wavelike deformities (probably a variation of a Beau line) have been described. A peculiar lilac-colored 0.5 to 1.0 mm discoloration behind and parallel to the free border of the nail was described by Milan in 1922 as very indicative, if not pathognomonic, of syphilis.

Nail signs of syphilis are as protean as are other skin lesions. A serum VDRL test is an important part of a workup for most nail dystrophies.

Acquired Immunodeficiency Syndrome

Flagrant and recalcitrant fungal infections of the nails, severe psoriatic nail changes, nail clubbing, blue nails, yellow nails, and Beau's lines have all been noted in patients with AIDS. Bluish discoloration of the nails may be seen in AIDS or may be a result of zidovudine (azidothymidine [Retrovir]) therapy.

OTHER CONDITIONS OF THE NAILS

The following rarer conditions of the nails will be defined briefly.

DRUG REACTIONS. Ingested drugs or chemicals can affect the nails in many ways. The changes can include pigmentation, Beau's lines, nail shedding (see onycholysis from tetracyclines), thickening of the plate, and vascular changes. Cancer chemotherapeutic agents can cause all of the above problems. Antimalarials can cause pigmentary changes.

ANONYCHIA. There is total congenital absence of the nail. Less drastic is partial presence of the nail or hypoplasia. These conditions may be hereditary or part of several congenital syndromes, including *fetal hydantoin syndrome.*

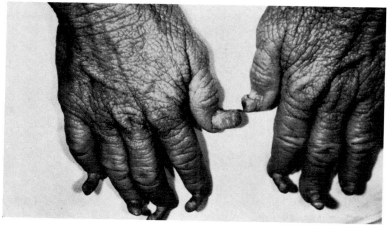

Figure 28–2. **Onychogryphosis (claw nails) of unknown cause.** (*Dr. C. Lessenden*)

MEDIAN CANALIFORM DYSTROPHY (see Plate 76). A fir-tree configuration appears in the middle of the nail plate. The cause is unknown, and the defect can spontaneously disappear.

ONYCHATROPHIA. Simple atrophy of the nails occurs, which may be congenital, hereditary, traumatic, or due to any severe local or systemic disease.

HABIT-TIC NAIL DEFORMITY (see Plate 75). This is seen on one or both thumbnail plates, where by habit, which may be denied by the patient, usually the middle fingernail is used to traumatize the cuticle area of the thumbnail. The result is a fir tree–like ridging of the nail plate.

SOFTENED NAILS (HAPALONYCHIA). This rare atrophic condition is usually concurrent with the aging process.

THICKENING OF THE NAIL PLATES (ON-YCHAUXIS). Usually due to continued trauma, it often occurs as a result of ill-fitting shoes.

CLAW NAILS (ONYCHOGRYPHOSIS). A marked thickening of the nails, particularly the toenails, occurs where the nail plate becomes elongated and twisted. Trauma is the most important cause (Fig. 28–2).

DISTAL SEPARATION OF THE NAILS (ONY-CHOLYSIS). A spontaneous separation of the nail plate from the underlying bed begins at the distal end and slowly progresses proximally. It occurs with systemic diseases and from irritating local causes. A *photosensitivity*

onycholysis can occur following systemic demeclocycline or other tetracycline therapy (see Plate 75).

YELLOW NAIL SYNDROME. A triad of lymphedema of the legs, pulmonary disease, and yellow nail plates occurs.

MISCELLANEOUS NAIL DISORDERS. Examples are nail picking (onychotillomania) (see Plate 75), racket nails, longitudinal single nail groove, enlargement and adherence of the cuticle (pterygium), reeded nails with longitudinal splitting (onychorrhexis), horizontal splitting of the nails (onychoschizia), and shedding of the nail (onychomadesis).

BIBLIOGRAPHY

Daniel CR (ed): The nail. Dermatol Clin, July 1985

Hanno R, Mathes BM, Krull EA: Longitudinal nail biopsy in evaluation of acquired nail dystrophies. J Am Acad Dermatol 14:803, 1986

Kechijian P: Twenty-nail dystrophy of childhood. Cutis 35:38, 1985

Kechijian P: Onycholysis of the fingernails: Evaluation and management. J Am Acad Dermatol 12:552, 1985

Kestenbaum T: Nail diseases. Kans Med 83:302, 1982

Norton ZA: Nail disorders: A review. J Am Acad Dermatol 2:451, 1980

Samman PD, Fenton DA: The Nails in Disease, 4th ed. Chicago, Year Book Medical Publishers, 1986

Scher RK: Brittle nails. Int J Dermatol 28:515, 1989

Zaias N: The Nail in Health and Disease, 2nd ed. East Norwalk, CT, Appleton & Lange, 1988

29

Diseases of the Mucous Membranes

The mucous membranes of the body adjoin the skin at the oral cavity, nose, conjunctiva, penis, vulva, and anus. Histologically, these membranes differ from the skin in that the horny layer and the hair follicles are absent. Disorders of the mucous membranes are usually associated with existing skin diseases or internal diseases.

Only the most common diseases of the mucous membranes are discussed here. At the end of the chapter is a listing of the uncommon affections of these areas.

GEOGRAPHIC TONGUE
(Plate 77)

Geographic tongue is an extremely common condition of the tongue that usually occurs without symptoms. Rarely, the lesions are sensitive to sour or salty foods. When these lesions are noticed for the first time by the individual, they may initiate fears of cancer.

CLINICAL APPEARANCE. Irregularly shaped (maplike or geographic) pale red patches are seen on the tongue. Close examination reveals that the filiform papillae are flatter or denuded in these areas. The patches slowly migrate over the tongue surface and heal without scarring.

COURSE. The disorder may come and go but may be constantly present in some persons.

ETIOLOGY. The cause is unknown, but the lesions seem to be more extensive during a systemic illness.

SUBJECTIVE COMPLAINTS. Some patients complain of burning and tenderness, especially on eating sour or salty foods.

Differential Diagnosis

Syphilis, secondary mucous membrane lesions: very similar, clinically, but acute in onset, usually more inflammatory; other cutaneous signs of syphilis; darkfield examination and serology positive (see Chap. 16).

Treatment

1. Reassure patient that these are not cancerous lesions.
2. There is no effective or necessary therapy. However, if patient complains of burning and tenderness, prescribe:
   Kenalog in Orabase   15.0
   Sig: Apply locally t.i.d.

APHTHOUS STOMATITIS
(Plate 77)

Canker sores are extremely common, painful, superficial ulcerations of the mucous membranes of the mouth.

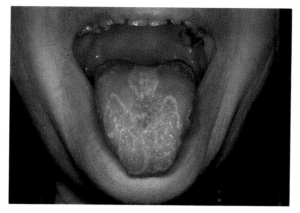

(A) Geographic tongue

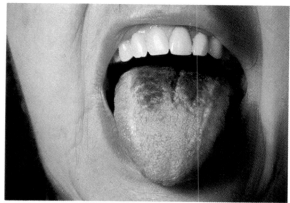

(B) Black tongue

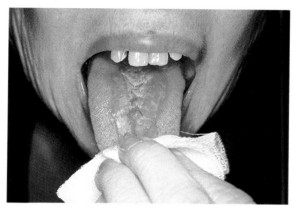

(C) Glossitis rhomboidea mediana

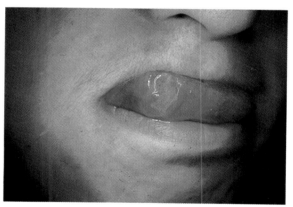

(D) Recurrent aphthous ulcer of tongue

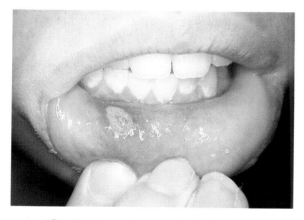

(E) Aphthous ulcer in patient with cyclic
neutropenia

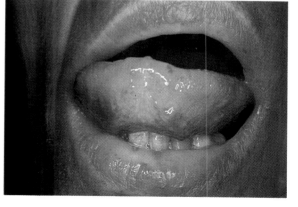

(F) Rendu-Osler-Weber disease of lips and
tongue

Plate 77. **Mucous membrane diseases.** (*Neutrogena Corp.*)

COURSE. One or more lesions develop at the same time and heal without scarring in 5 to 10 days. They can recur at irregular intervals.

ETIOLOGY. The cause is unknown, but certain foods, especially chocolate, nuts, and fruits, can precipitate the lesions or may even be causative. Some cases in women recur in relation to menstruation. A viral etiology has not been proved. A pleomorphic, transitional L-form of an α-hemolytic *Streptococcus* (*S. sanguis*) has also been implicated as causative.

Differential Diagnosis

Syphilis, secondary lesions: clinically similar; less painful; other signs of syphilis; darkfield examination and serology positive (see Chap. 16).

Treatment

Most persons who get these lesions have learned that very little can be done for them and that the ulcers will heal in a few days.

1. Toothpaste swish therapy. Brush the teeth and swish the toothpaste around in the mouth after each meal and at bedtime. If done soon after the onset of ulcers, extension of the lesions can be prevented and early healing can be effected in many cases.

SAUER NOTES:

1. I wish to emphasize the value of the toothpaste swish therapy for aphthous stomatitis. It is especially valuable if begun soon after lesions appear.
2. The toothpaste swish is also healing for self-inflicted tongue-bite sores.

---

2. Kenalog in Orabase (prescription needed) applied locally before meals will relieve some of the pain.
3. Tetracycline therapy. An oral suspension in a dosage of 250 mg per teaspoonful (or the powdery contents of a 250-mg capsule in a teaspoon of water) kept in the mouth for 2 minutes and then swallowed, four times a day, is healing.

HERPES SIMPLEX

Herpes simplex virus infection can occur as a group of umbilicated vesicles on the mucous membranes of the lips, the conjunctiva, the penis, and the labia. Frequently recurring episodes of this disease can be quite disabling. (See Chap. 17.)

FORDYCE'S DISEASE

This is a physiologic variant of oral sebaceous glands in which more than the normal number exist. When they are suddenly noticed, the person becomes concerned as to the diagnosis.

OTHER MUCOSAL LESIONS AND CONDITIONS

Causes

Mucosal lesions can also be due to the following:

PHYSICAL CAUSES. Sucking of lips, pressure sores, burns, actinic or sunlight cheilitis, factitial disorders, tobacco, other chemicals, and allergens are causative.

INFECTIOUS DISEASES (from viruses, bacteria, spirochetes, fungi, and animal parasites). Gangrenous bacterial infections are called *noma*. *Ludwig's angina* is an acute cellulitis of the floor of the mouth due to bacteria, abscesses, and sinuses and may be due to dental infection. *Trench mouth*, or *Plaut-Vincent's disease*, is an acute ulcerative infection of the mucous membranes caused by a combination of a spirochete and a fusiform bacillus.

SYSTEMIC DISEASES. These include lesions seen with *hematologic diseases* (e.g., leukemia, agranulocytosis from drugs or other causes, thrombocytopenia, pernicious anemia, cyclic or periodic neutropenia), *immunocompromised conditions* (such as the acquired immunodeficiency syndrome, organ transplants, lymphomas), *collagen diseases* (lupus erythematosus and scleroderma), *pigmentary diseases* (e.g., Addison's disease, Peutz-Jeghers syndrome) and *autoimmune diseases,* which cross over in several categories but include pemphigus and pemphigoid, and possibly benign mucosal pemphigoid.

DRUGS. *Phenytoin sodium* causes a hyperplastic gingivitis; *bismuth* orally and intramuscularly causes a bluish black line at the edge of the dental gum (see Plate 14); certain drugs cause hemorrhage and secondary infection of the mucous membranes.

METABOLIC DISEASES. Mucosal lesions are seen in primary systemic amyloidosis, lipoidosis, reticuloendothelioses, diabetes, and other disorders.

TUMORS, LOCAL OR SYSTEMIC. These include leukoplakia, squamous cell carcinoma, epulis, and cysts.

Rarer Conditions of Oral Mucous Membranes

HALITOSIS. Halitosis, or fetor oris, is a disagreeable odor of the breath.

PERIADENITIS MUCOSA NECROTICA RECURRENS (Fig. 29–1). Also known as Sutton's disease, this is a painful, recurrent, ulcerating disease of the mucous membranes of the oral cavity. The single or multiple deep ulcers exceed 10 mm and heal with scarring.

FOOT-AND-MOUTH DISEASE. This virus disease of animals and occasionally humans is characterized by a painful, self-limited vesicular stomatitis.

KOPLIK'S SPOTS. Bright red, pinpoint-size lesions on the mucous membranes of the cheek are seen in patients before the appearance of the rash of measles.

BURNING TONGUE (GLOSSODYNIA). This rather common complaint, particularly of middle-aged women is usually accompanied by no visible pathology. The cause is unknown, and therapy is of little value, but the many diseases and local factors that cause painful tongue must be ruled out from a diagnostic viewpoint.

BLACK TONGUE (HAIRY TONGUE, LINGUA NIGRA) (See Plate 77). Overgrowth of the papillae of the tongue, apparently caused by an imbalance of bacterial flora, is due to the use of antibiotics and other agents.

HAIRY LEUKOPLAKIA OF THE TONGUE. A slightly raised, poorly demarcated lesion with a corrugated or "hairy" surface appears on the sides of the tongue. It is seen mainly in immunosuppressed homosexual men infected with human T-cell lymphotrophic virus type III (HTLV-III). Human papillomavirus and Epstein-Barr virus have been identified in biopsy specimens. (See Chap. 18.)

MOELLER'S GLOSSITIS. This painful, persistent, red eruption on the sides and the tip of the tongue persists for weeks or months, subsides, and then recurs. The cause is unknown.

FURROWED TONGUE (GROOVED TONGUE, SCROTAL TONGUE). The tongue is usually larger than normal, containing deep longitudinal and lateral grooves of congenital origin or due to syphilis.

GLOSSITIS RHOMBOIDEA MEDIANA (See Plate 77). This rare disorder, characterized by a smooth reddish lesion, usually occurs in the center of the tongue. This term is poor because there is no inflammation and the reddish plaque may not always be in the center.

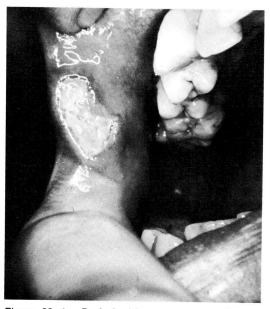

Figure 29–1. Periadenitis mucosa necrotica recurrens.

SJÖGREN'S SYNDROME. This rare entity is characterized by dryness of all of the mucous membranes and of the skin in middle-aged women. The primary form of this syndrome is in many cases associated with a cutaneous vasculitis. The secondary type of Sjögren's syndrome is associated with rheumatic and collagen diseases.

CHEILITIS GLANDULARIS APOSTEMA-TOSA. This chronic disorder of the lips is manifested by swelling and secondary inflammation, due to hypertrophy of the mucous glands and their ducts.

Rarer Conditions of Genital Mucous Membranes

FUSOSPIROCHETAL BALANITIS (Fig. 29–2). This uncommon infection of the penis is characterized by superficial erosions. It must be differentiated from syphilis by a darkfield examination and blood serology.

BALANITIS XEROTICA OBLITERANS (Fig. DI–2). (See Atrophies of the Skin, in the Dictionary-Index.) This whitish atrophic lesion on the penis is to be differentiated from leukoplakia. The female counterpart is *lichen sclerosus et atrophicus*.

LICHEN SCLEROSUS ET ATROPHICUS. A rare atrophy of the skin (usually around the neck) and of the genital mucous membranes occurs. In children (see Plate 92) it is the most common chronic genital dermatitis. (See Atrophies of the Skin, in the Dictionary-Index.)

ULCUS VULVAE ACUTUM. This rare self-limited disease, mainly of virgins, is charac-

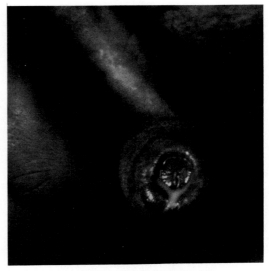

Figure 29–2. **Fusospirochetal balanitis.**

terized by shallow ulcerated lesions of the vulva. It is believed to be caused by *Bacillus crassus* or by a virus.

BIBLIOGRAPHY

Alexander E, Provost TT: Sjögren's syndrome. Arch Dermatol 123:801, 1987

Bell GF, Rogers RS III: Observations on the diagnosis of recurrent aphthous stomatitis. Mayo Clin Proc 57:297, 1982

Lupton GP, James WD, Redfield RR et al: Oral hairy leukoplakia. Arch Dermatol 123:624, 1987

30

Dermatoses Due to Physical Agents

Physical agents such as heat, cold, pressure, and radiant energy (x-rays, lasers, ultraviolet rays, gamma rays) can produce both irritative reactions and allergic reactions on the skin. The two common physical irritations of the skin are *sunburn*, due to ultraviolet radiation, and *radiodermatitis*, due to ionizing radiation. Allergic reactions can also develop from these two physical agents and from the other agents listed above.

Chapter 31 on *photosensitivity dermatoses* also covers some of the sun reactions mentioned here.

SUNBURN

A sunburn can be mild and desired or severe and feared. The most severe reactions come from prolonged exposure at swimming areas or when the unfortunate person falls asleep under an ultraviolet lamp. The degree of reaction depends on several factors, including length and intensity of exposure, the patient's complexion, and previous conditioning of the skin.

Sun-reactive "skin typing" of white-skinned persons became necessary when psoralen–ultraviolet light therapy (PUVA) was developed for the treatment of psoriasis. Type I persons always burn, never tan; type II persons usually burn and tan with difficulty; type III persons sometimes have a mild sunburn and tan about average; and type IV persons rarely burn and tan with ease. The

typing has been further expanded to type V for brown-skinned persons and type VI for black-skinned persons, both of whom never sunburn and do tan.

Certain drugs can increase the sensitivity of the skin to sunlight. The reaction can vary in intensity from a simple erythema to a measles-like rash or to a severe bullous eruption. Consult page 91 for a list of these *photosensitizing drugs.*

PRIMARY LESIONS. Varying degrees of redness develop within 2 to 12 hours after exposure to the ultraviolet radiation and reach maximum intensity within 24 hours. Vesiculation occurs, in severe cases, along with systemic weakness, chill, malaise, and local pain.

SECONDARY LESIONS OR REACTIONS. Scaling or peeling, although not desired by the sun devotee, is the aftermath of any overexposure. Vesiculation can be complicated by secondary infection. An increase in pigmentation is usually the desired end result, but this tanning is not accomplished by overzealous exposure.

Lupus erythematosus of either the systemic or the discoid type may be triggered by sun exposure in a susceptible person (see Chap. 25). *Sunlight allergy (polymorphic light eruption* or *actinic dermatitis)*, in susceptible persons, is manifested clinically by (1) plaquelike erythematous lesions, (2) contact dermatitis–like lesions, (3) papular pruritic lesions, and (4) erythema multiforme–like lesions. These cases may be difficult to distinguish from lupus erythematosus, especially the discoid type. Short-term oral chloroquine therapy combined with protection from sunlight is quite effective.

LATE REACTIONS TO SUNLIGHT. *Actinic* or *senile keratoses* appear mainly after the age of 50 but are seen in highly susceptible persons in their 30s. Chronic sun and wind exposure on the part of a light-complexioned farmer, sailor, or gardener will lead to the development of these superficial, red, scaling keratoses on exposed surfaces of the face, the lips (*actinic cheilitis,* Plate 78), the ears, the neck, and the dorsa of the hands.

Malignant melanomas, basal cell carcinomas, and *squamous cell carcinomas* can be the late result of excessive sun exposure. An increasing number of these cancers are being discovered. The light-complexioned person and those with *dysplastic nevi* are more susceptible. The genetic factor is important, as are other factors.

Wrinkling, freckling, and *aging* of the skin are promoted by injudicious chronic sun exposure.

Treatment

PROPHYLACTIC TREATMENT

The ultraviolet rays from the sun or from other sources can be either completely blocked or partially blocked from the skin surface by sunscreens.

Most sunscreens contain *p*-aminobenzoic acid (PABA), either esterified or nonesteri-

fied, but some are PABA-free. Products with the higher sun protective factor (SPF) ratings will screen out relatively more ultraviolet B, which comprises the wavelengths responsible for acute sun damage. Photoplex Sunscreen may be used when one also wants protection against ultraviolet A (the wavelengths responsible for most exogenous photosensitizations).

Sensible and gradual sun exposure of the skin is the best preventative for sunburn, but most persons learn this the hard way.

ACTIVE TREATMENT

A young woman presents with a painful, erythematous, vesicular skin reaction on her face, back, and thighs of 24 hours' duration following a holiday trip to the beach (first- and second-degree burns).

1. Burow's solution wet dressing
   Sig: 1 packet of Domeboro or Bluboro to 1 quart of cool water.
   Apply cloths wet with the cool solution to the affected areas for as long a time as necessary to keep comfortable.
2. Calamine lotion or Sarno Lotion
   Sig: Apply locally t.i.d. to affected areas.
3. Blisters can be drained but should not be débrided.
4. Systemic analgesics and even systemic corticosteroids may be used.
5. Ultraviolet injury to the cornea calls for expert ophthalmologic treatment.

Subsequent Care. A day or two later, to soften the scales and to prevent secondary infection, prescribe:

1. Polysporin or other antibiotic ointment
   15.0
   Sig: Apply locally t.i.d.
2. Warn the patient to exercise caution in resuming sun exposure to the now very sensitive skin.

SAUER NOTES:

1. The brand of sunscreen one uses is not as important as the fact that the sunscreen has an SPF of 15 or over.
2. The duration the sunscreen remains on the skin, especially after swimming or sweating, is also important.
3. Sunscreen preparations, especially for susceptible persons, should be applied every day, as if they were a cosmetic or shaving lotion.
4. For acne-prone persons it is best to avoid oily or greasy sunscreens.
5. The use of sunscreens on the skin of children is encouraged.

SAUER NOTES:

1. Dermatologists are not crying "wolf" when they implore people to avoid excessive sun exposure.
2. Millions of dollars are spent for wrinkle creams, bleaches for "liver spots," and "moisturizers," yet people continue to abuse their skin in the sun.

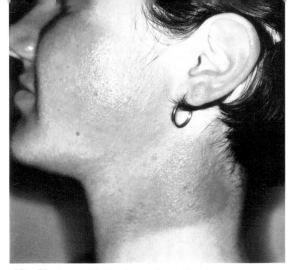

(A) Photosensitivity dermatitis following demeclocycline therapy

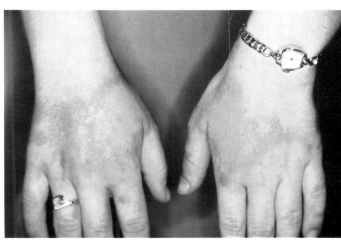

(B) Photosensitivity with residual hyperpigmentation from soap

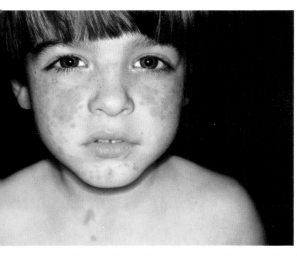

(C and D) Hydroa aestivale off and on for 4 years in 7-year-old boy; close-up of cheek

(E) Papular polymorphic light eruption off and
on for 15 years

(F) Porphyria cutanea tarda with blisters and
hyperpigmentation

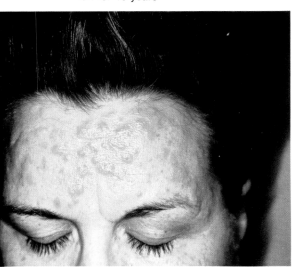

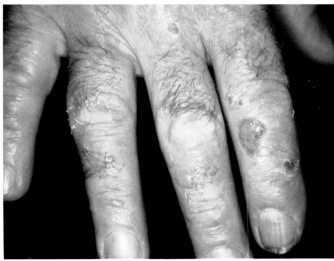

Plate 79. **Photosensitivity dermatoses.** (*Texas Pharmacal*)

common now than it once was, since halogenated salicylanilides were removed from the market. The fragrance musk ambrette has become an important cause of photoallergic dermatitis.

Topical *phototoxic* agents include tars and psoralens. Psoralens are found in many plants and a few colognes. Acute phototoxic dermatitis typically is followed by striking hyperpigmentation with bizarre configurations (*e.g., berlock dermatitis* (see Plate 67) and *phytophotodermatitis*).

Clinically, *photoallergic* contact dermatitis appears eczematous, whereas acute *phototoxic* contact dermatitis is edematous or bullous; erythema is common to both. Occasionally, photoallergy lingers for months or even years without further exposure to the allergen ("persistent light reactor").

Actinic reticuloid resembles the persistent light reactor state but gives different phototest results (see Table 31–1) and resembles cutaneous lymphoma histologically.

Treatment

1. The patient should avoid sunlight (even glass-filtered sunlight) and strong fluorescent lighting, if possible. Topical sunscreens as a rule are only partially effective, especially in chronic cases. The patient should select a sunscreen with the highest sun protection factor (SPF) that does not irritate, preferably one that also screens out ultraviolet A. Most sunscreens contain *p*-aminobenzoic acid (PABA) or PABA ester (padimate). It should be noted that PABA itself occasionally causes photoallergic reactions.
2. Topical corticosteroids may give some symptomatic relief.
3. The patient should avoid further exposure to the photosensitizer.

ENDOGENOUS PHOTOSENSITIVITY

After ruling out exogenous photosensitivity by means of the history and/or phototesting (see Table 31–1), the clinician may then consider the so-called *primary light-sensitive disorders*. Most often, this means one of the porphyrias or one of the collagen vascular disorders. (Photosensitivity caused by deficient melanin pigment, as in *vitiligo* and *albinism*, is discussed in Chapter 24, *Pigmentary Dermatoses*.)

Porphyrias

Porphyria Cutanea Tarda (Plate 79)

The most common porphyria with cutaneous manifestations is symptomatic porphyria, or porphyria cutanea tarda (PCT). Patients with this disorder are usually over 40, drink heavily, and frequently are unaware that they are sensitive to sunlight. Diabetes mellitus is found in 25% of cases of PCT; 90% or more have hepatic siderosis. Nearly all untreated patients with PCT show abnormal bromsulphalein (BSP) retention. PCT is relatively uncommon in women that are not taking estrogens. A PCT-like illness has been observed in patients undergoing hemodialysis for chronic renal failure. PCT also has been linked to several toxins (*e.g.*, hexachlorobenzene and dioxin).

LESIONS. Cutaneous lesions are prominent in PCT and include facial plethora, hyperpigmentation of exposed areas, hypertrichosis (this may be the presenting complaint in women, who sometimes are then treated with estrogen!), blisters, erosions (secondary to very fragile skin), milia, and localized areas of scleroderma (latter may occur in nonexposed areas). Acute abdominal crises or other neurologic attacks do not occur in PCT, even after drugs like barbiturates and sulfonamides. Such crises may occur, however, in the less common inherited disorder, *variegate porphyria*. The skin lesions in variegate porphyria are very similar to those in PCT.

Diagnosis

The diagnosis of PCT is made by demonstrating greatly elevated urinary uroporphyrin excretion (>500 μg/24 hours). Urinary coproporphyrin levels are variable. A tentative diagnosis may be made by finding the characteristic orange-pink fluorescence of a freshly voided acidified urine sample under Wood's illumination (may be "negative" if the uroporphyrin excretion is less than 1000 μg/liter).

Treatment

1. *Phlebotomy.* The treatment of choice for PCT is multiple phlebotomies over a period of months. The schedule is generally less aggressive than one would use for hemochromatosis. A lasting remission, both clinically and biochemically, usually is achieved by withdrawal of one pint of blood every few weeks until 10 to 20 to 30 pints have been withdrawn.
2. *Chloroquine.* An alternative treatment is low-dose chloroquine or hydroxychloroquine therapy (high doses may cause acute toxic hepatitis). A dose of hydroxychloroquine, 100 mg, is given twice weekly for several months.
3. *Abstinence from alcohol* (by the patient) is very important. Even though patients with PCT are not subject to acute attacks from drugs such as those mentioned previously, other foreign chemicals such as estrogens, iron, and possibly phenytoin (Dilantin) may aggravate the disease. Patients with variegate porphyria may experience severe crises (pain, paralysis) when given barbiturates, griseofulvin, and so on.

Protoporphyria

The second most common cutaneous porphyria, protoporphyria, is found in families and typically begins in childhood. It frequently is misdiagnosed as contact dermatitis, solar urticaria, or psychoneurosis. Patients complain bitterly of burning and stinging of the exposed areas after a very short time (minutes) in the sun. For several days after exposure, even through window glass, they may display erythema, edema, and purpura of the skin. Sometimes urticaria or vesicles occur. Photosensitivity may persist well into adult life, but between attacks there are usually few objective skin lesions. Cholelithiasis and hepatic failure occasionally occur as late complications.

Diagnosis

The diagnosis of protoporphyria rests on demonstrating elevated free erythrocyte protoporphyrin levels (>100 μg/dl packed red blood cells). Fluorescence microscopy may be used to screen blood smears for the disease.

Treatment

Oral carotene (Solatene) in a dosage of from 60 to 180 mg daily is the treatment of choice. Topical sunscreens generally are not very effective.

Collagen Vascular Disorders
(See also Chap. 25)

Polymorphous Light Eruption

Polymorphous light eruption (PMLE) is included here, although opinion is divided as to whether it is in fact related to lupus erythematosus. PMLE is characteristically seasonal (spring or summer), implying a threshold or dose-response relationship. It most commonly affects children or young adults.

The skin lesions, as the name implies, are variable, with papules and vesicles being most common (see Plate 79). Plaques, wheals (*solar urticaria* may be related to PMLE), and petechiae sometimes occur (*solar purpura* also may be a related condition). Subjective symptoms are less severe than those of protoporphyria. When blisters are prominent, "*hydroa*" (aestivale, vacciniforme) is the term often applied (see Plate 79 *C* and *D*).

Treatment

1. Topical sunscreens and corticosteroids offer some relief.
2. Oral antimalarials are usually effective but should be given in short courses because of the ocular risks.

Lupus Erythematosus
(Plates 68 and 69)

Both systemic and discoid lupus erythematosus may be exacerbated by sunlight, especially the former. If the diagnosis is not evident clinically, skin biopsy for routine and immunofluorescence microscopy and laboratory tests (more valuable in systemic lupus than in discoid lupus) will usually confirm it.

Treatment

Sunscreens, local corticosteroids (topical or intralesional), and systemic antimalarials have been used to treat the skin lesions of lupus with moderate success (see Chap. 25).

Dermatomyositis
(Plate 70)

Photosensitivity in dermatomyositis usually is less striking than it is in lupus, but occasionally it may be prominent. Laboratory studies often are necessary to confirm the diagnosis.

Treatment

Sunscreens may help the photosensitive component of the disease (see Chap. 25).

OTHER PHOTODERMATOSES

Examples of other photosensitive disorders are *solar purpura, solar urticaria, pellagra, Hartnup's disease, xeroderma pigmentosum, Bloom's syndrome, actinic reticuloid, actinic granuloma,* and *rosacea.* Poikiloderma approaching that seen in radiodermatitis also may be induced by ultraviolet light, both on an acquired basis (*poikiloderma of Civatte*) (see Fig. 35–2) and, less commonly, on an inherited basis (*poikiloderma congenitale of Rothmund-Thomson*).

Except for rosacea and pellagra, effective treatment for all of the foregoing conditions is severely lacking.

Actinic Keratoses
(Plate 83)

Also known as *solar keratoses* or *senile keratoses,* actinic keratoses are dry, gritty, yellowish-white (occasionally hyperpigmented) excrescences on a telangiectatic base typically located on the face, ears, and hands of patients with fair complexions who have spent years in the sun. Because a sizable number (over 25%) evolve slowly into *squamous*

cell carcinoma, they merit careful, thorough removal (see Chap. 33.)

Treatment

1. 5-Fluorouracil solution (Efudex 2% or 5%, Fluoroplex 1%) is a convenient, although uncomfortable, treatment for multiple actinic keratoses. It should be applied to *all* the sun-damaged areas b.i.d. for 2 to 6 weeks, or to the limits of tolerance, whichever occurs first. Patients should be well aware that a brisk inflammatory reaction will occur during treatment, and that this seems to be necessary for the treatment to "work" (see Chap. 33).
2. Cryosurgery, caustic acids, curettage, and electrodesiccation are alternative treatments.
3. Retinoic acid cream (Retin-A) in relatively high concentrations (0.1%) also may be effective against early, less developed keratoses.

Sunburn

Sunburn usually is the result not of disease but of indiscretion. Certain white persons, however, are markedly deficient in melanin, the principal physiologic sunscreen in humans. These persons burn with the briefest unprotected sun exposure.

The prophylactic and active management of a sunburn is covered in Chapter 30.

BIBLIOGRAPHY

DeLeo VA (ed): Photosensitivity diseases. Dermatol Clin 4:165, 1986

Haber LC, Bickers DR: Photosensitivity Diseases: Principles of Diagnosis and Treatment, 2nd ed. Philadelphia, BC Decker, 1989

Kalivas L, Kalivas J: Solar purpura. Arch Dermatol 124:24, 1988

32

Genodermatoses

Walter H. C. Burgdorf, M.D.* and Gordon C. Sauer, M.D.

The importance of genetics to dermatologists is obvious. Many common dermatoses, such as atopic dermatitis and psoriasis, have a genetic component. In addition, there are a number of inherited disorders in which a knowledge of dermatology aids diagnosis and treatment. For example, white macules on an infant's skin may be the first clue to tuberous sclerosis and help explain infantile seizures. Some simple dermatologic techniques may also aid the pediatrician or geneticist: the pigment-producing enzymes may be assayed from hair bulbs, many enzymatic abnormalities may be measured in fibroblasts grown from a skin biopsy, and fetal skin biopsy can identify some disorders of keratinization.

The patterns of inheritance are available in any genetics book and are reviewed below in Table 32–1. Once the mechanism of inheritance is understood, genetic counseling is possible. Nonetheless, we encourage physicians to refer patients to experienced genetic counselors. This new area of medicine is fraught with emotional overtones, misdiagnosis, and immense moral and medicolegal responsibilities.

DISORDERS OF KERATINIZATION

Dominant Ichthyosis Vulgaris
(Plate 80)

The most dramatic disorder of keratinization is ichthyosis, or fish skin. Patients are either born with or develop at an early age thick, often dark scales. Of the many types of ichthyosis, the autosomal dominant *ichthyosis vulgaris* form is the most common and is considered here. A discussion of some of the other forms of ichthyosis appears at the end of this section.

PRIMARY LESIONS. Small white scales, often in association with keratosis pilaris–type lesions, are seen.

SECONDARY LESIONS. These lesions are rare. The scaling may be deep enough in some areas, particularly on the palms and soles, to result in small fissures.

DISTRIBUTION. The arms and legs are the most severely affected, but the extent of involvement varies with individual cases. Some patients can have a considerable amount of scaling over the entire body.

COURSE. This common form of ichthyosis is worse in the winter. In most cases there is essentially no scaling in the summer. There is a tendency for improvement after puberty or in early adult life.

* Professor and Chairman, Department of Dermatology, The University of New Mexico School of Medicine, Albuquerque, New Mexico.

Table 32–1
Patterns of Inheritance

PATTERN	KEY FEATURES	RISK TO SIBLINGS		RISK TO CHILDREN*	SEX RATIO
Autosomal dominant	Often sporadic; passes through families without skipping generation		50%	50%	M = F
Autosomal recessive	Occurs more often in consanguineous families: unlikely to occur in subsequent generations		25%	0%	M = F
X-linked recessive	Limited to males, skips generations, female carriers	M F	50% 0%	0%	M
X-linked dominant	Involved males usually die	F M stillborn	50% frequently	50%	F

* Assuming normal spouse

Differential Diagnosis

Xerosis or *acquired ichthyosis:* the most common cause of this dry skin problem is aging. If generalized dry skin develops in young adults, it is an indication for a detailed investigation to rule out an internal malignancy such as Hodgkin's disease or adenocarcinoma. Hypothyroidism may also be a precipitating factor of dry skin. Clinically, severe xerosis and ichthyosis vulgaris appear similar.

Treatment

1. It is important in the management of ichthyosis to explain that there is no cure for the problem (a fact that the patient undoubtedly already suspects) but that there are ways to decrease the dryness of the skin.

   Advise the patient to bathe less frequently. Suggest an emollient soap such as Dove, Aveeno bar, Neutragena soap, Basis soap, or Oilatum soap. Suggest the following emollients, for example, to be applied liberally on the skin after bathing and as needed:

   Nivea Skin Oil or Cream
   Keri Lotion or Cream
   Eucerin Lotion or Ointment
   Lubriderm Lotion or Cream
   Complex 15
   Ultraderm Moisturizer
   Neutraderm Lotion

   White petroleum jelly, locally, is appreciated by many who have a more severe form of this ichthyosis.
2. Retinoic acid (Retin-A) topically is helpful, mainly for lamellar ichthyosis, but also in some cases of ichthyosis vulgaris. Warn the patient that this causes a rather marked scaling and even redness of the skin. Intermittent therapy is usually well tolerated.
3. α-Hydroxy acids locally are quite effective. This is true especially for lamellar ichthyosis but also for ichthyosis vulgaris and X-linked ichthyosis. Lachydrin, a 12% lactic acid lotion, is both potent and readily available.

Other Forms of Ichthyosis

X-LINKED ICHTHYOSIS VULGARIS. Only males are involved, since inheritance is sex-linked recessive. This type is characterized by large brown scales that begin in infancy and persist throughout life (Fig. 32–1).

LAMELLAR ICHTHYOSIS. This rare disorder, inherited in an autosomal recessive fashion, is characterized by large platelike scales and ectropion. Neonates may present as a "collodion baby" covered with sheets of plastic-like scale. An even more severe form of neonatal ichthyosis whose nosology is unclear is the *harlequin fetus* (see Plate 89).

NONBULLOUS ICHTHYOSIFORM ERYTH-RODERMA. Patients with this autosomal re-

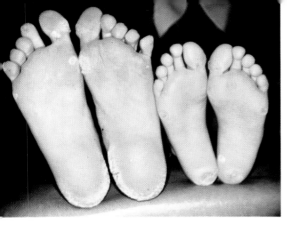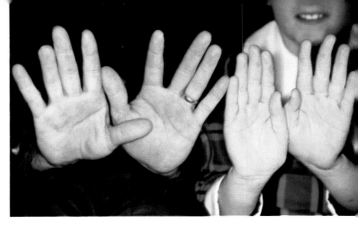

(*A* and *B*) Keratosis palmaris et plantaris of feet and hands of father and his 8-year-old daughter

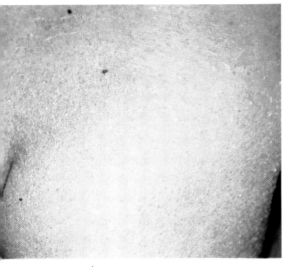

Ichthyosis vulgaris, dominant type, of buttocks

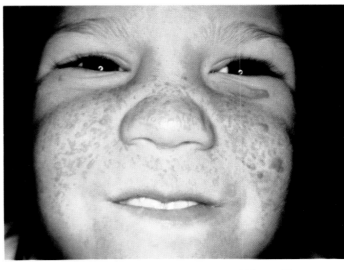

(*D*) Adenoma sebaceum in 4-year-old boy with epilepsy (tuberous sclerosis)

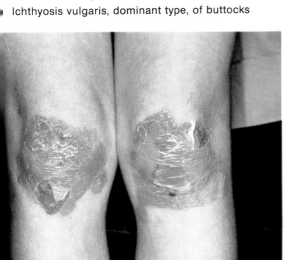

E) Epidermolysis bullosa dystrophica, dominant type, of knees in 5-year-old girl

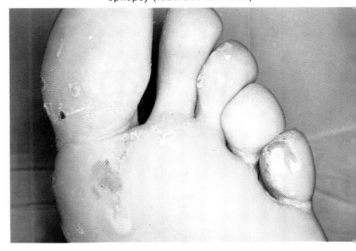

(*F*) Epidermolysis bullosa simplex, dominant type, in 23-year-old man

Plate 80. **Genodermatoses.** (*Westwood Pharmaceuticals*)

301

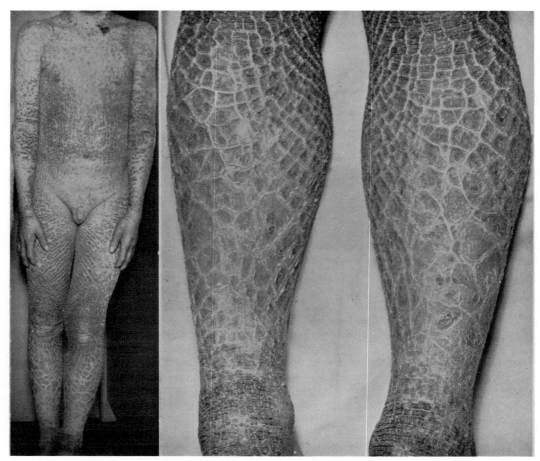

Figure 32–1. Ichthyosis, X-linked, showing full body and close-up of legs. (*Dr. D. Morgan, K.C.G.H.*)

cessive disorder have a fine diffuse scale and are more likely to have erythroderma than other ichthyosis variants.

BULLOUS ICHTHYOSIFORM ERYTHRODERMA. This rare ectodermal defect is characterized by generally thickened skin that is red, is shiny, and shows a tendency to lichenification over the larger joints. Flaccid bullae occur in most cases early in the course of the disease but may disappear later. The disease can be present at birth or develop later. This condition can be differentiated from other forms of ichthyosis in that it involves the flexural surfaces of the body and blisters. It is inherited in an autosomal recessive fashion.

All these other forms of ichthyosis are rare. They introduce the use of systemic retinoids (isotretinoin [Accutane] or etretinate [Tegison]) for keratinizing disorders. Since dryness

is the main side effect of isotretinoin in patients with acne, one wonders how the drug could help someone with intensely dry skin. If one thinks of the epidermis as being made of bricks and mortar, then forms of ichthyosis such as ichthyosis vulgaris with structural protein or "brick" problems, usually inherited in an autosomal dominant fashion, typically do not respond to retinoids. Those with a mortar problem, usually an abnormality of lipids and usually enzyme mediated, such as lamellar ichthyosis, which are inherited by a autosomal recessive pathway, may be helped by retinoids.

Other Disorders of Keratinization

KERATOSIS PALMARIS ET PLANTARIS (see Plate 80 *A* and *B*). Hereditary symmetrical thickening of the palms and the soles is no-

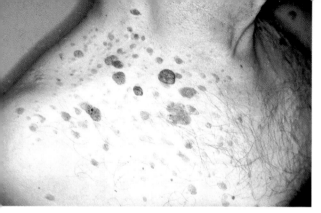

(A) Seborrheic keratoses on the neck

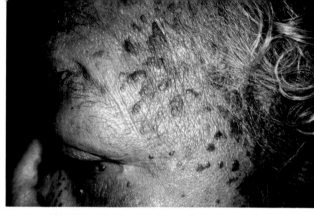

(B) Dermatosis papulosa nigra on temple area

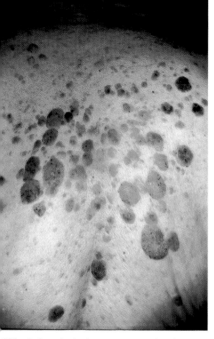

(C) Seborrheic keratoses on back

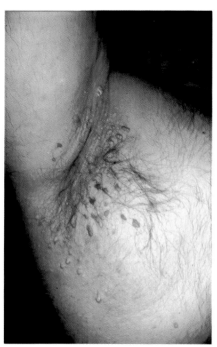

(D and E) Pedunculated fibromas in axilla

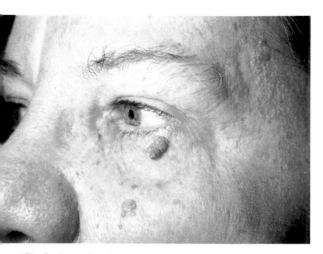

(F) Pedunculated seborrheic keratosis of eyelid

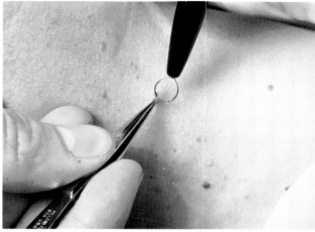

(G) A method of removal of pedunculated fibroma

Plate 81. **Epidermal tumors.** (*Stiefel Laboratories, Inc.*)

unattractive "moles" or "warts" that perturb the elderly patient, occasionally become irritated, but are otherwise benign.

Dermatosis papulosa nigra is a form of seborrheic keratosis of blacks that occurs on the face, mainly in women. These small, multiple tumors can be removed, but there is the possibility of causing keloids.

DESCRIPTION. The size of seborrheic keratoses varies up to 3 cm for the largest, but the average diameter is 1 cm. The color may be flesh-colored, tan, brown, or coal black. They are usually oval shaped, are elevated, and have a greasy, warty sensation to touch.

DISTRIBUTION. The lesions appear on the face, neck, scalp, back, and upper chest, and less frequently on arms, legs, and lower part of trunk.

COURSE. They become darker and enlarge slowly. Trauma from clothing occasionally results in infection, and this prompts the patient to seek medical care. Any inflammatory dermatitis around these lesions causes them to enlarge temporarily and become more evident, so much so that many patients suddenly note them for the first time. Malignant degeneration of seborrheic keratoses is doubted.

ETIOLOGY. Heredity is the biggest factor, along with old age. They are seen more commonly in patients with an oily, acne-seborrhea type of skin.

Differential Diagnosis

Actinic keratoses (Table 33-1).
Pigmented nevi: longer duration, smoother surface, softer to touch; may not be able to differentiate clinically (see later in this chapter).

Flat warts: in younger patients; acute onset, with rapid development of new lesions (see Chap. 17).
Malignant melanoma: very rare, usually with rapid growth, indurated; examine histologically (see later).

Treatment

A 58-year-old woman requests the removal of a warty, tannish, slightly elevated 2 × 2-cm lesion of the right side of her forehead.

1. Examine the lesion carefully. The diagnosis usually can be made clinically, but if there is any question, a scissors biopsy (p. 13) can be performed. It would be ideal if all of these seborrheic keratoses could be examined histologically, but this is not economically feasible or necessary.
2. A very adequate form of therapy is curettement, with or without local anesthesia, fol-

---

SAUER NOTES:

1. For many benign lesions it is best to err on the side of surgical undertreatment rather than overtreatment. You can always remove any remaining growth later, but you cannot put back what you took off.
2. Scarring should be kept to a minimum.
3. After any surgical procedure, I hand out the following information sheet. Skin surgery sites usually heal without any complication. However, there are always questions and concerns from the patient about aftercare.

Table 33–1
Differential Diagnosis

	ACTINIC OR SENILE KERATOSIS	SEBORRHEIC KERATOSIS
Appearance	Flat, brownish, reddish, or tan scale firmly attached to skin	Greasy, elevated, brown or black; scale is warty and can be easily scratched away
Location	Sun-exposed areas	Face, back, and chest
Complexion	Blue eyes, light hair, dry skin	Brown eyes, dark hair, oily skin
Subjective Complaints	Some burning and stinging	Occasional itching
Precancerous	Yes	No

SURGICAL NOTES

Minor surgery has been performed for the removal or biopsy of a skin lesion.

If liquid nitrogen was used to remove the growth, a blister or peeling at the growth site will develop in 24 hours; or

If electrosurgery or burning was used, a crust and scab will form.

The sites treated heal better if they are uncovered. Do not pick at the spot, and try to avoid accidentally hitting the area. One or more scabs will form in the course of healing.

You can wash over the area gently. Do not apply any creams to the lesions until the scabs have fallen off completely. If for cosmetic reasons you feel you must cover the site with a bandage, then apply alcohol or Betadine solution to the site twice a day.

A certain amount of redness and swelling around the surgery site is to be expected. Also you might have a small amount of drainage and crusting. A mild amount of redness and infection can be treated with alcohol, Betadine, or Polysporin Ointment locally three times a day.

If more drainage or infection develops, apply a wet dressing with sheeting or soak the area. Use a solution made with one Domeboro or Blueboro packet to one pint of cool water and apply for 20 minutes three times a day. These packets are available at a pharmacy without a prescription. Make a fresh solution every day.

If the infection becomes excessive, call me, or go to a hospital emergency department. This action should be necessary only very rarely.

If the scab is knocked off prematurely, bleeding may occur. This can be stopped by applying *firm* pressure with gauze or cotton for 10 minutes by the clock and then releasing pressure gradually.

Depending on the size of the surgery site, healing takes from 1 to 6 weeks. Some scarring or loss of pigment at the surgery site is possible. A few persons have a tendency to form thick or keloidal scars, which is not predictable.

If a biopsy was done, you will be receiving a bill for the pathology study from the laboratory. Call my office in 10 days for this report.

Return to the office for further care or follow-up as directed.

Gordon C. Sauer, M.D.
Phone (816) 444-5601

---

lowed by a light application of trichloroacetic acid, as outlined under actinic keratosis (p. 314). The resulting fine atrophic scar will hardly be noticeable in several months.

Electrosurgery can be used, but this usually requires anesthesia.

Liquid nitrogen freezing therapy works very well, if it is available. It is the therapy of choice of most dermatologists. *Do not freeze excessively.*

Surgical excision is an unnecessary and more expensive form of removal.

PEDUNCULATED FIBROMAS
(Plate 81)

Multiple skin tags are very common on the neck and the axillae of middle-aged, usually obese, men and women. The indications for removal are twofold: cosmetic, as desired and requested by the patient, and to prevent the irritation and the secondary infection of the pedicle that frequently develops from trauma of a collar or other article of clothing.

DESCRIPTION. Pedunculated pinhead-sized to pea-sized soft tumors or normal skin color or darker are seen. The base may be inflamed from injury.

DISTRIBUTION. The lesions occur on the neck, axillae, or groin, or less frequently on any area.

COURSE. These fibromas grow very slowly. They may increase in size during pregnancy. Some become infected and drop off.

Differential Diagnosis

Filiform wart: digitate projections, more horny; also seen on chin area (see Chap. 17).

Pedunculated seborrheic keratosis: larger lesion, darker color, warty, or velvety appearance (see preceding section).

Neurofibromatosis: lesions seen elsewhere, larger; can be pushed back into skin; also café-au-lait spots; hereditary (see Chaps. 26 and 32).

Treatment

A 42-year-old woman has 20 small pedunculated fibromas on her neck and axillae that she wants removed. This should be done by electrosurgery. Without anesthesia, gently grab the small tumor in a thumb forceps and stretch the pedicle (see Plate 81). Touch this pedicle with the electrosurgery needle and turn on the current for a split second. The tumor separates from the skin, and no bleeding occurs. The site will heal in 4 to 7 days.

For very small lesions, a short spark with the electrosurgical needle will suffice.

CYSTS
(Plate 82)

The three types are epidermal cyst, trichilemmal, pilar, or sebaceous cyst, and milium.

An *epidermal cyst* has a wall composed of true epidermis and probably originates from an invagination of the epidermis into the dermis and subsequent detachment from the epidermis, or it can originate spontaneously. The most common locations for epidermal cysts are the face, ears, neck and scalp, where tumors of varying size can be found.

Trichilemmal cysts were also known as *wens* and *pilar* or *sebaceous cysts (see Plate 82 B).* They are less common than epidermal cysts, occur mainly on the scalp, usually are multiple, and show an autosomal dominant inheritance. The sac wall is thick, smooth, and whitish and can be quite easily enucleated.

Milia (see Plate 82 D) are very common, white, pinhead-sized, firm lesions that are seen on the face. They are formed by proliferation of epithelial buds following trauma to the skin (dermabrasion for acne scars), following certain dermatoses (pemphigus, epider-

molysis bullosa, and acute contact dermatitis) or from no apparent cause.

Differential Diagnosis of Epidermal and Trichilemmal Cysts

Lipoma: rather difficult to differentiate clinically; more firm, lobulated; no cheesy material extrudes on incision; removal is by complete excision or by liposuction; clinically similar to *hibernoma.*

Dermoid cyst: clinically similar; can also be found internally; usually a solitary skin tumor; histologically, contains hairs, eccrine glands, and sebaceous glands.

Mucous cysts (see Plate 82 E): translucent pea-sized or smaller lesions on the lips, treated by cutting off top of the lesion and carefully lightly cauterizing the base with a silver nitrate stick or light electrosurgery.

Synovial cysts of the skin (see Plate 82 F): globoid, translucent, pea-sized swellings around the joints of fingers and toes.

Treatment of Epidermal and Trichilemmal Cysts

Several methods can be used with success. The choice depends on the ability of the operator and the site and the number of cysts. Cysts can regrow following even the best surgical care, because of incomplete removal of the sac.

1. A single 3-cm cyst on the back should be removed by surgical excision and suturing. This can be done in two ways: either by incising the skin and skillfully removing the intact cyst sac or by cutting straight into the sac with a small incision, shelling out the evacuated lining by applying strong pressure to the sides of the incision, and suturing the skin. The latter procedure is simpler, requires a smaller incision, and is quite successful.

2. A patient with several cysts in the scalp can be treated in another simple way. A 3- to 4-mm incision can be made directly over and into the cyst. The cheesy, foul-smelling contents can be evacuated by pressure and the use of a small curette. The sac can then be popped out of the hole with *very* firm pressure, or the sac can be grasped with a small hemostat and pulled out of the opening. No suturing or only a

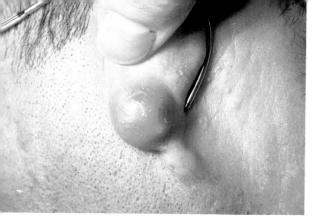

(A) Epidermal cyst of earlobe

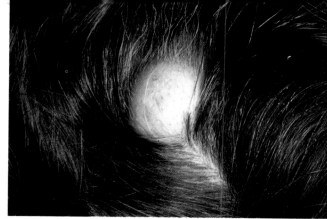

(B) Pilar or sebaceous cyst of scalp

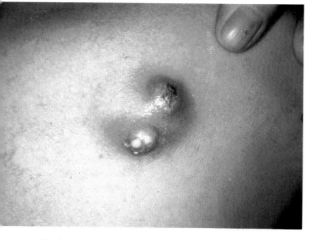

(C) Infected epidermal cyst on shoulder

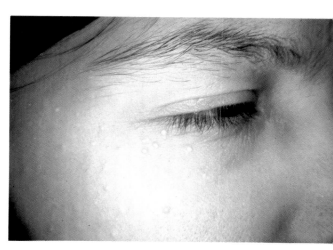

(D) Milia on upper cheek of 21-year-old woman

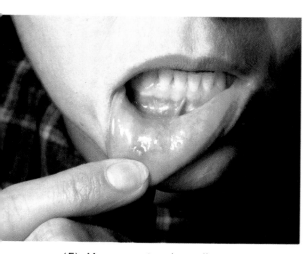

(E) Mucous cyst on lower lip

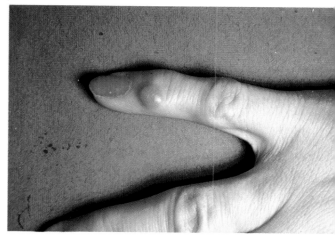

(F) Synovial cyst on finger

Plate 82. **Cysts of the skin.** (*Texas Pharmacal*)

single suture is necessary. The resulting scar will be imperceptible in a short time.

3. If, during incision by any technique, a solid tumor is found instead of a cyst, the lesion should be excised completely and the material studied histologically. This diagnostic error is very common because of the clinical similarity of cysts, lipomas, and other related tumors.

Treatment of Milia

1. Simple incision of the small tumors with a scalpel or a Hagedorn needle and expression of the contents by a comedone extractor is sufficient.
2. Another procedure is to remove the top of the milia lightly with electrodesiccation.

PRECANCEROUS TUMORS

Precancerous types of tumors include actinic keratosis and cutaneous horn, arsenical keratosis, and leukoplakia.

Actinic Keratosis
(Plate 83)

Actinic keratosis is a common skin lesion of light complexioned, older persons that occurs on the skin surfaces exposed to sunlight. A small percentage of these lesions develop into squamous cell carcinomas. Because of the popularity of sunbathing these lesions are seen also in persons in the 30- to 50-year age-group.

DESCRIPTION. Lesions are usually multiple, flat or slightly elevated, brownish or tan colored, scaly and adherent, measuring up to 1.5 cm in diameter. Individual lesions may become confluent. A *cutaneous horn* is a very proliferative, hyperkeratotic form of actinic keratosis that resembles a horn (Plates 84C and 86A).

DISTRIBUTION. Areas of skin exposed to sunlight, such as face, ears, neck, and dorsum of hands, are involved.

COURSE. The lesion begins as a faint red, slightly scaly patch that enlarges slowly, peripherally and deeply, over many years. A sudden spurt of growth would indicate a change to a squamous cell carcinoma.

SUBJECTIVE COMPLAINTS. Patients often complain that these lesions are sensitive or they burn and sting.

ETIOLOGY. Heredity and sun exposure are the two main causative factors. The blue-eyed, thin-skinned, light-haired person with a family history of such lesions is the best subject for multiple actinic keratoses.

SEX INCIDENCE. The disorder is most commonly seen in men.

Differential Diagnosis

Seborrheic keratosis (see Table 33–1)
Squamous cell carcinoma: any thickened lesion that has grown rapidly should be biopsied (see later in this chapter).
Arsenical keratosis: mainly on palms and soles.

Treatment

A 60-year-old farmer has three small actinic keratoses on his face.

Examine the lesions carefully. *If there is any evidence of induration or marked inflammation, the lesion should be biopsied.* (See scissors or surgical excision technique, p. 13.)

There are two methods of removal of these keratoses.

For a single lesion, or only three or four lesions, I prefer a one-visit surgical treatment.

SURGICAL METHOD

Liquid nitrogen, if available, applied very lightly to the lesion is an effective and rapid method of removal. This is the therapy of choice of dermatologists.

Curettement, followed by destruction of the base by acid or electrosurgery, is satisfactory. Local anesthesia is usually necessary. Firmly scrape the lesion with the dermal curette, which will remove the mushy, scaly keratosis and bring you down to the more fibrous normal skin. Experience will provide the necessary "feel" of the abnormal versus the normal tissue. Some of the bleeding can be controlled by pressure or use of either one of the two following procedures: (1) with a cotton-tipped applicator, apply a saturated solution of trichloroacetic acid cautiously to the

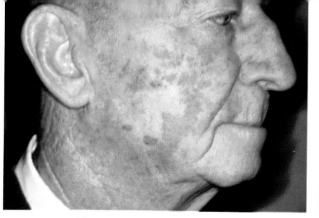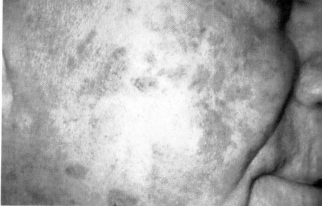

(A) Multiple actinic keratoses on face of 80-year-old, fair-complexioned farmer; (B) close-up

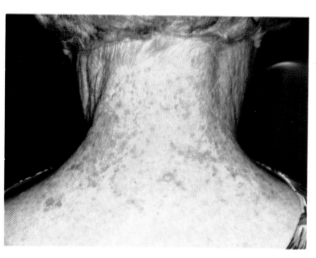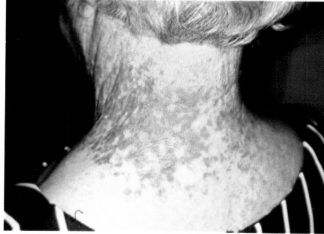

(C) Actinic keratoses of back of neck showing lesions before and (D) normal accentuation after therapy with 5-fluorouracil for 2 weeks

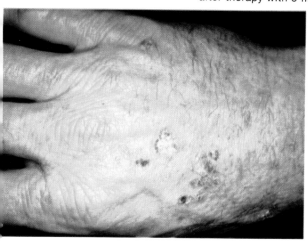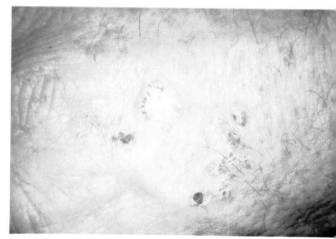

(E) Lesions on dorsum of hands; (F) close-up, in 44-year-old, blue-eyed outdoor worker

Plate 83. **Actinic or senile keratoses.** (*Dermik Laboratories, Inc.*) (*Owen Laboratories, Inc.*)

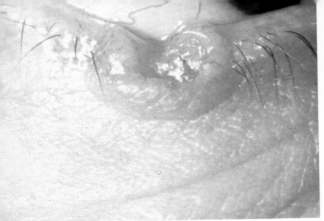

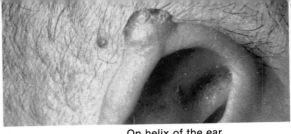

On helix of the ear

Of the lower eyelid. Note telangiectasia on the rolled edge of the ulcer. (*Drs. L. Calkins and A. Lemoine*)

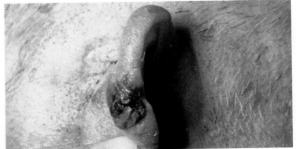

Hemorrhagic lesion on helix of ear

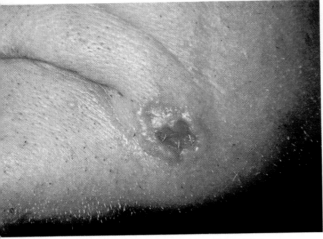

Ulcerated lesion on chin. (*K.U.M.C.*)

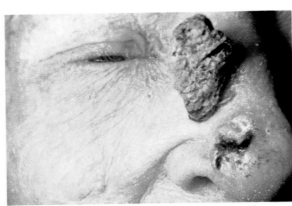

Cutaneous horn with basal cell carcinomatous degeneration of the base

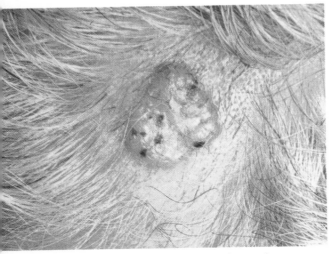

Basal cell carcinomatous change in a syringocystadenoma papilliferum nevus on the scalp.

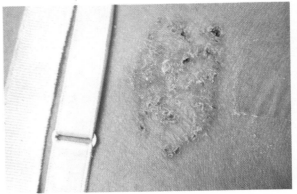

Superficial basal cell carcinoma on posterior aspect of shoulder. Patient took arsenic (Fowler's solution) for 3 months 30 years previously for psoriasis.

Plate 84.   **Basal cell carcinomas.** (*Texas Pharmacal*)

bleeding site, or (2) the bleeding base may be electrocoagulated. Small lesions will heal in 7 to 14 days. No bandage is required.

FLUOROURACIL METHOD

For the patient with multiple superficial actinic keratoses, fluorouracil therapy is very effective and will eliminate for some months or years the early damaged epidermal cells. Thus this fluorouracil therapy is really a cancer prevention routine.

Several preparations and strengths of solutions and creams are available, but the following are most commonly indicated:

Fluoroplex 1% solution	30.0

or

Efudex 2% solution	10.0

Sig: Apply to area to be treated twice a day, with fingers.

It is wise to treat only a small area on the face at a time. Give instructions carefully and warn that it is natural for the skin to get quite red and irritated and sore after 4 to 5 days. Most commonly the course of therapy is for 2 weeks. Some patients must stop therapy sooner, and some need more time to get the desired effect.

After completion of the course of therapy, the skin usually heals rapidly. A corticosteroid cream may be prescribed to hasten healing.

This therapy may have to be repeated in several months or years. If some keratoses are too thick to be removed by this fluorouracil method, then the liquid nitrogen or surgical method, as described first, is indicated for these lesions.

Treatment of a Cutaneous Horn
(Plates 84C and 86A)

The same surgical technique as for actinic keratosis is used. *To rule out cancer, most cutaneous horns should be sent with intact base for histopathologic examination.* The incidence of squamous cell carcinomatous change in the base of a cutaneous horn is appreciable.

Arsenical Keratosis

Prolonged ingestion of inorganic arsenic (*e.g.,* Fowler's Solution, Asiatic Pills) can result in the formation of many years later of small, punctate keratotic lesions, mainly seen

on the palms and the soles. Progression to a squamous cell carcinoma can occur but is unusual.

Treatment

Small arsenical keratoses can be removed by electrosurgery; larger lesions can be excised and skin grafted if necessary.

Leukoplakia
(Plate 85)

Leukoplakia is an actinic keratosis of the mucous membrane (Fig. 33–1).

DESCRIPTION. A flat, whitish plaque occurs localized to the mucous membranes of lips, mouth, vulva, and vagina. Single or multiple lesions may be present.

COURSE. Progression to squamous cell carcinoma occurs in 20% to 30% of chronic cases.

ETIOLOGY. Smoking, sunlight, and chronic irritation are the important factors in the development of leukoplakia. *Recurrent actinic cheilitis* may precede leukoplakia of the lips. The vulvar form may develop from *presenile* or *senile atrophy* of this area.

Differential Diagnosis

Lichen planus: a lacy network of whitish lesions, mainly on the sides of the buccal cavity; when on lips, it may clinically resemble leukoplakia; lichen planus elsewhere on body (see Chap. 14). Biopsy is often indicated.

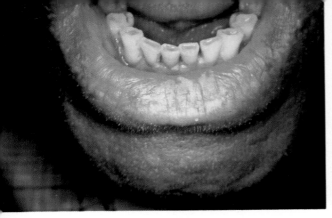

(A) Leukoplakia on lower lip, mild

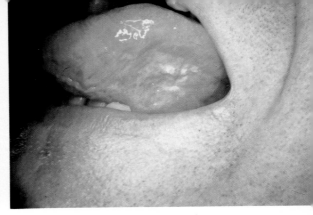

(B) Leukoplakia on tongue, from chronic biting

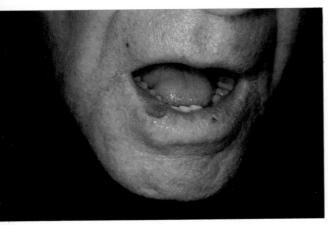

(C) Squamous cell carcinoma of lower lip

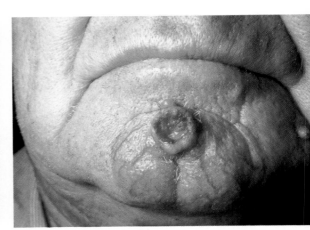

(D) Squamous cell carcinoma of chin

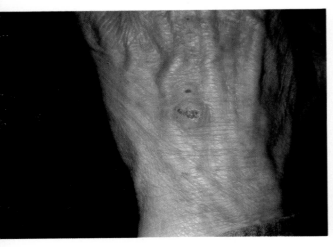

(E) Squamous cell carcinoma on dorsum of hand (compare with Plate 86C)

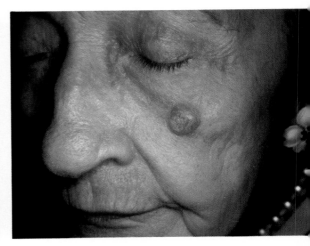

(F) Squamous cell carcinoma on cheek

Plate 85. **Leukoplakia and squamous cell carcinoma.** (*Westwood Pharmaceuticals*)

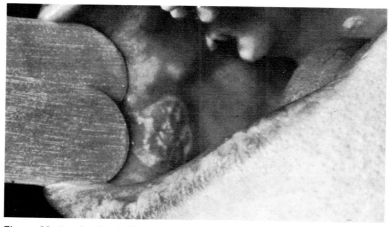

Figure 33–1. Leukoplakia. Biopsy-proved leukoplakia on the mucous membrane of the cheek. This was erroneously diagnosed, clinically, as lichen planus.

Pressure calluses from teeth or dentures: evidence of irritation; differentiation may be possible only by biopsy.

On the vulva, *lichen sclerosus et atrophicus* or *kraurosis vulvae:* no induration, as in leukoplakia of this area; can extend onto skin of inguinal folds and perianal region; pruritus may or may not be present. Biopsy is helpful.

Treatment

Small patch of leukoplakia is seen on lower lip of man who smokes considerably.

1. Examine lesion carefully. *Biopsy any questionable area that shows inflammation and induration.* If a squamous cell carcinoma is present, the patient should receive surgical or radiation therapy by a physician who is expert in this form of treatment.
2. Advise against smoking. The seriousness of continued smoking or other use of tobacco must be pointed out to the patient. Many early cases of leukoplakia disappear when smoking is stopped.
3. Eliminate any chronic irritation from teeth or dentures.
4. Protect the lips from sunlight with a sunscreen stick.
5. Electrosurgery, preceded by local anesthesia, is excellent for small, persistent areas of leukoplakia. The coagulating current is effective. Healing is usually rapid.

Liquid nitrogen freezing is also quite effective.

EPITHELIOMAS AND CARCINOMAS

Basal Cell Carcinoma
(Plates 1C, 3A, 84, 95, and 99)

This is the most common malignancy of the skin. Very fortunately, a basal cell epithelioma or carcinoma is not a metastasizing tumor, and the cure rate can be close to 100% if these lesions are treated early and adequately.

DESCRIPTION. There are four clinical types of basal cell carcinoma: (1) noduloulcerative, (2) pigmented, (3) fibrosing (sclerosing), and (4) superficial.

The *noduloulcerative basal cell carcinoma* is the most common type. It begins as a small waxy nodule that enlarges slowly over the years. A central depression usually forms that eventually progresses into an ulcer surrounded by the pearly or waxy border. The surface of the nodular component has a few telangiectatic vessels, which are highly characteristic.

The *pigmented type* is similar to the noduloulcerative form, with the addition of brown or black pigmentation.

The *fibrosing type* is extremely slow growing, is usually seen on the face, and consists of a whitish, scarred plaque with an ill-defined border, which rarely becomes ulcerated. This type is difficult to treat.

The *superficial form* may be single or multiple, is usually seen on the back and the chest, and is characterized by slowly enlarging red, scaly areas that, on careful examination, reveal a nodular border with telangiectatic vessels. A healed atrophic center may be present. Ulceration is superficial when it develops.

DISTRIBUTION. Over 90% of the basal cell carcinomas occur on the head and the neck, with the trunk next in frequency. These tumors are rarely found on the palms and the soles.

COURSE. The tumor is very slow growing, but sudden rapid growth periods do occur. Destructive forms of this tumor can invade cartilage, bone, blood vessels, or large areas of skin surface, and result in death. There are rare reports of metastasizing basal cell carcinomas.

ETIOLOGY. Basal cell carcinomas develop most frequently on the areas of the skin exposed to sunlight and in blond or red-haired persons. Trauma and overexposure to radium and x-radiation can cause basal cell carcinomas. Long-term ingestion of inorganic arsenic can lead to formation of superficial basal cell carcinomas. Most authors believe that a basal cell tumor is a carcinoma of the basal cells of the epidermis. Lever (see Bibliography) and others believe it not to be a carcinoma but a nevoid tumor (epithelioma) derived from incompletely differentiated embryonal cells.

AGE-GROUP. This tumor can occur from childhood to old age but is seen most frequently in men older than age 50.

Differential Diagnosis

<table>
<tr><td>

SAUER NOTE:

Whenever the clinical appearance of a skin tumor suggests a basal cell carcinoma, the lesion should be studied histologically.

</td></tr>
</table>

Squamous cell carcinoma: more rapid growth, firm, scaly papule or nodule, more

inflammation, no pearly telangiectatic border; biopsy is necessary.

Other lesions that can mimic a basal cell carcinoma are *sebaceous hyperplasias* (very common, have a central dell), *keratoacanthomas, sebaceous adenomas, large comedones, warts, nevi, small cysts,* and *scarring from injury or radiation.*

Superficial basal cell carcinomas can resemble lesions of *psoriasis, seborrheic dermatitis, lupus vulgaris,* and *Bowen's disease.*

If multiple basal cell carcinomas are found, one should consider the *basal cell nevus syndrome.* This is a rare hereditary condition characterized by multiple genetically determined basal cell carcinomas, cysts of the jaws, peculiar pits of the hands and feet, and developmental anomalies of the ribs, the spine, and the skull.

Treatment

A 48-year-old woman has an 8 × 8-mm basal cell carcinoma on her forehead.

1. Inform the patient that she has a cancer of the skin that needs to be removed. Tell the patient that this tumor cannot spread into the body, but if it is not treated it can spread on the skin. State that removal of the lesion is almost 100% effective but that periodic examinations will be necessary to check for any regrowth. If this tumor recurs, it will regrow only at is previous site. Tell the patient that a scar will result from the treatment.

2. If the diagnosis of the lesion is not definite clinically, a scissors biopsy, as described on page 13, may be done safely. Further treatment will depend on the laboratory report.

3. Surgical excision of a basal cell carcinoma is the only method of treatment that should be attempted by the physician who only occasionally is confronted with these tumors. (Some criticism will arise from this statement, but it is my belief that a great amount of experience is necessary to remove these tumors adequately by curettement, chemocautery, electrosurgery, radiation, or any combination of these methods. If the operator believes that he is qualified in these procedures, then this statement is not meant for him.) To excise the lesion, anesthetize the area, make an

elliptical incision with a scalpel to include a border of 3 to 4 mm around the tumor, tag one side of the excised skin with a piece of suture, close the incision, and submit the specimen for careful histologic examination. (See also Chapter 7, *Fundamentals of Cutaneous Surgery.*) If the pathologist states that the tumor extends up to the edge of the excision, a further, more radical excision should be performed.

4. Have the patient return for a checkup on a definite schedule, such as in 4 months, then every 6 months for four visits, then yearly, for a total of 5 years. Ten-year follow-ups are being suggested by some authors.

Treatment of deeply ulcerated, fibrosing or large superficial basal cell carcinomas should be in the domain of the competent dermatologist, surgeon, or radiologist. Mohs type surgery for these more difficult lesions is microscopically controlled and, unless the tumor is massive, results in a high cure rate.

Squamous Cell Carcinoma
(Plates 85, 95, and 99)

This rather common skin malignancy can arise primarily or from an actinic keratosis or leukoplakia. The grade of malignancy and metastasizing ability varies from grade I (low) to grade IV (high). Other terms for this tumor include prickle cell epithelioma and epidermoid carcinoma.

DESCRIPTION. The most common clinical picture is a rather rapidly growing nodule that soon develops a central ulcer and an indurated raised border with some surrounding redness. This type of lesion is the most malignant. The least malignant form has the clinical appearance of a warty, piled-up growth, which may not ulcerate. However, it is important to realize that the grade of malignancy can vary in the same tumor from one section to another, particularly in the larger lesions. This variation demonstrates the value of multiple histologic sections.

DISTRIBUTION. The lesion can occur on any area of the skin and mucous membrane but most commonly on the face, particularly lower lip and ears, tongue, and dorsa of the hands. Chronic trauma associated with certain occupations can lead to formation of this cancer on unusual sites.

COURSE. The course varies with the grade of malignancy of the tumor. Lymph node metastases may occur early in the development of the tumor or may never occur. The cure rate can be very high when the lesions are treated early and with the best-indicated modality.

ETIOLOGY. As in basal cell carcinomas, many factors contribute to provide the soil for growth of a squamous cell carcinoma. A simple listing of factors will be sufficient: hereditarily determined type of skin; age of patient; trauma from chemicals (tars, oils), heat, wind, sunlight, x-radiation, and severe burns; skin diseases that form scars, such as discoid lupus erythematosus, lupus vulgaris, and chronic ulcers; ingestion of inorganic arsenic; and in the natural course of xeroderma pigmentosum.

AGE AND SEX INCIDENCE. Most tumors are usually seen in elderly men, but exceptions are not rare.

Differential Diagnosis

> ### SAUER NOTE:
>
> Whenever the clinical appearance of a skin tumor suggests a squamous cell carcinoma, the lesion should be studied histologically.

Basal cell carcinoma: slower growth, pearly border with telangiectasis, less inflammation; biopsy may be necessary to differentiate (see preceding section).

Actinic keratosis: slow-growing, flat, scaly lesions; no induration; little surrounding erythema (see preceding section).

Pseudoepitheliomatous hyperplasia: primary chronic lesion, such as old stasis ulcer, bromoderma, deep mycotic infection, syphilitic gumma, lupus vulgaris, basal cell carcinoma, and pyoderma gangrenosum; differentiation often impossible clinically, and very difficult histologically.

Keratoacanthoma (Plate 86C and D): very fast-growing single or, more rarely, multiple lesion; clinically, this is a firm, raised

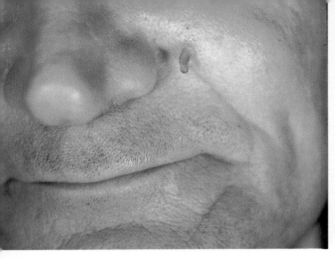

(A) Cutaneous horn, on cheek

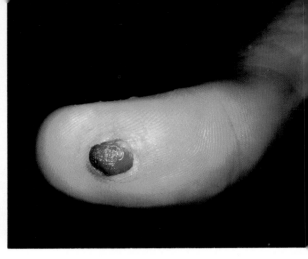

(B) Granuloma pyogenicum on thumb

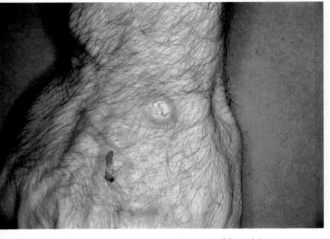

(C) Keratoacanthoma on dorsum of hand (compare with Plate 85E)

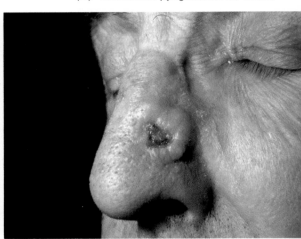

(D) Keratoacanthoma, on nose, that healed without therapy, except for biopsy

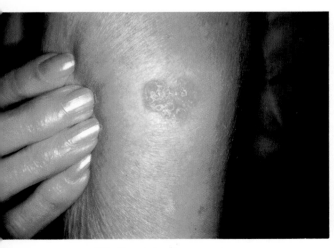

(E) Bowen's disease, on arm

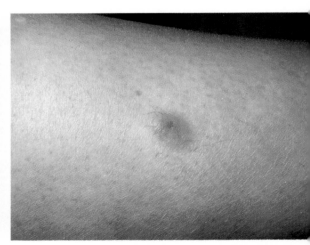

(F) Histiocytoma, on leg

Plate 86. **Miscellaneous tumors of the skin.** (*Syntex Laboratories, Inc.*)

nodule with a central crater; it should be studied histologically; it may disappear spontaneously.

Treatment

Because of the invasive nature of squamous cell carcinomas, intensive surgical and/or radiation therapy is indicated. A discussion of such procedures is beyond the scope of this text but consult Chapter 7, *Fundamentals of Cutaneous Surgery.*

HISTIOCYTOMA AND DERMATOFIBROMA

Histiocytomas and dermatofibromas are common, usually single, flat or very slightly elevated, tannish, reddish, or brownish nodules, less than 1 cm in size, that occur mainly on the anterior tibial area of the leg. These tumors have a characteristic clinical appearance and firm button-like feel that establishes the diagnosis. They occur in adults and are nonsymptomatic and unchanging.

The histologic picture varies with the age of the lesion. The younger lesions are called histiocytomas, and the older ones dermatofibromas. If the nodule contains many blood vessels it is histologically labeled a *sclerosing hemangioma.*

Differential Diagnosis

Fibrosarcoma: active growth with invasion of subcutaneous fat; any questionable lesions should be excised and examined histologically.

Treatment

No treatment is indicated. If there is any doubt as to the diagnosis, surgical excision and histologic examination are indicated.

For the female patient who shaves her legs and hits this lesion, liquid nitrogen applied lightly to the papule will flatten it.

KELOID
(Plate 3B)

A keloid is a tumor resulting from an abnormal overgrowth of fibrous tissue following injury in certain predisposed persons. Very unusual configurations can occur, depending on the site, the extent, and the variety of the trauma. This tendency occurs so commonly in blacks that one should think twice before attempting a cosmetic procedure on a black-skinned person or on any other person with a history of keloids. The face and the upper chest areas are especially prone to this proliferation.

SAUER NOTE:

Before any surgical procedure, the patient should be warned that a hypertrophic scar or keloid could follow the procedure. This is especially frequent following surgery on the chest or upper back.

Differential Diagnosis

Hypertrophic scar: initially same clinically and histologically as a keloid; flattens spontaneously in most cases after one or several years.

Treatment

Therapy is very unsatisfactory. Occasionally combined procedures using excision and intralesional corticosteroid injections have been successful.

HEMANGIOMAS
(Plates 1A and D and 87)

Hemangiomas are vascular abnormalities of the skin. Heredity is not a factor in the development of these lesions. There are nine types of hemangiomas, which vary as to depth, clinical appearance, and location (Fig. 33–2):

1. Superficial hemangioma
2. Cavernous hemangioma
3. Mixed hemangioma (when both superficial and cavernous elements are present)
4. Spider hemangioma
5. Port-wine hemangioma
6. Nuchal hemangioma

Two spider hemangiomas on the arm of a
pregnant woman

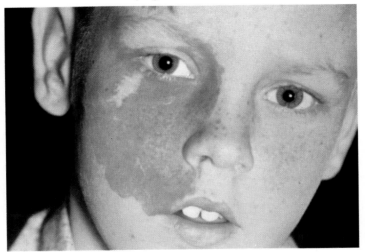

Port-wine stain on the face of a boy

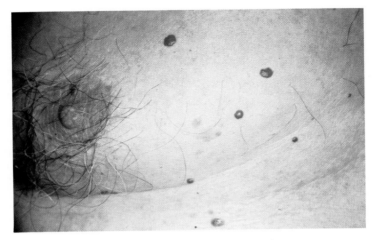

Capillary (senile) hemangiomas on the chest near
the nipple

Plate 87. **Hemangiomas.** (*Ortho Pharmaceutical Corp.*)

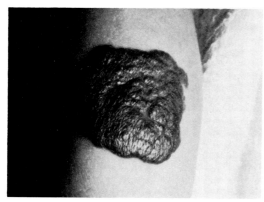

Superficial hemangioma on calf of the leg of a child

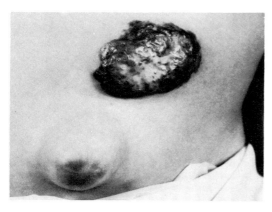

Mixed hemangioma on the abdomen above an umbilical hernia. (See Plate 1.)

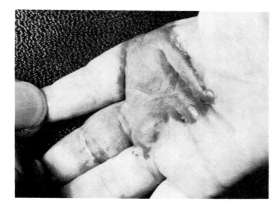

Cavernous hemangioma on the palm

Figure 33–2. **Hemangiomas.**

7. Capillary hemangioma
8. Venous lake
9. Angiokeratoma

Superficial and Cavernous Hemangiomas
(Plates 1 and 92)

The familiar bright-red, raised "strawberry" tumor has been seen by all physicians (See Fig. 33–2). Strawberries have to grow, and they start from a small beginning. The parents are usually the first to notice the small, red, pinhead-sized, flat lesions. They are noticed at, or soon after, birth. These red tumors can occur on any area of the body and can begin as small lesions and stay that way, remaining as *superficial hemangiomas,* or they can enlarge and extend into the subcutaneous tissue, forming a *cavernous type.* The enlargement can occur rapidly or slowly. Occasionally there can be multiple lesions.

Two aspects of the larger hemangiomas can be disturbing. First, the mere presence of the lesion or lesions will cause concern to parents. If the lesion is on an exposed area of the body, this will cause additional concern and comment by relatives, neighbors, and other well-meaning persons. This can be most disconcerting.

Second, if the lesion is large and near an eye, the nose, or the mouth, it can, by its physical size, cause an obstructive problem. Systemic corticosteroids have been used successfully. Surgery may be indicated. However, even some massive hemangiomas in these areas can be left alone and will resolve amazingly over a period of several months.

Treatment

The treatment of hemangiomas that are not of the obstructive type has been the subject of considerable discussion. To begin with, the size, the depth, and the location of the hemangiomas, and, I might add, the pressure on the physician from parents and relatives, are factors that must be considered for every case.

There are those who favor treating almost every superficial or cavernous hemangioma, and there are others who believe that all hemangiomas should be left alone to involute spontaneously. The latter group stand behind the studies of our English colleagues, Bowers, Simpson, and others, who showed that around

85% of hemangiomas disappeared without any appreciable scar by the age of 7 years. They also found that the hemangiomas usually stopped growing by the age of 1 year. Personally, I advocate the treatment of some hemangiomas, and I leave others alone. Let me illustrate by two case histories.

CASE 1

A 6-week-old child is brought in by her parents. She has a 4 × 4-mm slightly raised red lesion on her cheek. The parents first noticed it when she was 3 weeks of age, when it was of pinhead size.

1. Reassure the parents that this birthmark is not hereditary and that it will not turn into a cancer.
2. Inform them that you will treat this lesion, because it probably will enlarge and could become quite a deformity. If you wish, you can explain that the lesion, if left alone, might or might not enlarge, and if it does enlarge will probably disappear without much of a mark in 5 to 7 years. However, state that you would suggest treatment now to possibly abort any further growth.
3. Apply a solid dry ice "pencil" directly to the lesion for 4 to 8 seconds with firm pressure. The "pencil" tip should be shaped to conform exactly to, or be 1 mm larger than, the size of the tumor. Occasionally, second and third treatments are necessary in 3 to 6 weeks. Tell the parents that a blister will form within 24 hours at the site of the treatment but, if left alone, it will heal in 6 to 14 days. If any infection develops, have them contact you.

Dry ice can be purchased in blocks from any ice cream manufacturer and shaped to fit the lesion, or it can be made in a Kidde Dry Ice Kit (see p. 389).

A similar effect can be obtained with liquid nitrogen cryotherapy.

CASE 2

An 8-month-old girl is brought in by her parents. They state that she has a birthmark on her cheek that began at the age of 3 weeks. Their physician was consulted and stated that the lesion should be watched, since "a lot of them just go away."

At the age of 3 months, the lesion had grown further, but the physician still advised them to wait and watch.

Now at the age of 8 months the red hemangioma measures 12 × 12 × 5 mm and has a bluish mass at the base. It is a mixed hemangioma.

1. Reassure the parents that the lesion is not hereditary and that it will not turn into a cancer.
2. Since the child is now 8 months of age, and the lesion has in all probability reached its maximum growth, no treatment is indicated. The parents must be told in no uncertain terms *why* you are not going to treat the tumor. You should state that you believe it will not enlarge further and that you know from your experience, and that of others, that it will undoubtedly be gone by the age of 2 or 3 years and almost certainly by the age of 5 to 7. You can almost predict that the residual mark will be insignificant. However, if it does not disappear completely by that age, the remaining, usually insignificant lesion can be excised.

To *summarize*, the advantages of *early* treatment of *small* superficial or cavernous hemangiomas are as follows: (1) you eliminate the lesion completely, or almost completely; (2) you do not leave to chance the fact that it might or might not enlarge considerably; (3) you put a halt to apprehension on the part of the parents and relatives regarding the course of the lesion; and (4) with properly applied cryotherapy you leave no mark, or only a slight one that would be no worse than that resulting from leaving it alone.

The advantages of *not* treating one of these hemangiomas are as follows: (1) the residuum after 5 to 7 years may be better cosmetically than if the lesion had been treated with cryotherapy, or especially if x-ray therapy was used; and (2) the cost of therapy will be saved.

Spider Hemangioma
(Plate 87)

A spider hemangioma consists of a small pinpoint- to pinhead-sized central red arteriole with radiating smaller vessels like the spokes of a wheel or the legs of a spider. These lesions develop for no apparent reason or may develop in association with pregnancy or chronic liver disease. The most common location is on the face. The reason for removal is cosmetic.

Differential Diagnosis

Venous stars: small, bluish, telangiectatic veins, usually seen on the legs and the face but may appear anywhere on the body; these can be removed, if desired, by the same method as for spider hemangioma.

Hereditary hemorrhagic telangiectasis (Rendu-Osler-Weber) (see Plate 77): small, red lesions on any organ of the body that can hemorrhage; get familial history.

Treatment

A spider hemangioma is present on the cheek of a young woman who is 6 months post partum. This lesion developed during her pregnancy and has persisted unchanged.

Treat by electrosurgery. Use the fine epilating needle with either a very low coagulating sparking current or a low cutting current. Stick the needle into the central vessel and turn on the current for 1 or 2 seconds until the vessel blanches. No anesthetic is necessary in most patients. The area will form a scab and heal in about 4 days, leaving an imperceptible scar. Rarely, a second treatment is necessary to eliminate the central vessel. If the radiating vessels are large and persistent, they can be treated in the same manner as the central vessel.

SAUER NOTE:

It is advisable to tell the patient that it will be difficult to remove every vessel in a spider hemangioma. To attempt to do so might cause a scar.

Port-Wine Hemangioma
(Plate 87)

The port-wine hemangioma is commonly seen on the face as a reddish purple, flat, disfiguring facial mark. It can occur elsewhere in a less extensive form. Faint reddish lesions are often found on infants on the sides of the face, the forehead, the eyelids, and the extremities. The color increases with crying and alarms the mother, but most of these faint lesions disappear shortly after birth.

Treatment

An extensive port-wine hemangioma is present on the left side of the face of a man.

1. There is no satisfactory treatment for this defect. Tattooing, laser-beam therapy, and dermabrasion have been used by some with varied success.
2. Cosmetics, such as "Covermark," or any good pancake-type of makeup, are effective to a certain degree.

Nuchal Hemangioma

Nuchal hemangioma is a common, persistent, faint red patch on the posterior neck region, at or below the scalp margin. It does not disappear with aging, and treatment is not effective or necessary. Since the posterior neck area is also the site of the common neurodermatitis, it is well to remember that following the cure of the neurodermatitis a redness that persists could be a nuchal hemangioma that was present for years and not noticed previously.

Capillary Hemangioma
(Plate 87)

Capillary hemangiomas are also called *senile hemangiomas,* but this term obviously should not be used in discussing the lesion with the patient who is in the 30- to 60-year-old age-group. These pinhead, or slightly larger, bright red, flat or raised tumors are present in many young adults and in practically all elderly persons. They cause no disability except when they are injured and bleed.

Treatment is usually not desired, but if it is, light electrosurgery is effective.

Venous Lake

Another vascular lesion that occurs in older persons is a *venous lake.* Clinically, it is a soft, compressible, flat or slightly elevated, bluish red, 3- to 6-mm sized lesion, usually located on the lips or the ears. Lack of induration and rapid growth distinguish it from a *melanoma.* Lack of pulsation will distinguish a venous lake on the lower lip from a *tortuous segment of the inferior labial artery.*

Treatment is usually not desired, only reassurance concerning its nonmalignant nature.

Angiokeratomas

Three forms of angiokeratoma are known. The *Mibelli form* occurs on the dorsa of the fingers, the toes, and the knees; the *Fabry form* occurs over the entire trunk in an extensive pattern; and the *Fordyce form* occurs on the scrotum. The lesions are dark-red, pinhead-sized papules with a somewhat warty appearance.

Treatment is not indicated for the Mibelli and the Fordyce forms.

The Fabry form (angiokeratoma corporis diffusum), however, is the cutaneous manifestation of a systemic phospholipid storage disease in which phospholipids are deposited in the skin, as well as in various internal organs. Death usually occurs in the fifth decade from the result of such deposits in the smooth muscles of the blood vessels, in the heart, and in the kidneys.

NEVUS CELL TUMORS

Classification

I. **Melanocytic Nevi**
   A. Junctional or active nevus
   B. Intradermal or resting nevus
   C. Dysplastic nevus syndrome
II. **Malignant Melanoma**

Melanocytic Nevi
(Plates 88 and 96)

Nevi are pigmented or nonpigmented tumors of the skin that contain nevus cells. Nevi are present on every adult, but some persons have more than others. There are two main questions concerning nevi or moles. When and how should they be removed? What is the relationship between nevi and malignant melanomas?

Histologically, it is possible to divide benign nevi into *junctional* or *active nevi* and *intradermal* or *resting nevi*. Combinations of these two forms commonly exist and are labeled *compound nevi.*

In the *dysplastic nevus syndrome* (B-K mole syndrome), the nevi are larger than ordinary nevi (usually 5 to 15 mm in size), have an irregular border, and show a haphazard mixture of tan, brown, pink, and black. There is a propensity for this type of familial nevi to develop into malignant melanomas.

Clinically, one never can be positive with which histopathologic type of nevus one is dealing, but certain criteria are helpful in establishing a differentiation between the two forms.

DESCRIPTION. Clinically, nevi can be pigmented or nonpigmented, flat or elevated, hairy or nonhairy, warty, papillomatous, or pedunculated. They can have a small or a wide base. The brown- or black-pigmented, flat or slightly elevated, nonhairy nevi are usually *junctional nevi.* The nonpigmented or pigmented, elevated, hairy nevi are more likely to be the *intradermal nevi.*

A nevus with a depigmented area surrounding it is called a *halo nevus* or *leukoderma acquisitum centrifigum* (see Plate 88). The nevus in the center of the halo that histologically has an *inflammatory* infiltrate usually involutes in several months in contradistinction to the rarer *noninflammatory halo nevus.* Excision of the nevus is usually not indicated.

DISTRIBUTION. Nevi are very prevalent on the head and the neck but may be on any part of the body. The nevi on the palms, the soles, and the genitalia are usually junctional nevi.

COURSE. A child is born with no, or relatively few, nevi, but with increasing age, particularly after puberty, nevi slowly become larger, can remain flat or become elevated, and may become hairy and darker. A change is also seen histologically with age. A junctional-type active nevus, although it may remain as such throughout the life of the person, more commonly changes slowly into an intradermal or resting nevus. Some nevi do not become evident until adult or later life, but the precursor cells for the nevus were present at birth. A malignant melanoma can originate from a junctional nevus and from dysplastic nevi. A benign junctional nevus in a child can histologically look like a malignant melanoma. Known as a *Spitz nevus*, this poses a difficult diagnostic and management problem.

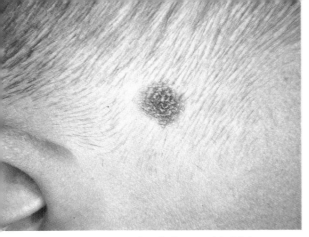

(A) Junctional nevus in scalp of 12-year-old child

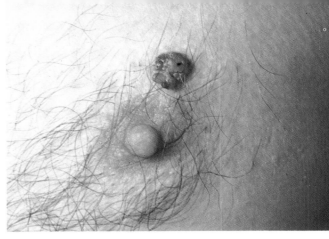

(B) Compound nevus, on chest above nipple

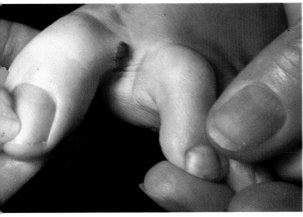

(C) Junctional nevus on web of toe of 8-year-old child

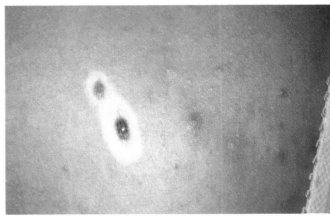

(D) Halo nevus, or leukoderma acquisitum centrifigum, on the back

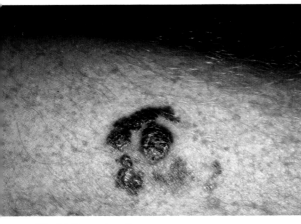

(E) Malignant melanoma, on arm

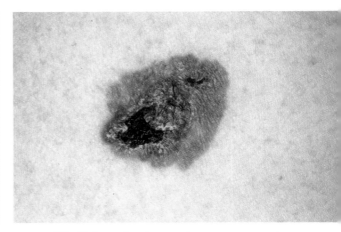

(F) Malignant melanoma in a nevus present since birth, on the scapular area

Plate 88. **Nevus cell tumors and malignant melanomas.** (*The Upjohn Company*)

HISTOGENESIS. The origin of the nevus cell is disputed, but the most commonly accepted theory is that it originates from cutaneous nerve cells.

Differential Diagnosis

IN CHILDHOOD

Warts: flat or common warts not on the hands or the feet may be difficult to differentiate clinically; should see warty growth with black "seeds" (the capillary loops), rather acute onset, and rapid growth (see Chap. 17).

Freckles: on exposed areas of the body; many lesions; fade in winter; not raised.

Lentigo: flat, tan or brown spot, usually on exposed skin surfaces; histologically, this is an early junctional nevus.

Blue nevus: flat or elevated, soft, dark bluish or black nodule.

Granuloma pyogenicum: rapid onset of reddish or blackish vascular tumor, usually at site of injury.

Molluscum contagiosum: one, or usually more, crater-shaped, waxy tumors (see Chap. 17).

Urticaria pigmentosa: single, but more commonly multiple, slightly elevated, yellowish to brown papules, that urticate with trauma (see Chap. 26).

IN ADULTHOOD

Warts: usually rather obvious; black "seeds" (see Chap. 17).

Pedunculated fibromas: on neck and axillae (see earlier in this chapter).

Histiocytoma (Plate 86): on anterior tibial area of leg; flat, button-like in consistency (see earlier in this chapter).

Other *epidermal* and *mesodermal tumors* are differentiated histologically.

IN OLDER ADULTS

Actinic or senile keratosis: on exposed areas; scaly surrounding skin usually thin and dry; not a sharply demarcated lesion (see earlier in this chapter).

Seborrheic keratosis: greasy, waxy, warty tumor, "stuck on" the skin; however, some are very difficult to differentiate clinically from nevus or malignant melanoma (see earlier in this chapter).

Malignant melanoma (see Plates 88 and 95): seen at site of junction nevus or can arise from normal-appearing skin, shows a change in pigmentation either by spreading, becoming spotty, or turning darker; may bleed, form a crust, or ulcerate (see following section).

Basal cell carcinomas and squamous cell carcinomas: if there is any question of malignancy, a biopsy is indicated (see earlier in this chapter).

Treatment

CASE 1

A mother comes into your office with her 5-year-old son, who has an 8 × 8-mm flat, brown nevus on the forehead. She wants to know if this "mole" is dangerous and if it should be removed.

1. Examine the lesion carefully. This lesion shows no sign of recent growth or change in pigmentation. (If it did, it should be excised and examined histologically.)
2. Reassure the mother that this mole does not appear to be dangerous and that it would be very unusual for it to become dangerous. If any change in the color or growth appears, the lesion should be examined again.
3. Tell the mother that it is best to leave this nevus alone at this time. The *only* treatment would be surgical excision, and you are quite sure that her boy would not sit tight for this procedure unless he was given a general anesthetic. When the boy is 16 years of age or older, the lesion can be examined again and possibly removed at that time by a simpler method under local anesthesia.

CASE 2

A 25-year-old, attractive woman desires a brown, raised, hairy nevus on her upper lip removed. There has been no recent change in the tumor.

1. Examine the lesion carefully for induration, scaling, ulceration, and bleeding. None of these signs is present. (If the diagnosis is not definite, a scissors biopsy may be performed safely and the base gently coagulated by electrosurgery. Further treatment will depend on the biopsy report.)
2. Tell the patient that you can biopsy and remove the mole safely but that there will be a residual, very slightly depressed scar, and that probably the hairs will have to be

removed separately after the first surgery has healed.

3. Surgical excision with tissue examination is the best method of removal. However, hairy, raised, pigmented nevi have been removed by electrosurgery for years with no real proof that this form of removal has caused a malignant melanoma.

First, following local anesthesia, perform a shave biopsy. Then electrosurgery can be performed with the coagulating or cutting current or with cautery. The site should not be covered and will heal in 7 to 14 days, depending on the size. If the hairs regrow, they can be removed later by electrosurgical epilation (see Chap. 6).

SAUER NOTES:
Do's and Don'ts Regarding Nevi

1. Don't remove a nevus in a child by electrosurgery; remove only by surgical excision and submit nevus for histopathological examination.

2. Do remember that in a child benign junctional nevus may resemble a malignant melanoma histologically. Don't alarm the parents unnecessarily, since these nevi are usually no threat to life.

3. Don't remove a flat pigmented nevus, particularly on the palm, the sole, or the genitalia, by electrosurgery. These should be excised surgically, if indicated, and should be examined histologically.

4. Don't remove any suspicious nevus by electrosurgery. Excise it and examine it histologically.

5. Don't perform a radical deforming surgical procedure on a possible malignant melanoma until the biopsy report has been returned. Many of these tumors can turn out to be seborrheic keratoses, granuloma pyogenicum, and so on.

MALIGNANT MELANOMA
(Plate 88)

The incidence of malignant melanoma has increased considerably in the past 2 decades. Predisposing factors for the development of malignant melanoma include heredity, complexion (fair skin, blue eyes), ultraviolet exposure (the incidence of melanoma in the United States is increased in those states nearer the equator), and the presence of large *bathing-trunk congenital nevi*. The person with hereditary dysplastic nevi is more prone to develop a malignant melanoma. Fifty percent of melanomas arise from preexisting nevi. Although melanomas make up only 1% of all skin cancers, they account for over 60% of the deaths due to skin cancer in the United States. The best chance for a cure lies in early diagnosis and prompt, adequate treatment of the primary lesion.

There are four major types of malignant melanomas. They differ in terms of mode of onset, course, prognosis, and incidence.

The most common melanoma is the *superficial spreading melanoma*, which develops from an *in situ* lesion. It grows slowly with a resulting good prognosis.

Nodular melanomas grow quite rapidly and have a poorer prognosis.

Acral lentiginous melanoma occurs, as the title signifies, on the palms, soles and around the nails, is the most common type seen in black patients, ulcerates, and metastasizes rapidly, so that it has the poorest prognosis.

Lentigo maligna melanoma, the least frequent type, develops from a lentigo maligna, occurs on the exposed areas of the body in the elderly, mainly on the forearms and face, grows slowly peripherally, and has a high survival rate.

DESCRIPTION. The classic malignant melanoma is a black or purple nodule, but it may be flat, or pedunculated, and may be pink, red, tan, brown, or black.

The changes in a recent or long-standing skin lesion that should arouse suspicion include change in the size or shape, change in pigmentation (particularly the development of pseudopodia or areas of satellite pigmentation), erythema surrounding the lesion, induration, friability with easy bleeding tendency, and ulceration.

DISTRIBUTION. The site of predilection for a melanoma varies with the type of lesion. The *superficial spreading melanoma* is seen most commonly on the backs of males and the legs of women. The *nodular melanoma* is seen in any location, more frequently in males. The *acral* type is seen, as indicated, on the palms and soles, and the *lentigo maligna melanoma* occurs mainly on face and arms.

COURSE. The greater the depth of involvement of the growth, the worse the prognosis. Clark has defined five levels of invasion, while Breslow measured the tumor thickness with a micrometer placed in the eye piece of the microscope. Risk groups have been defined using a combination of these measurements. For instance, a melanoma less than 0.76 mm thick and not invading the reticular dermis is in a low-risk group. Regional lymph node involvement or distant metastases gravely affect the prognosis.

HISTOPATHOLOGY. The histopathologic diagnosis of melanoma can be very difficult at times. An adequate biopsy, or better yet, an initial complete excisional biopsy provides the most information.

Differential Diagnosis

Benign nevus: no recent change in lesion, not black, no bleeding; hairy nevi are most frequently benign, but if there is any question as to the diagnosis, a biopsy, preferably by complete excision, is indicated.

The other lesions to be thought of in the differential diagnosis are the same as under nevi (see earlier section), with the addition of a *pigmented basal cell epithelioma* (biopsy indicated for diagnosis), and a *subungual hematoma* (history of recent injury; if in doubt, perform a biopsy).

Treatment

Rapid and adequate therapy is indicated after the diagnosis and staging are completed. The procedures include wide surgical excision, lymph node dissection, chemotherapy, and immunotherapy.

LYMPHOMAS

Mycosis Fungoides
(Plate 74)

This polymorphous lymphoma involves the skin only, except in some rare cases that terminally invade the lymph nodes and the visceral organs. As is true with most lymphomas, the histology may change gradually to another form of lymphoma, with progression of the disease. However, most cases of mycosis fungoides begin as such and terminate unchanged.

Mycosis fungoides is a T- (thymic-derived) lymphocyte dysplasia. The name *cutaneous T cell lymphoma* (CTCL) is an inclusive term grouping mycosis fungoides, Sézary syndrome, leukemia cutis, and reticulum cell sarcoma of the skin.

DESCRIPTION. The clinical picture of this disease is quite classic and is divided into three stages: the erythematous stage, the plaque stage, and the tumor stage. The course usually proceeds in order, but all stages may be evident at the same time, or the first two stages may be bypassed.

Erythematous stage: Commonly seen are scaly, red, rather sharply defined patches that resemble atopic eczema, psoriasis, or parapsoriasis. The eruption may become diffuse as an *exfoliative dermatitis.* Itching is usually quite severe.

Plaque stage: The red scaly patches develop induration and some elevation, with central healing that results in ring-shaped lesions. This stage is to be differentiated from tertiary syphilis, psoriasis, erythema multiforme perstans, mycotic infections, and other lymphomas.

Tumor stage: This terminal stage is characterized by nodular and tumor growths of the plaques, often with ulceration and secondary bacterial infection. These tumors are to be differentiated from any of the granulomas (see Chap. 20).

COURSE. The early stages may progress slowly, with exacerbations and remissions over many years, or the disease may be rapidly fulminating. Once the tumor stage is reached, the eventual fatal outcome is more imminent.

Treatment

The combined services of a dermatologist, an oncologist, a radiologist, and an internist or a hematologist are required for the management of this usually fatal disease.

Locally, for early cases, a tar cream (L.C.D. 5% in a water-washable base or in a corticosteroid cream) plus ultraviolet B therapy is quite beneficial. PUVA therapy (see Chap. 6) is also temporarily effective in resolving lesions. Local nitrogen mustard solution to the erythematous and plaque stage lesions has proved to be very effective for some cases.

Use of systemic therapy depends on the stage and extent of the disease. Most therapists believe that one should treat the symptoms and signs only as they appear. Corticosteroids are quite helpful, especially for the first two stages. Radiation therapy for the superficial type is very effective for plaque and small tumor lesions; electron beam radiation therapy can be administered to the total body, either early or late in the disease.

Systemic chemotherapeutic agents enter into the therapy routine in the plaque and tumor stages of mycosis fungoides. These include the alkylating agents cyclophosphamide (Cytoxan), chlorambucil (Leukeran), and nitrogen mustard; the plant alkaloid vincristine (Oncovin); the antimetabolite methotrexate; the antibiotic doxorubicin (Adriamycin); and the antibiotic derivative bleomycin (Blenoxane). Monoclonal antibodies are also being used for therapy, as is interferon alfa-2a. Photopheresis therapy is another recent therapeutic modality.

COMPLETE HISTOLOGIC CLASSIFICATION

A complete histologic classification of tumors of the skin is listed here. Those tumors discussed in the first part of this chapter are marked with an asterisk. The rarer tumors listed will be defined.

> ### SAUER NOTE:
>
> A histologic examination of tissue is indicated for a definite diagnosis of most growths of the skin.

I. **Epidermal Tumors**
   A. Tumors of the surface epidermis
      1. Benign tumors
         a. Linear epidermal nevus (Fig. 33–3). A rather common tumor usually present at birth, consisting of single or multiple lesions in various forms that give rise to several clinical designations, such as hard nevus, nevus verrucosus, nevus unius lateris, papilloma, and when systematized, ichthyosis hystrix. No nevus cells are present.
        *b. Seborrheic keratosis and dermatosis papulosa nigra
        *c. Pedunculated fibromas
         d. Cysts
           *1) Epidermal cyst
           *2) Trichilemmal, pilar, or sebaceous cyst
           *3) Steatocystoma multiplex. A dominantly inherited condition with small, moderately firm, cystic nodules adherent to the overlying skin, which on incision yield an oily fluid.

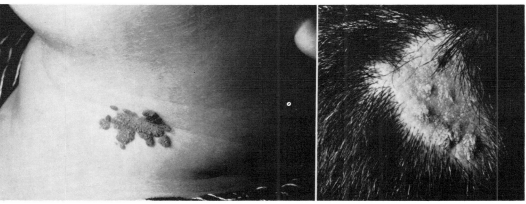

Figure 33–3. **Linear epidermal nevus** on the neck (*left*) and on the scalp (*right*).

*4) Milium
*5) Dermoid cyst
*6) Mucous retention cyst
  e. Clear cell acanthoma. A rare, usually single, slightly elevated, flat, pale red, scaling nodule less than 2 cm in diameter, nearly always located on the lower extremities.
  f. Warty dyskeratoma. A solitary warty lesion with a central keratotic plug, most commonly seen on the scalp, face, and neck.
  g. Keratoacanthoma
2. Precancerous tumors
  *a. Senile or actinic keratosis and cutaneous horn
  *b. Arsenical keratosis
  *c. Leukoplakia
3. Epitheliomas and carcinomas
  *a. Basal cell carcinoma
  *b. Squamous cell carcinoma
  c. Bowen's disease and erythroplasia of Queyrat. Bowen's disease is a single red scaly lesion with a sharp but irregular border that grows slowly by peripheral extension. Histologically, it is an intraepidermal squamous cell carcinoma (see Plate 86). Erythroplasia of Queyrat (see Plate 99) represents Bowen's disease of the mucous membranes and oc-

curs on the glans penis, and rarely on the vulva. The lesion has a bright red, velvety surface.
  d. Paget's disease (see Plate 99). A unilateral scaly red lesion resembling a dermatitis, usually present on the female nipple. The early lesion is an intraepidermal squamous cell carcinoma that also involves the mammary ducts and deeper connective tissue.
B. Tumors of the epidermal appendages
  1. Nevoid tumors
    a. Organic nevi or hamartomas
      1) Sebaceous nevi
        a) Nevus sebaceus (Jadassohn) (Fig. 33–4). Seen on the scalp or face as a single lesion present from birth, slightly raised, firm, yellowish, with furrowed surface. Large examples are associated with a "neurocutaneous syndrome" of epilepsy and mental retardation. Basal cell and squamous cell carcinomas can develop within these growths.
        b) Adenoma sebaceum (Pringle). Part of a triad

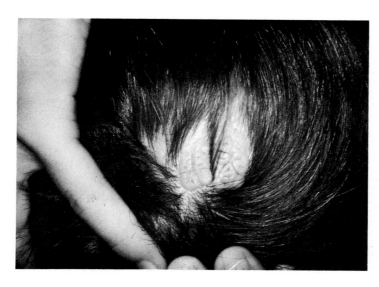

Figure 33–4. **Nevus sebaceus (Jadassohn) on the scalp.**

of epilepsy, mental deficiency, and the skin lesions of adenoma sebaceum. The skin lesions occur on the face and consist of yellowish brown, papular, nodular lesions with telangiectases.

c) Sebaceous hyperplasia. *Very common* on the face in older persons and consists of one or several small, yellowish, translucent, slightly umbilicated nodules.

d) Fordyce's disease (see Chap. 29). A rather common condition of pinpoint-sized yellowish lesions of the vermilion border of the lips or the oral mucosa.

b. Adenomas or organoid hamartomas

1) Sebaceous adenoma. A very rare solitary tumor of the face or the scalp, smooth, firm, elevated, often slightly pedunculated, and measuring less than 1 cm in diameter.

2) Apocrine adenomas

a) Syringocystadenoma papilliferum. This adenoma of the apocrine ducts appears as a single verrucous plaque, usually seen on the scalp. Basal cell epitheliomatous change does occur.

b) Hidradenoma papilliferum. This adenoma of the apocrine glands occurs almost exclusively on the labia majora and the perineum of women, as a single intracutaneous tumor covered by normal epidermis.

c. Benign epitheliomas or suborganoid hamartomas

1) Sebaceous epithelioma. A rare, solitary small nodule or plaque that has no characteristic clinical appearance.

2) Apocrine epithelioma

a) Syringoma. This is characterized by the appearance of pinhead-sized soft, yellowish nodules at the age of puberty in women, developing around the eyelids, the chest, the abdomen, and the anterior aspects of the thighs.

b) Cylindroma. These appear as numerous smooth, rounded tumors of various size on the scalp in adults, and resemble bunches of grapes or tomatoes. These tumors may cover the entire scalp like a turban and are then referred to as turban tumors.

3) Hair epitheliomas

a) Trichoepithelioma. Also known as epithelioma adenoides cysticum and multiple benign cystic epithelioma. This begins at the age of puberty, frequently on a hereditary basis, and is characterized by the presence of numerous pinhead- to pea-sized, rounded, yellowish or pink nodules on the face and occasionally on the upper trunk. Ulceration occurs when these lesions change into a basal cell epithelioma.

b) Calcifying epithelioma (Malherbe) or pilomatrixoma. A rather rare, solitary, hard, deep-seated nodule of the face or the upper extremities. Malignant degeneration does not occur.

4) Eccrine epitheliomas
  a) Eccrine spiradenoma. A rare, usually solitary, intradermal, firm, tender nodule.
  b) Clear cell hidradenoma. A rare, well-circumscribed, often encapsulated tumor of dermis and subcutaneous tissue.
  c) Eccrine poroma. This occurs as an asymptomatic solitary tumor on the soles and the palms.

2. Carcinomas of sebaceous glands and eccrine and apocrine sweat glands (rare)

C. Metastatic carcinoma of the skin. Occurs frequently from carcinoma of the breast but rarely from other internal carcinomas.

Metastatic carcinoid nodules may appear in the skin, as well as in lymph nodes and the liver. The primary tumor and the metastases produce excess 5-hydroxytryptamine (serotonin), which in turn produces attacks of flushing of the skin.

II. Mesodermal Tumors
A. Tumors of fibrous tissue
  *1. Histiocytoma and dermatofibroma
  *2. Keloid
  3. Fibrosarcoma
    a. True fibrosarcoma. A rare tumor that starts most commonly in the subcutaneous fat, grows rapidly, causes the overlying skin to appear purplish, and finally ulcerates.
    b. Dermatofibrosarcoma protuberans. A small tumor that grows slowly in the corium and spreads by the development of adjoining reddish or bluish nodules that may coalesce to form a plaque that can eventually ulcerate.
B. Tumors of mucoid tissue

1. Myxoma. Clinically seen as fairly well circumscribed, rather soft intracutaneous tumors with normal overlying epidermis.
2. Myxosarcoma. Subcutaneous tumors that eventually ulcerate the skin.
*3. Synovial cyst of the skin

C. Tumors of fatty tissue
  1. Nevus lipomatosus superficialis. A rare, circumscribed nodular lesion, usually in the gluteal area.
  2. Lipoma. A rather common tumor which may be multiple or single, lobulated, of varying size, and in the subcutaneous tissue.
  3. Hibernoma. A form of lipoma composed of embryonic type of fat cells.
  4. Liposarcoma
  5. Malignant hibernoma

D. Tumors of nerve tissue and mesodermal-nerve sheath cells
  1. Neuroma. Rare. Single or multiple small reddish or brown nodules that are usually tender as well as painful.
  2. Neurofibromatosis (see Plates 72E and F and 92F). Also known as von Recklinghausen's disease, this hereditary disease classically consists of pigmented patches, pedunculated skin tumors, and nerve tumors. All of these lesions may not be present in a particular case.
  3. Neurolemmoma
  4. Granular cell schwannoma or myoblastoma. From neural sheath cells, this appears usually as a solitary tumor of the tongue, the skin, or the subcutaneous tissue.
  5. Malignant granular cell schwannoma or myoblastoma

E. Tumors of vascular tissue
  *1. Hemangiomas
  2. Granuloma pyogenicum (see Plate 86). Also known as "proud flesh," this is a rather common end result of an injury to the skin that may or may not have been apparent. Vascular proliferation, with or without infection, produces a small red tumor that

bleeds easily. It is to be differentiated from a malignant melanoma. Mild electrocoagulation is curative if the known cause is removed.

3. Osler's disease. See Rendu-Osler-Weber disease in Dictionary-Index.

4. Lymphangioma. A superficial form, lymphangioma circumscriptum, appears as a group of thin-walled vesicles on the skin surface, whereas the deeper variety, lymphangioma cavernosum, causes a poorly defined enlargement of the affected area, such as the lip or the tongue.

5. Glomus tumor. A rather unusual small, deep-seated, red or purplish nodule that is tender and may produce severe paroxysmal pains. The solitary lesion is usually seen under a nail plate, on the finger tips, or elsewhere on the body.

6. Hemangiopericytoma

7. Kaposi's sarcoma (multiple idiopathic hemorrhagic sarcoma) (Fig. 33–5). Most commonly seen on the feet and the ankles as multiple bluish red or dark brown nodules and plaques associated with visceral lesions. Sarcomatous malignant degeneration can occur.

Kaposi's sarcoma is also seen as part of the *acquired immunodeficiency syndrome* (AIDS) (see Chap. 18). In this complex, the sarcoma lesions are small, oval, red or pink papules that occur on any area of the body.

8. Hemangioendothelioma

9. Postmastectomy lymphangiosarcoma

F. Tumors of muscular tissue
   1. Leiomyoma. Solitary leiomyomas may be found on the extremities and on the scrotum, whereas multiple leiomyomas occur on the back and elsewhere as pinhead-to pea-sized, brown or bluish, firm, elevated nodules. Both forms are painful and sensitive to pressure, particularly as they enlarge.
   2. Leiomyosarcoma. Very rare.

G. Tumors of osseous tissue
   1. Osteoma cutis
      a. Primary. The primary form of osteoma cutis develops from embryonal cell rests. These may be single or multiple.
      b. Secondary. Secondary bone formation may occur as a form of tissue degeneration in tumors, in scar tissue, in scleroderma lesions, and in various granulomas.

H. Tumors of cartilaginous tissue
   1. Nodular chondrodermatitis of the ear. A painful, hyperkeratotic nodule, usually on the helix of the ear of elderly males.

III. **Nevus Cell Tumors**
   A. Melanocytic nevi
      *1. Junctional (active) nevus
      *2. Intradermal (resting) nevus

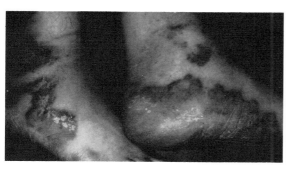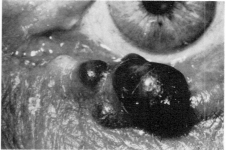

Figure 33–5. **Kaposi's sarcoma.** (*Left*) Of feet (*Dr. David Morgan*). (*Right*) Of lower eyelid (*Drs. A. Lemoine and L. Calkins*).

*3. Dysplastic nevus syndrome

4. Lentigines. These represent early junctional nevi, which are to be differentiated from freckles (ephelides). A *freckle* histologically shows hyperpigmentation of the basal layer but no elongation of the rete pegs and no increase in the number of clear cells and dendritic cells. *Juvenile lentigines* begin to appear in childhood and occur on all parts of the body. *Senile lentigines* (see Plate 95), also known as "liver spots," occur in elderly persons on the dorsa of the hands, the forearms, and the face. *Lentigo maligna melanoma* (see Plate 95) is a dark brown or black macular, malignant lesion, usually on the face or arms of elderly persons, that has a slow peripheral growth (see under Malignant Melanoma earlier).

5. Mongolian spots (see Plate 89). These are seen chiefly in Asian or black infants, usually around the buttocks. They disappear spontaneously during childhood.

Related bluish patchy lesions are the *nevus of Ota*, seen on the side of the face, and the *nevus of Ito*, located in the supraclavicular, scapular, and deltoid regions.

6. Blue nevus. Clinically, the blue nevus appears as a slate blue or bluish black, sharply circumscribed, flat or slightly elevated nodule, occurring on any area of the body. It originates from mesodermal cells.

*B. Malignant melanoma

IV. **Lymphomas** (see Plate 74)

A. Monomorphous group. The non-Hodgkin's lymphomas are referred to as monomorphous lymphomas because, in contrast to Hodgkin's disease, they lack a significant admixture of inflammatory cells and are composed almost entirely of lymphoma cells largely derived from B lymphocytes. A classification follows:

1. Lymphocytic type, well differentiated
2. Lymphocytic type, poorly differentiated ("lymphosarcoma")
3. Histiocytic type ("reticulum cell sarcoma")
4. Mixed lymphocytic-histocytic type
5. Undifferentiated, pleomorphic stem cell type
6. Undifferentiated Burkitt type

Lymphomas may have specific skin lesions containing the lymphomatous infiltrate, or nonspecific lesions may be seen. These latter consist of macules, papules, purpuric lesions, blisters, eczematous lesions, exfoliative dermatitis, and secondarily infected excoriations.

B. Polymorphous group
1. Hodgkin's disease. Specific lesions are very rare, but nonspecific dermatoses are rather commonly seen.
*2. Mycosis fungoides

Sézary syndrome. This is a very rare form of exfoliative dermatitis (see Chap. 23) that occurs at an early stage of a lymphoma. It is diagnosed by finding unusually large monocytoid cells (so-called Sézary cells) in the blood and in the skin. This cell is indistinguishable from the mycosis cell, both of which are derived from the T cell.

V. **Myelosis**

A. Leukemia. Refers to circulating abnormal blood cells. May be seen along with lymphomas, but it is almost always associated with myelosis, such as myeloid leukemia. Cutaneous lesions are quite uncommon but may be specific or nonspecific.

VI. **Pseudolymphoma of Spiegler-Fendt**

A benign, localized erythematous, nodular dermatosis, usually on the face, with histologic features that make a distinction from lymphoma very difficult.

BIBLIOGRAPHY

Abel EA, Sendagorta E, Hoppe RT et al: PUVA treatment of erythrodermic and plaque-type mycosis fungoides. Arch Dermatol 123:897, 1987

Barnes LM, Nordlun JJ: The natural history of dysplastic nevi. Arch Dermatol 123:1059, 1987

Bowers RE, Graham EA, Tomlinson KM: The natural history of the strawberry nevus. Arch Dermatol 82:667, 1960

Cassileth BR, Temoshok L, Frederick BE et al: Patient and physician delay in melanoma diagnosis. J Am Acad Dermatol 18:591, 1988

Goette DK: 5-Fluorouracil. J Assoc Milit Dermatol 15(No. 1):22, 1989

Hail WN, Farber L, Cadman E: Non-Hodgkins lymphoma for the nononcologist. JAMA 253:1431, 1985

Jansen GT: Commentary: Use of topical fluorouracil. Arch Dermatol 119:784, 1983

Kopf AW, Welkovich B, Frankel RE et al: Thickness of malignant melanoma: Global analysis of related factors. J Dermatol Surg Oncol 13:345, 1987

Lee CP: Keloids: Their epidemiology and treatment. Int J Dermatol 21:504, 1982

Lever WF, Schaumburg-Lever G: Histopathology of the Skin, 7th ed. Philadelphia, JB Lippincott, 1989

Olsen EA, Rosen ST, Vollmer RT et al: Interferon alfa-2a in the treatment of cutaneous T-cell lymphoma. J Am Acad Dermatol 20:395, 1989

Reymann F, Ravnborg L, Schou G et al: Bowen's disease and internal malignant diseases. Arch Dermatol 124:677, 1988

Rowe DE, Carroll RJ, Day CL: Long-term recurrence rates in previously untreated (primary) basal cell carcinoma: Implications for follow-up. J Dermatol Surg Oncol 15:315, 1989

Scheibner A, Wheeland RG: Argon-pumped tunable dye laser therapy for facial port-wine stain hemangiomas in adults. J Dermatol Surg Oncol 15:277, 1989

Simpson JR: Natural history of cavernous hemangiomata. Lancet 2:1057, 1959

Sina B: The spectrum of cutaneous pseudomalignancy. Cutis 34:381, 1984

Swanson NA: Mohs surgery. Arch Dermatol 119:761, 1983

Tuyp E, Burgoyne A, Aitchison T et al: A case-control study of possible causative factors in mycosis fungoides. Arch Dermatol 123:196, 1987

Vonderheid EC, Tan ET, Kantor AF et al: Long-term efficacy, curative potential, and carcinogenicity of topical mechlorethamine chemotherapy in cutaneous T-cell lymphoma. J Am Acad Dermatol 20:416, 1989

Yamada M, Takigawa M, Iwatsuki K et al: Adult T-cell leukemia/lymphoma and cutaneous T-cell lymphoma: Are they related? Int J Dermatol 28:107, 1989

34

Pediatric Dermatology

The skin and the skin problems of infants and children are different enough from adult skin and skin problems to warrant special consideration of the subject of pediatric dermatology (Figs. 34–1 and 34–2).

Certain skin problems are seen *only* in infants and children (*e.g.*, cradle cap and diaper dermatitis). Other dermatoses are seen in both children and in adults, but in children these dermatoses clinically appear different from the adult counterpart (*e.g.*, the infantile form of atopic eczema).

Pediatric dermatology can be divided into the dermatoses at birth, dermatoses of infancy, and dermatoses of childhood.

DERMATOSES AT BIRTH
(Plate 89)

There are really very few problems found on the skin at birth. The phrase "babies' skin" conveys an image and sensation of smooth, soft skin.

AMNIOCENTESIS MARKS. The transabdominal insertion of a needle into the amniotic sac can occasionally scar the skin or produce dimple-like lesions.

BIRTHMARKS. Of the many so-called birthmarks, only the superficial erythematous *hemangiomas* at the nape of the neck (*nuchal*) and center of the brow (*glabellar*) are commonly seen at birth. Most of the glabellar hemangiomas disappear in later childhood, while the nuchal ones can persist. The disfiguring *port-wine type of hemangioma* may also

be present at birth, but it is a rare defect. The well-known *strawberry* and *cavernous hemangiomas* usually are noticed at birth as only a small red spot on the skin surface and do not appear as obvious skin defects until the age of 3 or 4 weeks.

Neonatal erythema is quite common but rather unimportant. At birth, but more frequently a few days after birth, a blotchy, macular erythema with minute pustules can arise most profusely on the trunk. Rarely, papules or hives are seen. These lesions fade without treatment in 2 to 3 days. The cause is unknown.

Mongolian spots on the buttocks and sacral area are also commonly seen in yellow and black races.

Neonatal jaundice, from several causes, is very commonly seen and can prove to be a diagnostic problem.

GROWTHS. A few growths, such as *linear epidermal hamartomas*, are present on the skin at birth, but the more common true *melanocytic nevi* or "moles" found on the skin of almost every adult are rarely seen at birth. An exception is the *congenital giant pigmented nevus*, which fortunately is extremely rare. If extensive it can have a "bathing trunk" distribution.

DERMATITIS. A true dermatitis is rarely seen at birth; even *cradle cap* takes a few days after birth to develop.

INFECTIONS. Of the infections, candidiasis, syphilis, and viral herpetic lesions are rarely seen at birth. Pyodermas usually are not

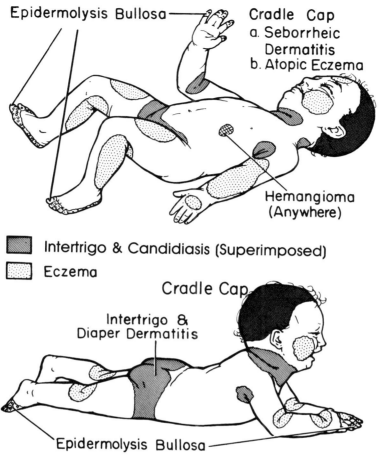

Figure 34–1. **Pediatric dermograms (infancy).**

present at birth but can begin in the nursery. Scalp abscesses can occur from fetal electrodes implanted transvaginally on the presenting scalp. The electrodes are used to monitor the fetal heart rate during labor.

ACNE AND MILIA. Both of these conditions can be present at birth. The acne, as small comedones or pustules, may be related to the administration of progesterone to the pregnant mother.

The remaining list of the dermatoses present at birth consists of a very rare group of congenital and/or hereditary defects of the skin, such as *ichthyosis* in several forms, *congenital aplasias* (absence of nails, hair, glands, or areas of skin), *congenital ectodermal dysplasias, incontinentia pigmenti* in the blister stage, and *epidermolysis bullosa.*

Thus, while the only *common* defects of the skin at birth are the flat, superficial nuchal and glabellar hemangiomas, neonatal jaundice, neonatal erythema, and Mongolian spots, there are quite a number of *rarer* abnormalities that can be present on the skin at birth.

For the sake of completeness, the following dermatoses are listed as being present at birth (consult the Dictionary-Index for additional page references for these conditions).

1. Neonatal erythema is common. (See previous discussion.)
2. Infectious dermatoses:
   a. Candidiasis (see Chap. 19 and Plate 89*E* and *F*), clinically, is an intertriginous eruption with small, red, pustule-like lesions.
   b. Syphilis (see Chap. 16 and Plate 89*D*)

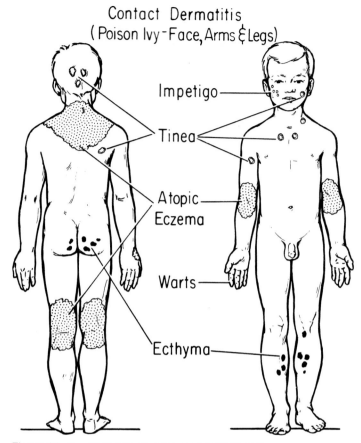

Figure 34–2. **Pediatric dermograms (childhood).**

can mimic almost any dermatosis with macules, papules, or bullae. It is rare in infants.

c. Herpes simplex (see Chap. 17), seen usually as vesicles, in clusters. It is rare in infants.

d. Acquired immunodeficiency syndrome (AIDS) in newborns. AIDS fetopathy is a unique dysmorphic syndrome with growth retardation and many other defects (see Chap. 18).

e. Rubella syndrome. This syndrome is very rare in newborns. There can be purpuric and eczematous lesions of the skin, along with other defects. Purpura can also be due to several other causes.

f. Cytomegalic inclusion disease syndrome. Skin changes include jaundice, petechiae, purpura, "blueberry muffin" lesions, and generalized maculopapular eruptions.

g. Cat-scratch disease. An uncommon disease, it is caused by a pleomorphic gram-negative bacillus. The scratch site in 1 to 2 weeks can develop an erythematous papule, vesicle, or pustule. A morbilliform rash of short duration can occur. Lymphadenopathy, in local or generalized sites, is present.

3. Neonatal acne and milia are rather commonly seen.

4. Psoriasis and discoid lupus erythematosus have been reported only rarely at birth.

5. Bullous dermatoses:

a. Epidermolysis bullosa (see Plate 80) is seen mainly as denuded bullae on toes, fingers, elbows, or entire body in the severe forms (dystrophic and letalis). All forms are rare.

b. Incontinentia pigmenti (Plates 90 and 91) is seen in the first stage with red-based vesicles or bullae, most com-

(*text continues on page 346*)

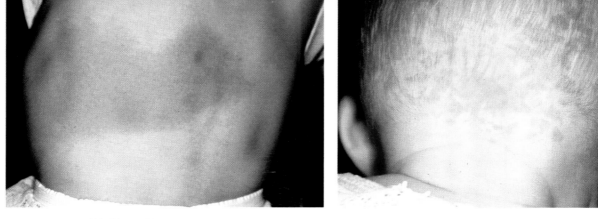

(A) Mongolian spot on back

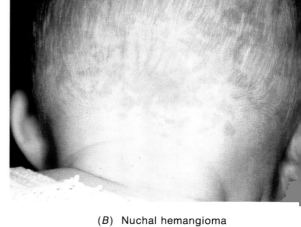

(B) Nuchal hemangioma

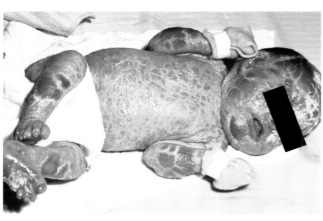

(C) Ichthyosiform erythroderma or Harlequin fetus, fatal

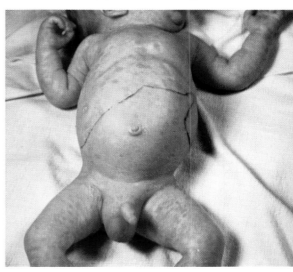

(D) Congenital syphilis with hepatomegaly and splenomegaly

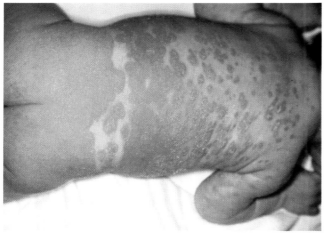

(E and F) Generalized candidiasis in 5-week-old child from diabetic family

Plate 89. **Dermatoses of newborns and infants.**

343

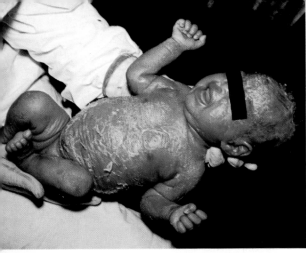

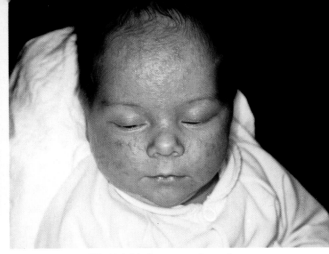

(A) Bullous impetigo or Ritter's disease; no thymus on autopsy

(B) Prickly heat, age 3 weeks

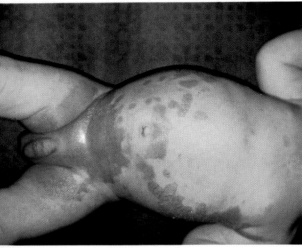

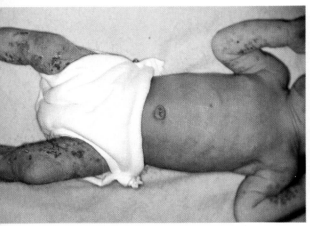

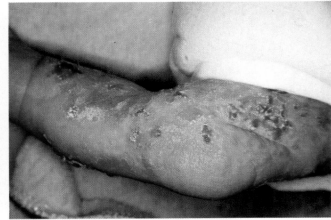

(C and D) Psoriasis of 2½-month-old child of body and scalp that began in diaper area

(E and F) Incontinentia pigmenti of 1-month-old girl in vesicular and warty stage, with (F) close-up

Plate 90.   **Dermatoses of newborns and infants** (Continued).

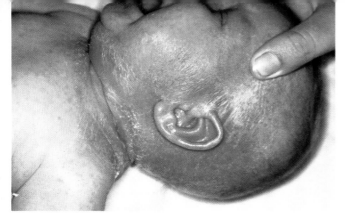

(*A*) Bacterial intertrigo and seborrheic dermatitis

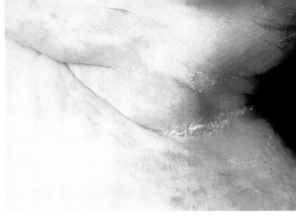

(*B*) Candidal intertrigo of neck

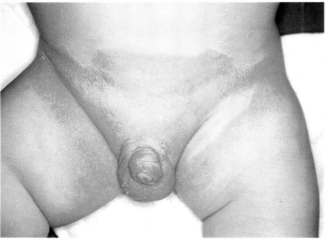

(*C*) Diaper dermatitis due to seborrhea

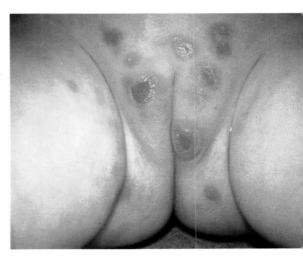

(*D*) Diaper erythema of Jacquet

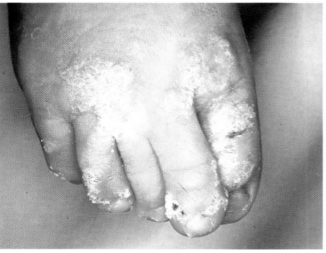

(*E*) Incontinentia pigmenti of foot in warty stage at age 2 months; (*F*) of back, in pigmented stage, at age 14 months in same girl

Plate 91. **Dermatoses of newborns and infants** (Continued).

monly on the dorsum of the hands and feet. It is rare in infants.

6. Pigmentary changes:
   a. Albinism, very rare, with entire loss of pigment.
   b. Piebaldism, very rare, with patchy loss of pigment.
   c. Neurofibromatosis (von Recklinghausen's syndrome) (Plate 92F) can be anticipated if macular café-au-lait spots are found.
   d. Adenoma sebaceum (see Plate 80D) can also be diagnosed at birth if there is depigmentation in an ash-leaf configuration.
   e. Mongolian spots (see Plate 89A) are more common in the yellow and black races.
   f. Jaundice is commonly seen at birth and can be due to several causes.
7. Congenital ectodermal dysplasias or defects (Plate 93D). The extent and involvement of the defects of the skin and/or glands, and/or nails, and/or hair accounts for the existence of a multiplicity of complicated syndromes. These are rare.
8. Ichthyosis, (see Chap. 32). The two vulgaris types (see Plate 80 and Fig. 32–1) are not present at birth, but the rarer lamellar form and the erythroderma forms are present at birth. The harlequin fetus (see Plate 89C) is a severe, lethal type of the erythroderma form. Rarely, palmar and plantar keratodermas occur.
9. New growths:
   a. Hemangiomas (see previous discussion).
      1) Superficial flat type of neck (nuchal) (see Plate 89B) or brow (glabella) are common.
      2) Port-wine type.
      3) Superficial strawberry or cavernous types (see Fig. 33–2 and Plate 92B).
   b. Epidermal tumors. Linear warty growths (hamartomas) or pigmented, noncellular nevi are rarely seen. Bathing trunk nevi can cover large areas.

DERMATOSES OF INFANCY (BIRTH TO 2 YEARS)

From the protected, quite sterile, temperature- and humidity-controlled environment of the uterus, the newborn is launched into a less protected, contaminated, 30° to 40° cooler, and much drier environment. That the body, and the skin in particular, can adjust so rapidly and without apparent abnormal reaction is a miracle. There is some toll, however.

The newborn is usually washed gently with a mild soap and then oiled daily. A skin problem can develop if the mother is too fastidious and bathes the skin *excessively*. This can cause *dry skin (xerosis)* or even a *contact dermatitis*. If there is a familial tendency toward *atopic eczema* (see Plates 9 and 10), then excess and too frequent bathing, especially in the winter, is definitely very harmful. For the atopic child, the lanolin in baby oils can also be irritating, and a switch should be made to nonlanolin oils such as Allercreme Special Formula Dry Skin Lotion, Curel Lotion, Moisturel Lotion, or Nutraderm Lotion. Other management techniques for atopic eczema are listed in Chapter 9.

A problem from *lack* of daily bathing and adequate drying of the skin is that debris can accumulate in the intertriginous areas of the neck, axilla, and groin. This can lead to a *bacterial or candidal intertrigo* (see Plate 92A). The fatter the child, the greater this problem. (See Chaps. 15 and 19.)

Cradle cap (see Plate 20) is a yellowish, greasy, and crusted collection of vernix caseosa and shedding skin, caught around the hairs of the scalp. If the inherited tendency for the child is to have a seborrheic or atopic diathesis, this also contributes to the mess. But another, more common contributing factor is the tendency on the part of the mother to want to avoid damage to the "soft spot" on the scalp, so that she avoids adequate cleansing of it. When the child's body skin is oiled, the scalp is oiled also, and this adds to the accumulation of the debris. Thus, many factors lead to the development of cradle cap.

Treatment consists of explaining to the mother the causative factors, prescribing a 1% hydrocortisone cream twice a day to cut down on inflammation and epidermal shedding, and the use of a mild shampoo two to three times a week, followed by gentle physical removal of the scaling with a comb.

Neonatal erythema, seen at birth, is more commonly seen 2 to 3 days later (see at beginning of chapter).

Diaper area dermatitis (see Plates 89 through 91) can be caused by many factors also. It can be a manifestation of a *contact*

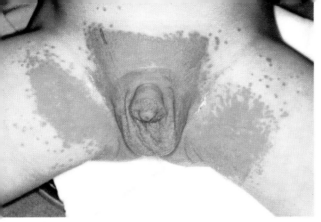

(A) Candidal intertrigo following oral antibiotics, age 1 year

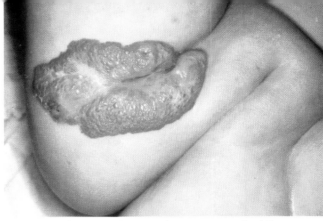

(B) Compound hemangioma, untreated, of the crural area, age 4 months

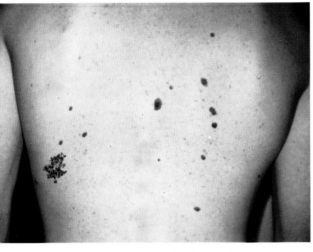

(C) Junction nevi of the back, age 16 years

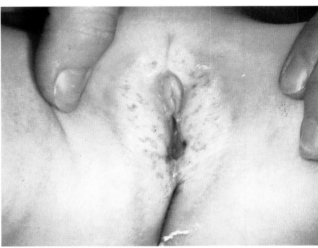

(D) Lichen sclerosus et atrophicus of labia, age 3 years

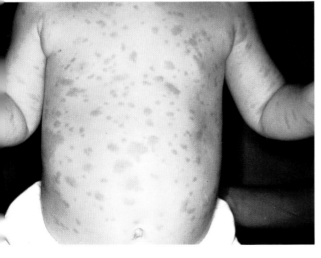

(E) Urticaria pigmentosa of chest, age 2 years (note the red, urticating lesion below left nipple)

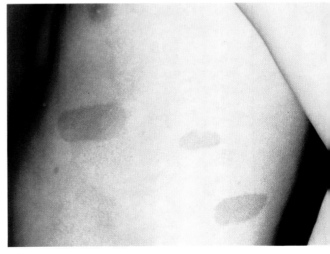

(F) Neurofibromatosis with early oval café-au-lait lesions, age 5 years

Plate 92.   **Dermatoses of children.** (*Owen Laboratories, Inc.* [in part])

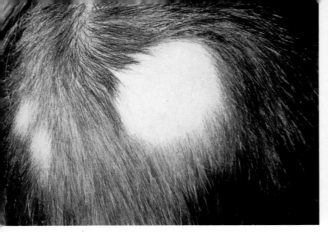

(A) Tinea of scalp due to *M. audouini*

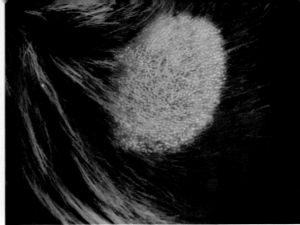

(B) Tinea hairs fluorescing under Wood's light

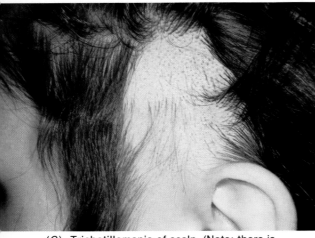

(C) Trichotillomania of scalp. (Note: there is no complete baldness in area, as in alopecia areata.)

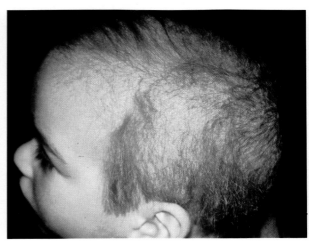

(D) Diffuse alopecia with general ectodermal defect in 3-year-old child

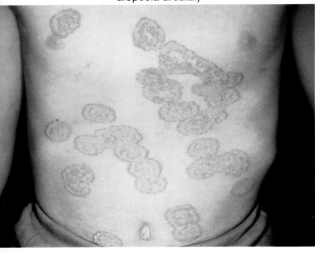

(E) Tinea of body due to *M. Canis*

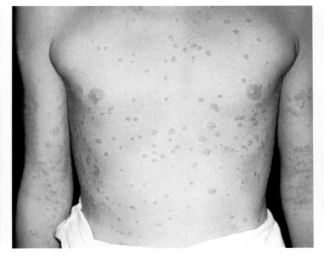

(F) Guttate psoriasis following streptococcal throat infection

Plate 93. **Dermatoses of children** (Continued).

dermatitis from too enthusiastic bathing of the diaper area, with inadequate rinsing of the soap, or, conversely, it can be an *intertrigo* caused by accumulation of debris because of too little bathing, inadequate cleansing of the skin folds, and infrequent changing of soiled diapers. By proper questioning, a physician can determine which of these divergent factors apply to a given case of diaper area irritation.

Seborrheic dermatitis (see Plates 20 and 91*C*), and, rarely, *psoriasis* (see Plate 90*C* and *D*), can be found in infants, usually as an intertriginous type of dermatitis.

Prickly heat (see Plate 90*B*) is another one of the problems caused by the wrong environment—in this case, too many clothes and/or too warm a room. One sees small, pinpoint-sized vesicles or pustules localized in the intertriginous areas or even quite generalized. Treatment consists of removing the cause (fewer clothes or lower room temperature) and application of a calamine-type lotion three or four times a day.

A list of the common, less common, and rare dermatoses and skin problems of infants follows. (Consult the Dictionary-Index for additional page references on these conditions.)

Common Dermatoses of Infants

Neonatal erythema
Cradle cap dermatitis
    Greasy and scaly debris
    Seborrheic dermatitis
    Atopic eczema
Dry skin (xerosis)
Contact dermatitis
Atopic eczema
Intertrigo
    Bacterial
    Candidal
Diaper area dermatitis
    Contact dermatitis
    Intertrigo
    Erythema of Jacquet is an uncommon form of diaper dermatitis characterized by discrete papuloerosive lesions (see Plate 91*D*).
Seborrheic dermatitis
Prickly heat
New growths
    Hemangiomas, strawberry and cavernous types

Exanthems
    Roseola
    Chickenpox

Less Common Skin Problems of Infants

Burns
Pyodermas
    Omphalitis. Infection of the umbilical cord site is common, but usually self-limiting.
    Furuncles (boils) (see Plate 36). These infections can develop as a nursery epidemic.
    Impetigo. A more severe form, with large bullae quite extensive on the body, is called *bullous impetigo, Ritter's disease,* or *staphylococcal scalded skin syndrome* (see Plates 90 and 35*A*).
Fungal infections
Insect bites and stings. The term *papular urticaria,* which is nosologically incorrect, is used to describe the chronic excoriation of old bites. This is most often seen in hereditary families of "pickers."
Pediculosis
Scabies
Icthyosis, and congenital and hereditary defects (see Plate 80).
Other exanthems

Rare Skin Diseases of Infants

GENERALIZED ERYTHRODERMAS. The following conditions can be difficult to differentiate, and prolonged observation is helpful in ascertaining the final diagnosis. Most of these conditions are rare.

Atopic eczema, as an erythroderma, is rare but can occur in the first few weeks of life. With the passage of time, it assumes the more typical pattern of eczema (see Chap. 9).

Candidal erythroderma is rare but can spread out from the intertriginous areas (see Plates 89*E* and *F*).

Leiner's disease is a severe form of generalized exfoliative dermatitis of infants that presents in different cases varying degrees of atopy, seborrhea, and perhaps infectious eczematization. It is accompanied by a peculiar systemic reaction that is most evident in its gastrointestinal manifestations. Secondary infection results in mortality in over 10% of cases.

Staphylococcal scalded skin syndrome is a rare, severe problem where large bullae form, and the skin peels off in sheets. Another name for this condition is *Ritter's disease* or *bullous impetigo* (see Plate 90A). It occurs predominantly in infants and children. The cause is usually from infection with *Staphylococcus*. Treatment is supportive, with antibiotics and corticosteroids, as the severity warrants.

Lamellar desquamation or *collodion baby* is a syndrome of generalized erythema, scaling, peeling, and cracking of the skin. Mild physiologic cases are transitory. Severe forms are seen as the early stage of *lamellar ichthyosis*, *bullous* and *nonbullous ichthyosiform erythroderma*, and *sex-linked ichthyosis*. These conditions are discussed in Chapter 32.

DISORDERS OF THE SUBCUTANEOUS FAT. *Neonatal cold injury* is relatively frequently seen in infants born at home and exposed to cold temperature. The skin is pallid, cool to touch, edematous, and immobile. The hands, feet, and cheeks are red. Sclerema or hardening may occur on the limbs and cheeks. Most patients recover with careful rewarming.

Sclerema is an extremely rare condition of premature or debilitated infants affected by a preexisting respiratory or gastrointestinal infection. Progressive hardening, spreading from the buttocks and thighs, occurs. The mortality is around 50%.

Fat necrosis in the newborn is a benign, self-limited, localized process occurring over the bony prominences in infants born after a difficult labor. Nodular thickening of the subcutaneous tissue is detected, usually in the second or third week of life. The nodules may coalesce to form large plaques. In a few months they disappear, but some lesions may become calcified.

Scleredema and *scleroderma* are rare in children and not related to the above conditions.

Localized scleroderma or *morphea* develops occasionally in older children.

ACRODERMATITIS ENTEROPATHICA. This rare serious disease of infants is characterized by pustular and psoriasiform lesions around body orifices, on the face, the perineum, and also the limbs. It is associated with recurrent episodes of diarrhea. Systemic zinc therapy is effective.

ACRODYNIA (PINK DISEASE). This rare disease due to hypersensitivity to mercury is characterized by weight loss, anorexia, and painful hands and feet. Death can occur from secondary infection.

DUKE'S DISEASE. A mild exanthem occurring usually in the spring or summer months, with an incubation period of from 9 to 21 days. The eruption becomes generalized within a few hours, is bright red, and is accompanied by a low-grade fever.

GRANULOSIS RUBRA NASI. This chronic, rare disease is characterized by increased sweating of the nose and surrounding skin, with development of reddish, maculopapular lesions.

LICHEN STRIATUS. A rare skin condition of infants and children, this condition is characterized by acute onset of linear bands of papular and lichenified lesions that usually do not itch. This occurs mainly on the arms or the legs and disappears spontaneously in a few months. It is to be differentiated from *lichen planus* and *nevus unius lateris*.

XANTHOGRANULOMA (Fig. DI–10). This rather frightening condition consists of small, discrete, yellowish tan papules that can cover the body. They develop in the first year of life and without therapy disappear by the age of 5 or so.

DERMATOSES OF CHILDREN

Children seem to fall heir to most of the skin diseases of their adult counterparts, especially those problems that also affect their parents or other relatives. A discussion of the skin diseases of children aged 2 to 12 years would really cover the majority of all dermatologic ills in this book.

Here is a list of the most common children's skin problems, along with a short note about pertinent points. For more complete coverage in this book, refer to the chapters listed, or to the Dictionary-Index.

Dermatologic Allergy (see Chap. 9)
Contact dermatitis: very common; *poison plant (ivy or oak) dermatitis* is seen (see Plate 6).
Atopic eczema (see Plates 9, 10, and 94): in children, eczema of the feet or toes and depigmented, scaly, eczema lesions on the cheeks and arms (pityriasis simplex type).

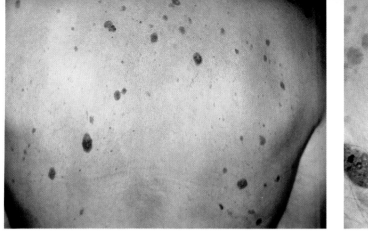

(A) Seborrheic keratoses over back of 71-year-old man

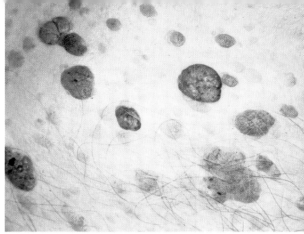

(B) Seborrheic keratoses, close-up

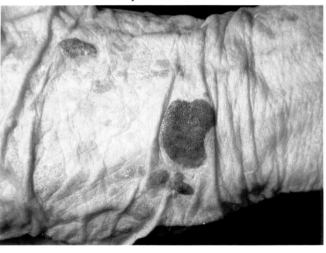

(C) Large seborrheic keratosis on hand in 84-year-old woman

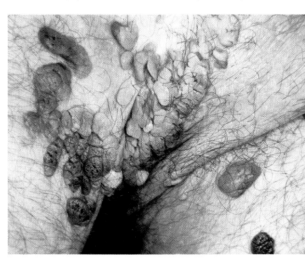

(D) Multiple seborrheic keratoses of crural area

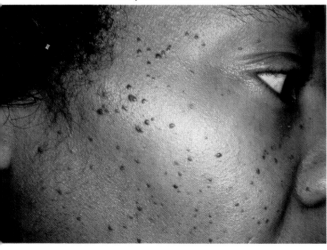

(E) Seborrheic keratoses or dermatosis papulosa nigra on face

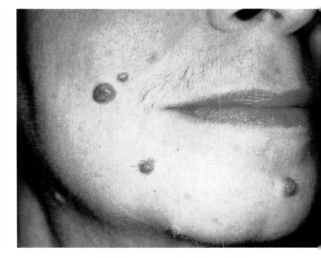

(F) Compound nevi on face

Plate 96. **Geriatric dermatoses** (Continued).

357

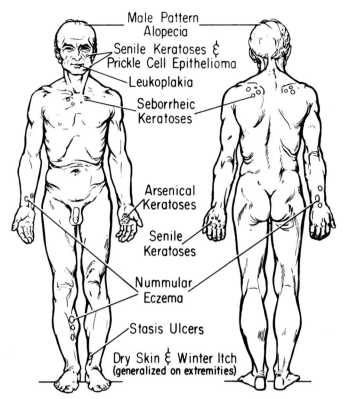

Figure 35–1. **Geriatric dermograms.**

In general, the *color* of the entire skin becomes pale and opaque.

The **appendages** of the skin change also. The most obvious and common changes are in the scalp, where the **hair** develops varying shades, from *grayness* to *pure white color* in certain persons.

The *male-pattern alopecia*, which can begin in the late teens, becomes more progressive through life. For the elderly patient, though, who has not had this hereditary balding problem, another form of hair loss, manifested as a diffuse thinning of the scalp hair, can develop. This *senile alopecia* can occur in both males and in females. Diffuse hair loss is also obvious in the axillae and the pubic area.

Excess facial hair is quite commonly seen in the elderly woman and can require shaving.

The **nails** do not change tremendously with age, but there is an increase in the longitudinal ridging. The toenails commonly become discolored, usually yellowish or brownish.

The **sebaceous glands** and **sweat glands** become less active in the older person. For the unfortunate persons who have had *acne* for years, age can be pleasant for them, with a clearing of this problem. If a patient does present with a complaint of the recent development of acne, question him carefully regarding the administration of *testosterone*, either orally or by injection.

The decrease in the secretion of oil and sweat glands contributes directly to the development of the *dry skin* or *xerosis* mentioned earlier.

The **mucous membranes** become drier. Patients complain of dry lips and tongue. The mucous membranes of the vaginal orifice also become dry, atrophic, and fragile.

Thus, essentially every elderly person has some evidence, however mild, of a skin problem.

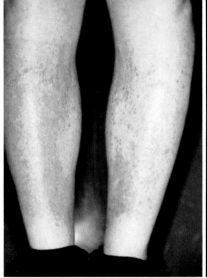
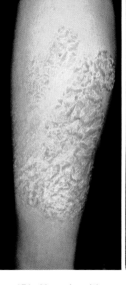
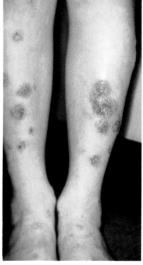

(A) Redness of winter itch on legs

(B) Xerosis with secondary infection on legs

(C) Nummular eczema of legs and
(D) of arm of same patient

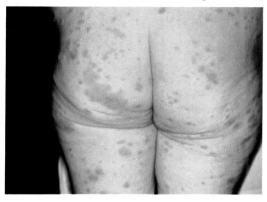

(E) Nummular eczema of buttocks

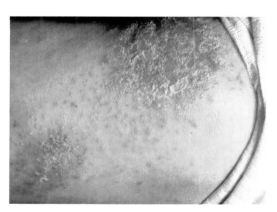

(F) Close-up showing oozing in nummular eczema of leg

(G) Stasis dermatitis of leg aggravated by contact allergy to neomycin

(H) Stasis ulcer of leg with varicose veins

(I) Senile pruritus in 74-year-old woman

(J) Drug eruption from phenacetin

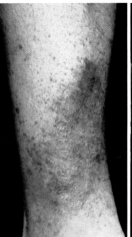
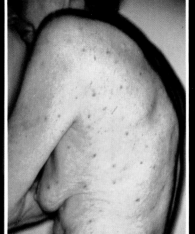

Plate 97. **Geriatric dermatoses** (Continued). (*Johnson & Johnson*)

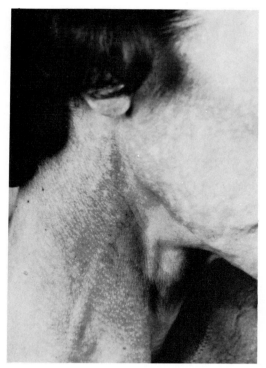

Figure 35–2. Poikiloderma of Civatte. Very common reddish brown discoloration on sides of neck seen mainly in women.

Pigmented nevus	143
Discoloration of the toenails	133
Seborrheic keratosis	84
Plantar hyperkeratosis	36
Stasis dermatitis of the legs	31
Seborrheic dermatitis	27
Dermatitis of the legs (unspecified)	23
Marked atrophy of the skin	19
Xanthelasma	12
Capillary hemangiomas	10

The numbers of cases refer to the total number of dermatologic disorders found in the 286 men and women examined.

They attributed the majority of the cases of discoloration of the nails as being due to bacterial and fungal infections, related to air content of the nail plate, or due to hemorrhage.

MANAGEMENT OF GERIATRIC SKIN PROBLEMS

INCIDENCE OF GERIATRIC SKIN DISEASES

For a study of the incidence of true skin diseases in a group of geriatric patients, here is a summary of a report in a classic study by Gip and Molin (see Bibliography).

These investigators studied 286 patients over the age of 60 who were hospitalized in a Swedish geriatric clinic. The skin of each patient was examined carefully. Histopathologic, bacteriologic, or mycologic examinations were undertaken in some cases.

In the 107 men there were 231 skin diagnoses (2.2 per person), and in the 179 women 372 skin diagnoses were found (2.1 per person). The number of skin diagnoses per person ranged from 1 to 5. No skin diagnoses were registered in 22 cases (only 8%) (5 men and 17 women).

All of the skin diagnoses were recorded. The following list contains the ten most frequent dermatologic disorders registered:

SAUER NOTES:

1. Nowhere is the the broadness of the term *management* more meaningful than when it is used in reference to the handling of the skin problem for an elderly patient.

2. Management implies the imparting of much more information and instruction than the simple prescribing of "treatment."

The dermatologic management of an elderly patient is considerably complicated, however, by the patient's physical and mental inability to understand and carry out instructions. The correct application of wet dressings, coping with tub bathing, and even the simple application of creams and ointments are more complex processes for the elderly. And as age progresses and debility increases, this care is further complicated by having to be administered by another person, such as a family member or nurse; this, additionally, has aesthetic and economic limitations.

Most elderly patients can be treated at home, but some of the more severe skin problems are seen in institutionalized persons.

Depending on the care available and the extent of the dermatosis, hospitalization may be necessary. The role of both corticosteroids and antibiotics in decreasing the number of elderly patients needing hospitalization is enormous and is most fortuitous.

CLASSIFICATION OF GERIATRIC DERMATOSES
(Plates 95 through 98)

The elderly patient is subject to the regular skin ills. However, as with the other age extreme, the child, there can be a different reaction by the aged skin to a given skin problem by virtue of the presence of fragility, dryness, and atrophy.

It would be unusual to see certain skin problems in the aged, such as *atopic eczema, acne, pityriasis rosea, impetigo, primary* and *secondary syphilis, herpes simplex, warts, exanthems, chloasma,* and *sunburn.*

A compilation of the more common problems of the geriatric patient is as follows, listed according to chapter groupings:

DERMATOLOGIC ALLERGY (see Chap. 9). *Contact dermatitis:* For the geriatric patient this commonly is a dermatitis caused by the use of too harsh a local medication. This is seen quite frequently where too strong a salve is used in the treatment of itching legs.

Nummular eczema (see Plate 97): This is quite a common problem, seen particularly in the winter and characterized clinically by coin-shaped vesicular areas on the arms, the legs, and less frequently, the buttocks.

Drug eruptions (see Plates 14 and 97J): Drug eruptions are not too common but can be seen as a *photosensitivity-type* dermatitis when the patient is on a diuretic or a phenothiazine-type tranquilizer, or as an *acne-like picture*, due to the administration of testosterone.

PRURITIC DERMATOSES (see Chap. 11). *Generalized pruritus:* This is quite common and can defy adequate therapy. Careful examination of the patient is necessary to rule out any internal cause of the generalized pruritus. Rather frequently, and rather unfortunately, no apparent cause is ascertainable. Scalp and face itching can be a real problem.

Xerosis (see Plate 97): As a cause of the generalized itching in the winter this is rather easily managed by decreasing bathing and applying an emollient lotion or even a mild corticosteroid cream or ointment. See p. 103 for a more detailed discussion of this problem in the elderly patient.

Localized pruritic dermatoses: These are not as common as the more generalized pruritus.

VASCULAR DERMATOSES (see Chap. 12). *Urticaria* is not commonly seen.

Stasis dermatitis (see Plate 97G and *H*): This is rather commonly seen in elderly patient and is almost always associated with venous insufficiency due to varicose veins or other circulatory problems. It is important to stress that circulatory support is indicated on a *continuing basis* after the dermatitis has responded to therapy. This can prevent the development of *stasis ulcers.*

Atrophie blanche: Arterial insufficiency of the legs from several causes can produce redness, scaling, ulcers, and eventually, stellate scars. It occurs mainly over the ankles.

SEBORRHEIC DERMATITIS, ACNE, AND ROSACEA (see Chap. 13). *Seborrheic dermatitis:* This becomes less bothersome with age but can recur following a cerebrovascular accident or stroke.

Acne: Acne is rarely seen in the elderly patient.

Testosterone and related drugs: These drugs can produce an acne-like picture, so be sure to ascertain whether such drugs are being administered.

PAPULOSQUAMOUS DERMATOSES (see Chap. 14). *Psoriasis* (see Plates 22 and 23): It is rare to see psoriasis develop as a new problem in an elderly person. Thus most elderly persons who have psoriasis have learned to live with the disease.

DERMATOLOGIC BACTERIOLOGY (see Chap. 15). *Furuncles and carbuncles:* These lesions are not too common.

Decubital ulcers: The alternate term, *bedsores*, describes the pathogenesis of these chronic, painful, and debilitating ulcerations. They occur on pressure sites, mainly buttocks and posterior aspect of heels. The patient is usually bedridden.

Prophylactic measures are extremely important. Good nursing care can prevent some of these ulcers. The care should include turning the patient frequently, keeping the pa-

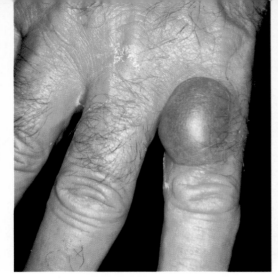

(A) Fixed bullous drug eruption due to tetracycline

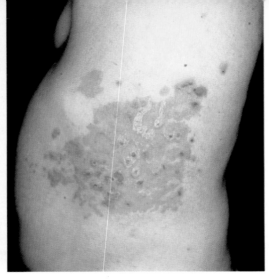

(B) Pemphigoid on lateral abdominal area

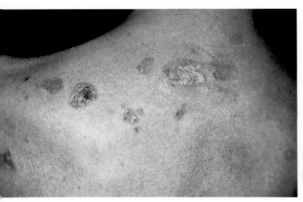

(C) Pemphigus vulgaris of upper back area

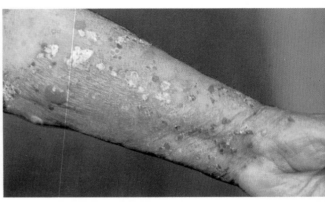

(D) Pemphigus vulgaris of forearm

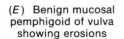

(E) Benign mucosal pemphigoid of vulva showing erosions

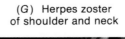

(F) Lichen sclerosus et atrophicus of vulva (*not* leukoplakia)

(G) Herpes zoster of shoulder and neck

(H) Discoid lupus erythematosus of cheek in 77-year-old woman

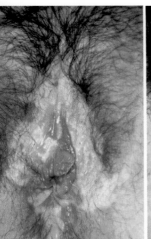

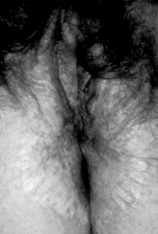

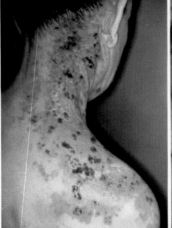

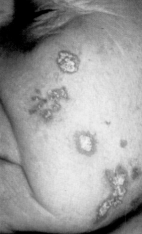

Plate 98. **Geriatric dermatoses** (Continued).

tient clean and dry, and applying powder to the bed. Once an ulcer has developed, the care is compounded. Donut-type sponge cushion supports are indicated, with local application of Betadine solution and continued good nursing care.

Secondary bacterial infections: Stasis ulcers (see Plate 97*H*) are the cause of marked disability in the elderly patient. The ulcers heal slowly and can be very painful. The care required to heal these ulcers, or even prevent them from spreading, can be considerable. More often than not, other members of the family, or nursing personnel must take over the management of these chronic sores.

SYPHILOLOGY (see Chap. 16). Tertiary syphilis of the skin or other organs is now rarely seen. The most common problem seen in the elderly patient in relation to syphilis is the persistently positive serology following adequate therapy. Some syphilologists are alarmed that dormant but persistent spirochetal infections can become clinically significant, with involvement of the eye and central nervous system.

DERMATOLOGIC MYCOLOGY (see Chap. 19). *Candidal infections* are the most common mycologic infections seen in the elderly patient, particularly if the patient is obese. Lack of bathing and cleansing is a major factor.

DERMATOLOGIC PARASITOLOGY (see Chap. 21). *Scabies* as an epidemic in a nursing home can be a difficult management problem. The elderly, especially if mentally confused, present a challenge for basic hygiene. When they itch, this itch is usually attributed to *dry skin* or *senile pruritus.* Only when several residents in the nursing home, and the personnel, begin to itch, does one think of scabies as a cause. Then the therapy is difficult because so many persons are affected (and for personnel, possibly their families), so that a basic simple therapy becomes a major management problem. All persons affected must be treated at the same time.

BULLOUS DERMATOSES (see Chap. 22). *Pemphigoid* (see Plate 90*B*) is probably the most common bullous condition seen in the elderly patient.

Dermatitis herpetiformis in the elderly should prompt a careful workup to rule out an *internal malignancy.*

EXFOLIATIVE DERMATITIS (see Chap. 23 and Plate 66) is a miserable disease, and the etiology can be difficult to ascertain. An axiom is that 50% of the patients older than age 50 with an exfoliative dermatitis have a *lymphoma.*

PIGMENTARY DERMATOSES (see Chap. 24). Hyperpigmentation or hypopigmentation of the skin can occur in the elderly from many causes. Aside from a simple change in pigmentation of the skin due to age, other pigmentary problems are uncommon.

COLLAGEN DISEASES (see Chap. 25). Discoid lupus erythematosus can begin in old age (see Plate 68).

THE SKIN AND INTERNAL DISEASE (see Chap. 26). *Diabetes mellitus* causes a degeneration of the vascular supply, and skin changes in the diabetic are progressive with age. *Ulcers, gangrene of the digits,* and *ulcerations of the mal perforans-type* are most commonly seen (see Plate 73).

DISEASES AFFECTING THE HAIR (see Chap. 27). *Graying of the hair* and *thinning of the hair* have been discussed earlier.

Hypertrichosis, or excessive growth of hair, is common on the face of women.

DISEASES AFFECTING THE NAILS (see Chap. 28). Other than the development of increased ridging of the nail plates and the discoloration of the toenails, mentioned earlier, there are no major nail changes in the aged individual.

DISEASES OF THE MUCOUS MEMBRANES (see Chap. 29). The mucous membranes become dry and fragile with age.

DERMATOSES DUE TO PHYSICAL AGENTS (see Chap. 30). Sunlight effects on the skin are extremely common and can result in simple hyperpigmentation and atrophy of the skin or can produce *actinic keratoses* (see Plate 83) that can occasionally eventuate as *squamous cell carcinomas* (see Plate 99*D*).

PHOTOSENSITIVITY DERMATOSES (see Chap. 31). Photosensitivity problems are rarely seen unless triggered by drugs.

GENODERMATOSES (see Chap. 32). The genetic inheritance of the person has considerable influence on the aging of the skin, including wrinkling, the effect of sunlight, the

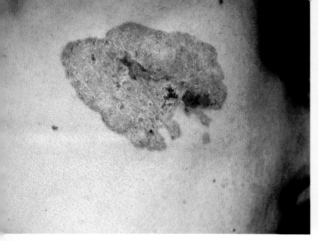

(A) Lateral view of large superficial basal cell carcinoma on back

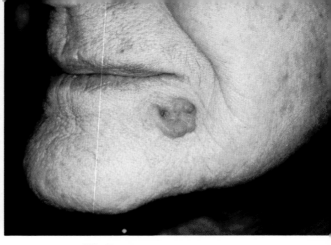

(B) Basal cell carcinoma on chin

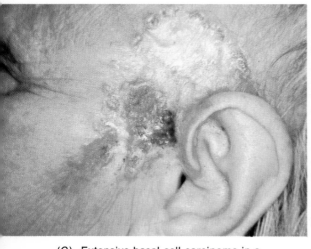

(C) Extensive basal cell carcinoma in a 79-year-old patient

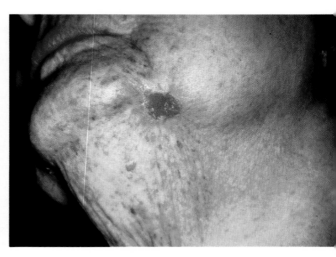

(D) Squamous cell carcinoma in area of chronic radiodermatitis for hypertrichosis of skin

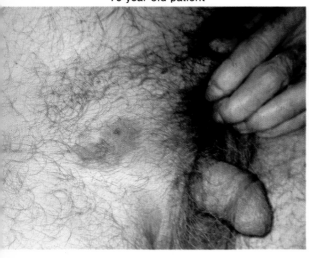

(E) Paget's disease of crural area

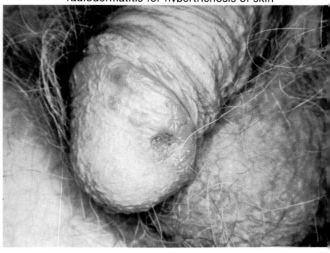

(F) Erythroplasia of Queyrat on penis

Plate 99. **Geriatric dermatoses** (Continued).

activity of the oil and sweat glands, and hair changes.

TUMORS OF THE SKIN (see Chap. 33). *Seborrheic keratoses* (see Plates 81 and 96), as mentioned earlier, are very common, and seen in almost every elderly person. The number of these lesions is genetically determined.

Pedunculated fibromas of the neck and axilla are quite common, and again, there is a familial tendency for these to develop.

Precancerous tumors, such as *senile* or *actinic keratoses*, develop in relation to earlier sun exposure and the genetic makeup of the skin complexion.

Squamous cell carcinoma can develop by itself or from degeneration of actinic keratoses.

Basal cell carcinomas (see Plates 84, 95, and 99) are the most common malignancy of the skin in the elderly patient. These are characterized by waxy nodular lesions, with or without ulceration in the center.

Hemangiomas of the lips are not uncommon and frighten the patient into thinking that he or she has a *melanoma*.

Capillary hemangiomas (see Plate 87) on the chest and back are present in almost every elderly person.

Nevi mature with age, and many seem to disappear. Junctional elements are rarely seen in nevi in the geriatric patient.

Malignant melanoma is an uncommon malignancy, but it can develop from a brownish black, flat lesion known as a *lentigo*, which is usually seen on the face and arms. The result is a *lentigo maligna melanoma* (see Plate 95E).

BIBLIOGRAPHY

Arlian LG, Estes SA, Vyszenski-Moher DL: Prevalence of *Sarcoptes scabiei* in the homes and nursing homes of scabietic patients. J Am Acad Dermatol 19:806, 1988

Beauregard S, Gilchrest BA: A survey of skin problems and skin care regimens in the elderly. Arch Dermatol 123:1638, 1987

Gip L, Molin L: Skin diseases in geriatrics. Cutis 6:771, 1970

Kligman AM: Psychological aspects of skin disorders in the elderly. Cutis 43:498, 1989

Leveque JL et al: *In vivo* studies of the evolution of physical properties of the human skin with age. Int J Dermatol 23:322, 1984

Marks R: Skin Disease in Old Age. Philadelphia, JB Lippincott, 1987

Rossman I (ed): Clinical Geriatrics, 3rd ed. Philadelphia, JB Lippincott, 1986. Good sections on skin diseases and skin aging.

Rousseau P: Pressure sores in the elderly. Geriatr Med Today 7(February):28, 1988

Smith L: Histopathologic characteristics and ultrastructure of aging skin. Cutis 43:414, 1989

Weiss JS, Ellis CN, Headington JF et al: Topical tretinoin improves photoaged skin. JAMA 259:527, 1988

36

Geographic Skin Diseases

NORTH AMERICA

Most common skin diseases of North America are universal in geographic distribution, but a few are confined to, or more prevalent in, certain regions. In my attempt to cover completely the common skin diseases, I have called on other dermatologists from representative areas of the United States (including Alaska and Hawaii) and Canada to list their geographic skin diseases (Fig. 36–1). A list of the dermatologists consulted follows. I am taking the liberty of quoting certain parts of their letters because they add interest to this question of geographic dermatoses.

Canada

VANCOUVER, BRITISH COLUMBIA—DR. STUART MADDIN. "It is quite generally agreed that we do not have any important or common dermatologic problem out here that is unusual due to our geographic location. However, the coastal region of the Pacific Northwest differs from other areas in that there is no poison ivy or poison oak to cause this form of *contact dermatitis*."

WINNIPEG, MANITOBA—DR. SAUL BERGER. "We do have a fungus condition here which is called *suppurative ringworm*. It is contracted from cattle and is a rather common infection in rural Manitoba." (The majority of cases of *suppurative ringworm* seen in rural areas of Manitoba are due to *Trichophyton faviforme*.) "The other condition which we

think is perhaps more common here than elsewhere is *hereditary polymorphic light eruption* of the North American Indian."

United States

ANCHORAGE, ALASKA—DR. THOMAS MCGOWAN. In a long, informative letter Dr. McGowan stated that the data he had gathered in Alaska had not yet been completely tabulated or evaluated and should be considered as his personal clinical impression, based on examination and interviews of several thousand natives: ". . . these impressions actually apply only to the Aleuts, resident in the Aleutian Islands and Alaska Peninsula, and to the Indians resident in Southeastern Alaska. Among these two groups I found that the only skin diseases seen with any frequency were *impetigo, scabies, pediculosis capitis,* and *pruritus ani* associated with pinworms, and all of these were almost completely limited to children. *Acne vulgaris* was quite common in the Indian but very rare in the Aleut. Very rare in both groups were *allergic infantile eczema*, vesicular *eczematoid dermatoses* of the hands, and *fungus infections* of the nails and of the scalp. I found no cases of fungus infection of the skin, of psoriasis, of skin malignancy or of tuberculosis cutis (other than old healed scars of scrofuloderma), nor did I find any active venereal disease. One condition of interest, common among children of both groups in the springtime, was an acute *dermatitis venenata*, similar to poison ivy, occurring on the face and

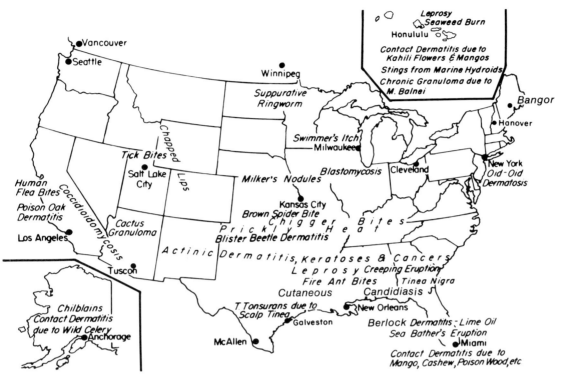

Figure 36–1. **Predominant localization of geographic dermatoses of United States and Canada.**

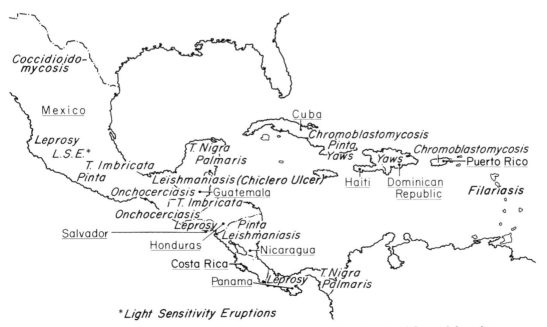

Figure 36–2. **Predominant localization of geographic dermatoses of Central America.**

hands after contact with the juice of the outer skin of the local "wild celery.'"

Dr. John Schultz, of Anchorage, wrote that he "occasionally sees a patient with *phytophotodermatitis* due to cow-parsnip."

SEATTLE, WASHINGTON—DR. HARVEY ROYS. "I know of no skin disease that is peculiar to the Northwest. Some cases of *contact dermatitis* from forestry products may be more common."

MILWAUKEE, WISCONSIN—DR. THOMAS J. RUSSELL. "*Swimmer's itch* is seen only occasionally and in a multiyear, cyclical pattern. *Milker's nodules* are now seldom seen in livestock workers, but *tinea infections* in these occupations must be considered in differential diagnoses of all skin disease because of the protean manifestations and potential for initial misdiagnosis and treatment."

NEW YORK, NEW YORK—DR. A. I. WEIDMAN. "There is no specific, regional dermatologic condition prevalent in New York City, but we should consider the varied nature of the population in this city where individuals derive from every country in the world (even when we disregard the large staff of the U.N.). These individuals may carry with them a vast array of skin conditions specific for their genetic make-up and place of origin. I would list among them *sickle cell anemia* and *leg ulcers* (black population 1,784,000); *lichen simplex chronicus* (localized neurodermatitis) among Orientals (124,000 Chinese); and *Hansen's disease* (among the new arrivals from the Caribbean, South America and Asia). Even *AIDS* (*acquired immunodeficiency syndrome*), very prevalent in New York City, gives testimony to the specific nature of the population (tens of thousands of homosexuals, large Haitian community). I would also venture to speculate that skin conditions having their origin primarily in stress in this financial, cultural and artistic capital of the world, could be listed." (From my limited experience in New York City I feel that *exudative discoid and lichenoid chronic dermatosis* should be listed. This will be discussed later in this chapter.)

BANGOR, MAINE—DR. ROBERT W. HAEBERLEIN, JR. "This region is endemic for *Lyme disease* due to the population of deer and the deer tick. Publicity about this rash, which can be associated with cardiac and neu-

rological damage, is of great concern to our hikers and campers. Our many lakes are only an occasional source of *swimmer's itch*. Outbreaks rarely produce office visits because of the familiarity with the bite-like rash, its symptomatic treatment and self-limited nature.

"Our cold winters are famous here in New England and regularly produce acute and chronic forms of *pernio*. Also associated with the cold winters is a keen interest in wood burning as a primary and supplemental source of heat. Hardwoods are plentiful in the region and back yard chain saw cutting as well as professional cutting is very common. The involved exposure to wood chips and chain saw oil commonly produce forms of *irritant* and *allergic contact dermatitis*.

"Small farms are common in Maine. Barnyard animals are an interesting source of infections, like *Milker's nodules* and *orf*."

LOS ANGELES, CALIFORNIA—DR. SAMUEL AYRES, III. In addition to *human flea bites*, which will be discussed more fully later, Dr. Ayres listed *actinic keratoses* and *skin cancers*, and, as an uncommon condition, *coccidioidomycosis* of the San Joaquin Valley. He also stated, "On the negative side, we do not have *chiggers, chilblains*, or *miliaria*."

Water skiers, skin divers, waders, and swimmers in southern California waters are frequently bitten by the crustaceans of the *Cymothoid* suborder. This has been called *sea louse dermatitis*. The small punctate bites heal in 5 to 6 days time.

There are many persons with *AIDS* in California.

SALT LAKE CITY, UTAH—DR. ARTHUR M. BURTON. "The *exanthem of Rocky Mountain spotted fever* is characteristic and well documented. The *tick bite* itself, however, does not leave a characteristic cutaneous lesion. This I have observed from personal observation on myself. The tick burrows into the skin with its head, engorges itself with blood, then withdraws and drops off the body. There is actually very little, if any, evidence remaining at the site of the tick bite." (Plate 100*F*)

KANSAS CITY, MISSOURI—AUTHOR. The two most common geographic dermatoses of the Midwest are *chigger bites* and *prickly heat*. These will be referred to later in the chapter. *Milker's nodules, grain itch, bites*

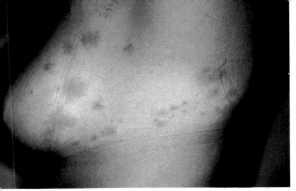

(A) Chigger bites collected under a bra

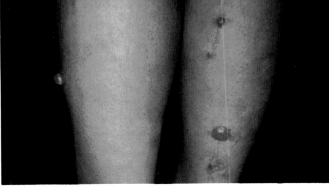

(B) Bullous chigger bites on the legs

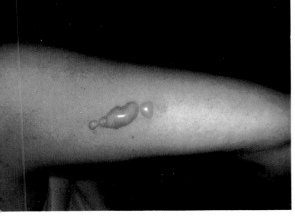

(C) Blister beetle bullous reaction on arm

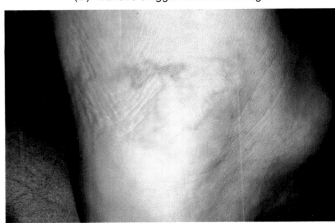

(D) Creeping eruption on plantar surface of heel

Plate 100. **Geographic skin diseases.**

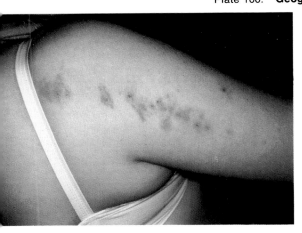

(E) Bedbug bites on the arm

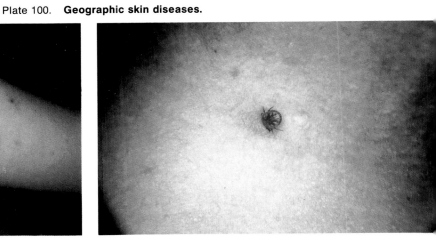

(F) Tick imbedded in the skin, presented as a tumor by patient

(G) Brown recluse spider bite on leg

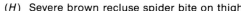

(H) Severe brown recluse spider bite on thigh

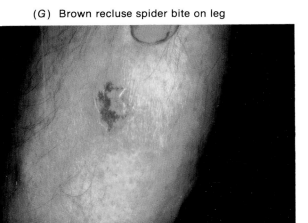

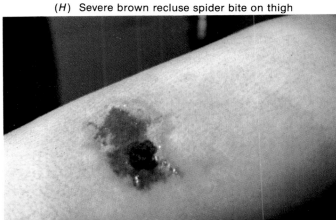

from the brown spider (see Plate 100G and H), and *tick bite granulomas* are peculiar to this area but not common.

CLEVELAND, OHIO—DR. GEORGE H. CURTIS AND DR. WILMA F. BERGFELD. "We know of no common skin disease endemic to this area." Dr. Curtis proceeded to list the most common skin conditions seen and treated at the Cleveland Clinic. At the top of the list were *neurodermatitis circumscripta* (including pruritus ani), *superficial fungal infections*, and *pyogenic infections*.

TUCSON, ARIZONA—DR. OTIS MILLER AND DR. PETER J. LYNCH. I requested information concerning *atopic eczema*, since so many of these patients improve when in Tucson or Phoenix. Dr. Miller's reply was, "There is little question that the warm climate of Arizona is beneficial to many, but not all, cases of *atopic dermatitis*. In the acute and angry stage, sunlight and heat make the condition considerably worse. There are many children who are born in Arizona with familial histories of allergies, who develop atopic dermatitis right here in Tucson. Many of these are highly allergic to pollens which are peculiar to this neck of the woods. One of the most common trouble-makers is Bermuda grass."

He continued with a discussion of *cactus granuloma*. "This is a tissue reaction which is found principally on the exposed areas of the body, due to the penetration of the stickerweed into the skin. It's conceivable that the same type of reaction is produced by small thorns found on various cacti." Dr. Lynch added, "There is no new material on *cactus granulomas* but certainly we continue to see them. Generally, they are simply left untreated though occasionally a punch biopsy is used to remove the foreign body particularly when it is on a pressure point over the hands."

Dr. Lynch continued, "Bites due to *kissing bugs* (*Triatoma* species) are a real problem for us. The bite is painless and usually occurs at night. As a result the patients are unaware how or why they have developed the lesion. Generally, the lesions are quite large (2–3 cm in diameter) and they can be quite pruritic. They last for about 10 days. A few cases in which anaphylaxis develop have been recognized."

Cutaneous coccidioidomycosis also continues to be a problem according to Dr. Lynch. "In fact, we are probably recognizing it more often now. These lesions are cutaneous granulomas but sometimes they are amazingly innocuous in appearance. I am impressed that the face is commonly involved, where they are often mistaken for acneiform or rosacealike lesions. In almost all cases these are not primary inoculation granulomas but instead occur as a result of disseminated disease. Unfortunately, usually the lung disease has disappeared by the time the patient sees the dermatologist. The only real indication of systemic involvement is the fact that complement fixation titers are usually positive, though in low dilution. Ketoconazole is quite good from a standpoint of suppression, but most lesions recur once the ketoconazole has been stopped."

Dr. Lynch also mentioned that *brown recluse spider bites* are quite commonly seen in Arizona, also many *skin cancers*, including *melanomas*, and occasional cases of *leprosy*.

"The Mexican-American population appears to have a higher incidence of *lupus erythematosus* than do Anglos. *Photosensitivity reactions* are quite common in our Indian population. This, of course, has been reported before for other American-Indian groups."

McALLEN, TEXAS—DR. IVAN KUHL. Dr. Kuhl listed *tinea capitis* due to *Trichophyton tonsurans, keratoses,* and *skin cancers, leprosy, contact dermatitis* due to mango fruit, *candidiasis* of all forms, and *flea bites.* "The flea bites are more prevalent in January through April. We do not have *fire ant bites*, as yet, but have *creeping eruption* after rains in the surrounding sandy ranch country to the north of us. Chiggers, rodent and bird mites, blister bugs, stinging caterpillars, and ticks keep us interested in *bites* although they are not common. Tineas and other fungus and yeast infections, plus keratoses and skin cancers probably constitute about 60% of my practice."

GALVESTON, TEXAS—DR. EDGAR BEN SMITH. "The island city of Galveston, Texas, is a port and seaside resort. As might be expected *actinic keratosis, basal* and *squamous cell carcinoma,* and *malignant melanoma* are relatively common in those who have lived in the area for some time. *Tinea versicolor* and *dermatophyte infections* are also quite common. Most *tinea capitis* in the area is caused by *Trichophyton tonsurans. Insect bites* and *papular urticaria* are also common. Fleas cause a significant proportion of these problems. The imported fire ant is now quite common in Galveston and we frequently see the pustular lesions of *fire ant stings. Creeping eruption* (see Plate 100*D*) was once quite common but is now only occasionally seen. We also occasionally see the linear punctate lesions of *stings* due to *jelly fish* and the *Portuguese man-of-war*."

NEW ORLEANS, LOUISIANA—DR. LARRY E. MILLIKAN. "In the New Orleans Gulf Coast area we see a great deal of fungal and yeast infections. *Tinea corporis, tinea cruris,* and *candidiasis* are all extremely common. Even more of a problem is *tinea capitis* due to *T. tonsurans.* It is responsible for more than 75% of all cases of tinea capitis and is extremely polymorphic in appearance, ranging from that resembling seborrhea to scarring alopecia. Fire ants are another major problem and some cases of allergy to fire ant venom have occurred. *Sarcoidosis* is extremely common in the population at Charity Hospital.

"The city has more than its share of venereal diseases. All phases of *syphilis* are seen not infrequently, in both charity clinics and private offices, in spite of the existence of very busy venereal disease clinics. These syphilis cases of course provide very interesting clinical challenges. Other common conditions are *berlock dermatitis* from limes, *Rhus dermatitis, actinic skin damage, keratoses, carcinoma,* and *atypical acid fast infections.*"

MIAMI, FLORIDA—DR. HARVEY BLANK. Dr. Blank listed *creeping eruption, cutaneous candidiasis, Portuguese man-of-war stings, contact dermatitis* due to various members of the Anacardiaceae, not only *Rhus,* but also mango, cashew, poison wood (*Metopium toxiferum*), and Brazilian pepper tree (*Schinus terebinthifolius*), *eczema solare, berlock dermatitis* due to lime oil, and *actinic skin with keratoses and carcinomas.* Quite a few cases of *drug-induced photodermatitis* are seen, usually from antihypertensives. The *acquired immunodeficiency syndrome* (AIDS) with *Kaposi's sarcoma* is now being seen not uncommonly.

HONOLULU, HAWAII—DR. HARRY L. ARNOLD, JR. "There is no basis at all for the prevailing impression that exotic tropical diseases are commoner in Hawaii than on the North American continent; only *leprosy,* of them all, is endemic in Hawaii, and its incidence is now down to around 2 cases per 100,000 population per year—with one of these being imported, usually from the Far East.

"Of perhaps greatest interest is the negative difference between Hawaii and the 'mainland' U.S.A. In Hawaii, not a single case of *sarcoidosis* has as yet been encountered; not a single case of *tinea capitis* due to *Microsporon audouini; larva migrans* is mysteriously extremely rare; not a single case of *chiggers,* or *coccidioidomycosis,* or *blastomycosis.*

"A few diseases familiar to other tropical or subtropical areas do occur here. *Leprosy* (Plate 101) has been mentioned. *Stings* produced by marine hydroids—*Halecium beani, Physalia* (the Portuguese man-of-war), *Syncoryne mirabilis* and others—occur occasionally. The Australian bottle-brush or *kahili* flower, *Grevillea banksii,* produces an occasional case of *dermatitis venenata* (the leaf of the plant, uniquely, is harmless), and visitors (but almost never natives, even as in Mexico and Cuba) may sometimes get a rash from handling or eating mangoes.

"Unique in Hawaii but happily infrequent is a *dermatitis escharotica* produced by contact with a rare seaweed, a blue green marine alga, *Lyngbya majuscula.*

"The '*seaweed burn*', reported by Grauer and Arnold in 1962, is an acute chemical burn produced by contact of the most dependent portion of the scrotum or the perianal area with fragments of the threadlike blue green alga *Lyngbya majuscula,* broken up by heavy surf on swimming beaches and held against the skin by the wet swimming suit for some minutes after the victim emerges from the water. Prompt removal of the suit, and thorough bathing, effectively prevent it. Several score cases have been encountered, every one from a swimming beach on the northeast or windward shore of the island of Oahu—though the offending seaweed is found on all the beaches in the state and indeed throughout the world."

These letters corroborated my feeling that in addition to certain skin diseases we as dermatologists know to be endemic to a particular area, such as swimmer's itch in Wisconsin and creeping eruption in the Gulf States, there are a few other common but less well-known geographic dermatoses.

The accompanying map (see Fig. 36–1) lists some of these geographic skin diseases. A few will be discussed in greater detail.

Bites Due to the Human Flea

The following is quoted from Dr. Ayres's letter regarding dermatoses localized to the California area: "I would first list human flea bites, that is, those due to *Pulex irritans.* These seem to be more or less limited to the Pacific coast and more particularly to San Francisco. They are not to be confused with dog or cat fleas, which may occasionally bite humans but prefer their natural hosts. Inhabitants of the area frequently are immune to the effect of the bites so that only newcomers are aware of the infestation. Interestingly enough this was my own experience when I went to medical school in San Francisco (Stanford). I had grown up in Southern California and had never known anything about human flea bites but I was nearly eaten alive by them during my years in San Francisco, while those of my fellow students who were native San Franciscans had no trouble at all. This is a widely recognized phenomenon in these areas. The manifestations are typically grouped, highly pruritic papules with central punctae, more prevalent over the covered portion of the body."

Certain cases of *"papular urticaria"* have been found to be due to the bites of insects such as fleas, bedbugs, chiggers (a mite larva), flies, and mosquitoes. This form of *"urticaria"* represents a chronic pruritic reaction to such bites that develops in children who have not been previously sensitized.

Treatment

Treatment of flea bites consists of preventive measures to destroy the insects. This is done best by spraying the home environment with an insecticide. Some insecticide powders can also be used directly on the patient and clothing.

Chigger Bites
(Plate 100)

Chigger bites, or trombiculiasis, is a very common summer eruption in inhabitants of the southern United States. The small urticarial papule is caused by the bite of the larva of the chigger. The larva does not burrow into the skin but drops off, after engorging itself on blood. Due to its almost microscopic size, it is rarely seen on the skin.

Clinically, the markedly pruritic papules occur where the larva meets resistance as it climbs up the legs, such as around the tops of the socks, the beltline, and the neckband area. Excoriation of the lesions leads to secondary infection. An allergic papulovesicular eruption is seen occasionally in sensitive persons following extensive generalized chigger bites. Papular urticaria has been mentioned previously.

In children, particularly, chigger bites are a common cause of *secondary impetigo,* especially in the scalp. For the first two summers that we lived in Kansas City, my two youngest children developed recurrent crops of impetiginous lesions on the scalp from the chigger bites. It was difficult to eradicate the lesions because of continued reinfestation and recurrent secondary infection. In later summers the bites became milder. This may be another example of the development of immunity following repeated exposure, similar to that seen from the flea bites of the San Francisco area.

Treatment

Preventive measures that are partially successful consist of applying repellants such as "Off" or Flowers of Sulfur powder to the feet and the stockings, and, if desired, spraying the infested lawn with insecticide.

Active therapy includes the use of 1% hydrocortisone lotion for the pruritus. For infected scalp lesions, sulfur (5%) in an antibiotic cream, such as Neo-Synalar Cream or Bactroban Ointment, is beneficial.

Swimmer's Itch

Bathers in the freshwater lakes of Wisconsin, Michigan, and Minnesota are prone to periodic attacks of inflammatory papular, urticarial, and vesicular eruptions on the uncovered areas of the body, mainly the legs. This pruritic eruption, which usually subsides within a week, is caused by the invasion of the skin by the cercariae of the schistosomes of ducks and mammals. The life cycle of these various species of schistosomes includes the snail as an intermediate host. On invasion of the abnormal definitive host, the human skin, the cercariae die, and the resulting skin eruption is the skin's reaction in ridding itself of the foreign bodies. Repeated attacks are met with stronger resistance, and the dermatitis becomes increasingly more severe. Secondary infection, edema, and lymphangitis can occur.

Seabather's eruption is a similar clinical entity, but its cause is unknown. Two main differences separate it from swimmer's itch: (1) the predominance of the seabather's eruption on the bathing suit area and (2) the limitation of this dermatosis to saltwater areas, particularly around the Florida coast.

Treatment

Prevention of swimmer's itch is accomplished best by destruction of the snails through careful addition to the lake water of a combination of copper sulfate and hydrated lime. Rapid drying of the swimmer with a towel apparently prevents penetration of the cercariae. Active therapy is directed toward the relief of the itching and secondary infection.

Creeping Eruption
(Plate 100D)

Larva migrans is a dermatosis of the southeastern United States, characterized by the presence of a serpiginous, advancing ridge overlying the tunnel of a migrating *Ancylostoma* larva. The advancing ridge is slightly behind the larva and is the skin's reaction to the foreign body. Itching and secondary infection are common.

The larva most commonly is derived from the roundworms of the genus *Ancylostoma* but occasionally from various species of botflies. The natural reservoir of the *Ancylostoma* hookworm is the intestines of dogs and cats. Infected feces on sand provide an excellent source for the passage of the larvae to the unsuspecting sunbather or barefoot child. Humans are not the natural host, so the parasite remains in the skin until destroyed.

Treatment

Thiabendazole effectively controls and treats creeping eruption. One routine is 50 mg/kg in a single oral dose, which may be repeated 24 to 48 hours later. The pruritus begins to subside within 4 to 6 hours. Rarely, side-effects of nausea and dizziness have been observed.

Most cases of creeping eruption can be effectively treated using the thiabendazole suspension (Mintezol, 500 mg per teaspoon, 120 ml) applied locally four times a day for a week or so.

Prickly Heat
(Plate 90B)

Prickly heat, or miliaria rubra, is a common disease of hot and humid climates. The physiologic pathology of the disease is the constant maceration of the skin, which leads to a blockage of the sweat duct opening. Continued exercise and further maceration of the skin results in dilatation of the epidermal portion of the sweat duct and rupture into the midepidermis. The result is a tiny vesicular papule that itches and burns. Pustular and deep forms of miliaria are observed mainly in the tropics and in particularly susceptible persons.

The distribution of the eruption is predominantly on the neck, the back, the chest, the sides of the trunk, the abdomen, and the folds of the body. Infants commonly show prickly heat confined to the diaper area. The eruption under adhesive tape is a form of localized miliaria due to blockage of the sweat pores.

Treatment

Prevention is of paramount importance. If the cycle of maceration and heat can be broken for a few hours each day, the eruption will not develop. Rest under fans or air conditioning for some hours of the day or the night is of great value. When these conditions are not available, application of a mild lotion or powder gives relief from the itching and may eliminate some of the skin maceration. A good example is

A calamine-type shake lotion q.s.   120.0

Exudative Discoid and Lichenoid Chronic Dermatosis

Oid-oid disease of Sulzberger and Garbe is probably a variant of atopic eczema or nummular eczema but with several important additional characteristics. It is seen predominantly among Jewish males in the New York City area and is a very chronic, disabling, markedly pruritic, lichenoid, and exudative dermatitis. Characteristic penile lesions are a diagnostic feature.

Treatment

Treatment is similar to that for a severe case of atopic eczema. A vacation or permanent change in residence of the patient to the southwestern part of the United States is quite often beneficial.

CENTRAL AND SOUTH AMERICA

Central and South America have extremes of climate and a mixture of ethnic groups that combine to produce some exotic and unique geographic skin diseases (Figs. 36–2 and 36–3).

As in the section on North America of this chapter, representative dermatologists of Central and South America were consulted for information on geographic skin diseases of these areas. Fortunately, the task of compilation of such information did not need to be

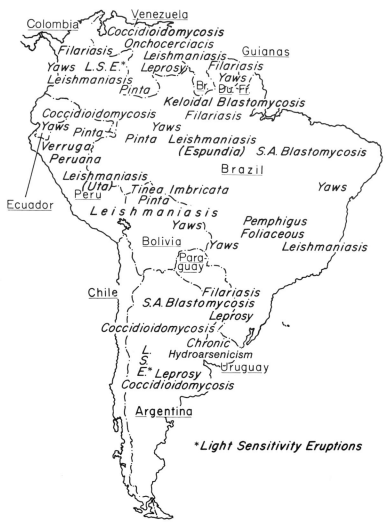

Figure 36–3. **Predominant localization of geographic dermatoses of South America.**

done by me, since it had already been done for a pioneer series of papers on this subject by Dr. Orlando Canizares. I therefore asked Dr. Canizares to submit material on this subject for this section, and also maps of the two areas. He graciously complied, and I am greatly indebted to him.

The experience of Dr. T. Charles Fail-mezger in a survey he made of skin diseases in selected Latin American countries is also acknowledged. He contributed comments and additional information for this section on geographic skin diseases.

It is my hope that those who are interested in these areas or these geographical diseases will contact me regarding changes, so that future editions can be kept up to date. This request applies especially to the readers of the Spanish edition of this book.

Epidemiology in Central and South America
(Contributed by Dr. Orlando Canizares)

FACTORS INFLUENCING EPIDEMIOLOGY. The factors that influence the epidemiology of skin diseases in Central and South America can be roughly divided, following the concepts of John Paul, into two types: the *macroclimate* and the *microclimate*. The macroclimate is the climate in its geographic sense that refers to temperature, humidity, rainfall, and so on. The microclimate refers to the environment and to the sum of conditions that affect the person—his origin, his socioeconomic status, his occupation, his home, his diet, and so on.

Macroclimate of Skin Diseases in Central and South America

ALTITUDE. One of the most important physical characteristics affecting the pattern of diseases in Central and South America is the altitude. Within the tropical belt, between sea level and about 2000 feet of altitude, the warm weather and the high humidity predispose to *pyogenic* and *fungal infections, candidiasis, miliaria, contact dermatitis, "tropical eczema"* and *tinea versicolor.* Between 2000 and 5000 feet, the pattern of disease encountered changes. Fungal and pyogenic infections, although present, are not as frequent as at lower altitudes. This elevation is within the

flying range of the phlebotomus and the simulium, the former transmitting *leishmaniasis* and *verruga peruana*, and the latter *onchocerciasis. Deep mycoses* are more common at this elevation.

At higher altitudes the climate is colder, regardless of the distance from the equator. Large cities such as Mexico City, Bogotá, Quito, and La Paz are on elevated plateaus, where *light-sensitivity eruptions, "winter eczemas,"* and other conditions encountered in colder Nordic climates are common.

SOIL. The soil is another factor in the epidemiology of the skin diseases. In the northern deserts of Mexico, *coccidioidomycosis* is abundant. The high content of arsenic in the drinking water near Cordoba, Argentina, causes the skin changes characteristic of *chronic arsenic ingestion.*

FAUNA. The fauna is important and varies in the different regions. Insect bites are common during the rainy season, causing a variety of *zoonoses. Tunga penetrans*, spiders, and so on may cause severe local or systemic reactions.

FLORA. The flora is an important factor in the epidemiology of skin diseases. *Contact dermatitis* is caused by the leaves or fruits of plants and the causative agents vary in different regions.

Microclimate: Humans and Their Environment

RACE. One of the main characteristics of the population of Central and South America is its racial and cultural diversity. More than half the population is of mixed ancestry. The role of race in the development of skin diseases is extremely difficult to determine. *Psoriasis* and *atopic eczema* have been found to be rare in pure-blooded Indians. *Actinic keratosis* and other actinic changes appear to be less common in those presenting with hyperpigmented skin. Some diseases are probably more common in the native Indians owing to their lower socioeconomic status and, therefore, greater exposure to infections.

DIET. Diet plays an important role, since the majority of the population of Central and South America is in a chronic state of malnutrition. The basic diet of the working class is corn, yucca, rice, and beans, which are starches with very little protein.

HOUSING. Crowded living conditions promote the spread of contagious diseases, such as *scabies*. The housing of the farmer and worker usually lacks the most elementary hygienic requirements. Bathing facilities are inadequate. Construction in the country is usually of wood or adobe, which harbors many insects that cause and transmit diseases.

OCCUPATION. The increased industrialization of Central and South America has resulted in a noticeable increase in *occupational dermatoses*. The farmers also develop dermatoses related to their work, such as *leishmaniasis* in woodcutters, *onchocerciasis* in the workers of the coffee plantation, and *sporotrichosis* in carpenters and packers.

Regional Survey of Epidemiology of Skin Diseases in Central and South America
(Also Contributed by Dr. Orlando Canizares)

REGION I—MIDDLE AMERICA, MEXICO, AND CENTRAL AMERICA. Mexico City is located on a plateau at 10,000 feet above sea level and presents the characteristic metropolitan high-altitude type of skin pathology. Some sections of Guatemala and Costa Rica, also at high altitudes, present a similar pattern of skin diseases. Bands of lowlands cut across with the typical hot and humid type of pathology. *Pinta* prevails at the basin of the river Balsas in Mexico. There are foci of *rhinoscleroma* and *onchocerciasis*. *Leishmaniasis* predominates in Yucatan and in some countries of Central America. There is a high incidence of deep mycosis, especially *mycetomas* and *sporotrichosis*. *Erythema dyschromicum perstans* is present in El Salvador and Hondoras.

REGION II—THE CARIBBEAN ISLANDS. The islands of the Caribbean include the Greater Antilles, the Lesser Antilles, and the Bahamas. In all, the climate is warm, with rather high humidity.

The characteristic of this region is a negative one. It is the absence of many serious skin diseases affecting the continent. Leishmaniasis, cutaneous tuberculosis, onchocerciasis, and deep mycoses, with the exception of *chromoblastomycosis*, are absent. *Pinta* is rare. *Yaws*, previously exceedingly common in Haiti and parts of Cuba and Jamaica, has been almost entirely eradicated.

REGION III—CARIBBEAN SOUTH AMERICA. This region includes Colombia, Venezuela, and the Guianas. The Caribbean coast of this region is the heat belt of South America, with the highest temperature and humidity. In the northern cities of Colombia, in the Maracaibo lowlands of Venezuela, and along the coast of the Guianas, we find the diseases common to this type of climate.

It has already been shown that Colombia is an excellent example of vertical zonation in dermatology. In the regions of the interior, west of the Andes, *leishmaniasis* is highly endemic. Recently, foci of *rhinoscleroma* and *onchocerciasis* have been isolated in Venezuela.

REGION IV—EASTERN SOUTH AMERICA: BRAZIL. In the jungles of the Amazon and in the northeast, *yaws, filariasis, keloidal blastomycosis of Lobo* (lobomycosis), and *leishmaniasis* are frequent. Due to an effective campaign, the incidence of yaws is being greatly reduced. *Leprosy* is endemic in Brazil.

The large cities of Rio de Janeiro, Belo Horizonte, and São Paulo present a metropolitan type of skin pathology with a noticeable increase in *industrial dermatoses*.

Endemic pemphigus foliaceus (fogo selvagem), a typical Brazilian skin disease, has its highest prevalence in the subtropical region of central Brazil, primarily at an altitude of 1500 feet.

In Brazil, as in most regions of Central and South America, *sarcoidosis* and *lymphoblastomas* are exceedingly rare.

REGION V—INTERIOR SOUTH AMERICA: BOLIVIA AND PARAGUAY. Bolivia and Paraguay share the common handicap of isolation from the sea. La Paz, the highest capital in the world, lies at an altitude of over 12,000 feet, showing the characteristics of a high-altitude type of cutaneous pathology. *Leishmaniasis* and *yaws* predominate in the plains of the Gran Chaco, and occasional foci of *pinta* are found.

REGION VI—PACIFIC SOUTH AMERICA: ECUADOR, PERU, AND CHILE. The high mountains of the Andes form the backbone of these countries. In the canyons of these high mountains, isolated foci of the typical Peruvian disease, *verruga peruana*, exist.

Chile, a long ribbon of land along the Pacific, has its population concentrated in the center. It has a mild climate, low-altitude type of skin pathology. As if walled off by the Andes, the inhabitants of Chile are free of most of the serious diseases affecting their neighbors, including *leprosy*.

REGION VII—SOUTHEASTERN SOUTH AMERICA: ARGENTINA AND URUGUAY. This region, with a middle-altitude climate, is geographically and ethnologically uniform. Its dermatologic pathology, because of the European origin of the population and the moderate climate, is similar to that of northern United States or continental Europe. In the northern region, the Chaco, some of the characteristic cutaneous pathology of warm and humid climate is seen. The city of Mendoza, at the foot of the Andes, shows evidence of the higher-altitude pattern of diseases. In the Cordoba region, a peculiar characteristic of the soil makes the drinking water high in arsenic content. This is called by Argentinean dermatologists "regional, chronic, endemic, *hydroarsenicism*" and causes melanoderma, keratoses, and multiple carcinomas.
(Conclusion of sections by Dr. Canizares)

Specific Skin Diseases

The various geographic skin diseases can be grouped into *bacterial infections, fungal infections, protozoal diseases, helminthic diseases, spirochetal diseases,* and *miscellaneous* conditions. They are elaborated on in the sections that follow.

Bacterial Infections

Warm weather, high humidity, insect bites, and poor hygiene predispose the skin to many of the pyodermas, such as impetigo, ecthyma, furunculosis, abscesses, ulcers, and secondary infection of the other skin diseases.

ULCERS OF THE LEGS. Ulcers of the legs are especially common and prove resistant to therapy. The causative factors are usually multiple and include trauma, malnutrition, and poor hygiene. A severe type with a rather distinct clinical pattern is the *tropical phagedenic ulcer.*

Management of tropical pyodermas is in general the same as that for the pyodermas discussed in Chapter 15. But, in addition,

greater stress must be laid on improvement of general hygiene and diet.

LEPROSY (see Plates 41 and 101). Leprosy is quite common in Mexico, especially in an area on the central west coast. The distribution of cases of leprosy in Mexico apparently has no relationship to climate, latitude, humidity, or altitude. *Diffuse lepromatosis* (Lucio's leprosy) is a form of lepromatous leprosy with rather definite characteristics of a diffuse, nonnodular, generalized skin infiltration and a necrotic lepra reaction. This variant is especially common in the Mexican state of Sinaloa.

More information on leprosy appears in Chapter 15.

Fungal Infections

Superficial fungal infections and candidal infections are very common in a humid climate.

TINEA. *Tinea versicolor* is common in the 15- to 19-year age-group, according to Dr. Failmezgar.

Tinea pedis is less common in the poorer classes who are barefoot or wear sandals, according to Failmezgar.

Tinea imbricata is a unique superficial fungal infection of the smooth skin caused by *Trichophyton concentricum.* It occurs primarily in Brazil, Colombia, Guatemala, and the state of Puebla, Mexico. Clinically, it is characterized by concentric rings of overlapping scales. It is extremely pruritic. Treatment with oral griseofulvin is apparently successful.

Deep fungal infections are relatively frequent in Central and South America.

SPOROTRICHOSIS (Plate 102). Sporotrichosis is one of the most common deep mycotic diseases and is seen especially among workers in the sugar cane fields and coffee plantations. Facial primary lesions are not uncommon and occur especially frequently in children (see Chap. 19).

MYCETOMAS (Fig. 36–4). Mycetomas have been reported as being the most common deep mycotic infection in Central America. Clinically, one sees granulomatous nodules, pustules, ulcers, and sinuses of the feet, with destruction of the bones, in severe cases. The

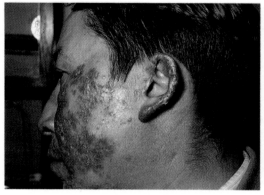

(A) Lepromatous leprosy

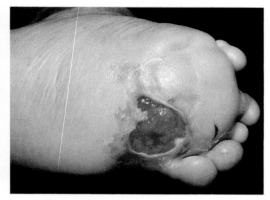

(B) Lepromatous leprosy on the foot

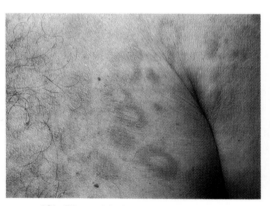

(C) Dimorphic leprosy on the chest

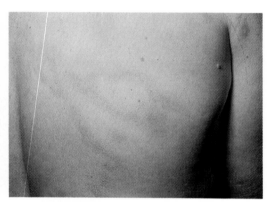

(D) Dimorphic leprosy on the back

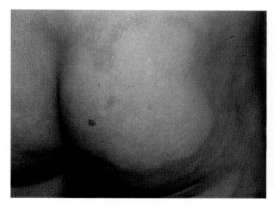

(E) Tuberculoid leprosy on the
buttocks

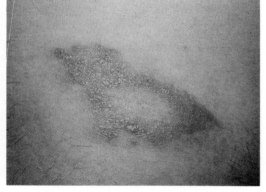

(F) Tuberculoid leprosy on the
chest

Plate 101. **Leprosy.** (*A and E from Dr. A. Gonzalez-Ochoa, Mexico; B and F from Dr. M. Rico, Durham, NC; C from Dr. R. Caputo, Atlanta; D from Drs. W. Schorr, Wisconsin, and F. Kerdel-Vegas, Venezuela*)

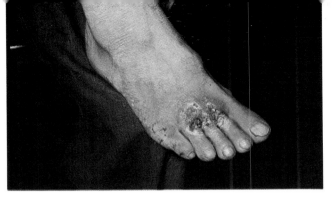

(A) Verrucous sporotrichosis on dorsum of foot

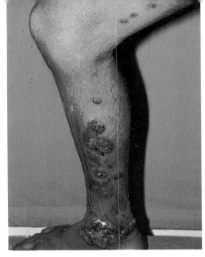

(B) Sporotrichosis with lymphatic spread on leg

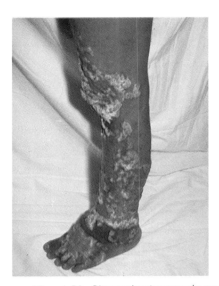

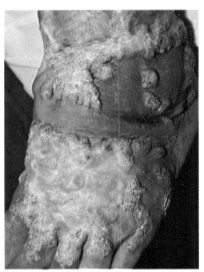

(C and D) Chromobastomycosis cauliflower-like leg lesion, with close-up of foot

(E) Cutaneous amebiasis with deep ulcers of the buttocks caused by direct extension following amebic dysentery

(F) Pinta showing early hyper-pigmented and depigmented patches on the back

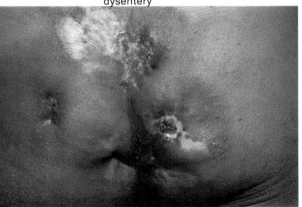

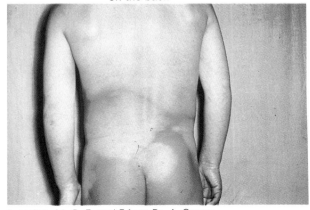

Plate 102. **Geographic skin diseases of Central and South America.** (*A, B, E, and F from Dr. A. Gonza-lez-Ochoa, Mexico; C and D from Drs. W. Schorr, Wisconsin, and F. Kerdel-Vegas, Venezuela*)

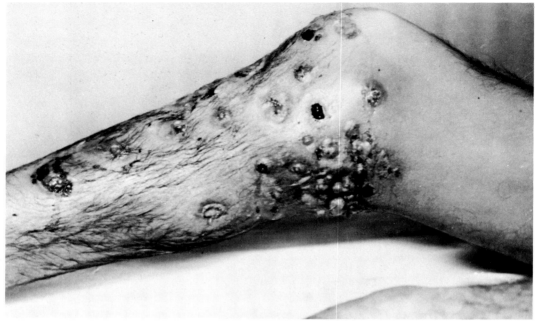

(A) Draining ulcers of leg and thigh

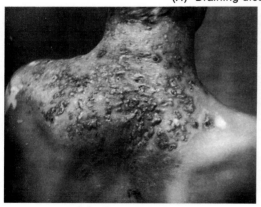

(B) Ulcers and nodules of back   *(C)* Ulcers of foot

Figure 36–4. **Mycetoma due to *N. brasiliensis*.** (*Dr. A. Gonzalez-Ochoa, Mexico*)

infection is caused by several species of Acti-nomycetes (*Nocardia* or *Streptomyces*) and fungi (*Madurella* species). The latter type of infection is called *maduromycosis*. Cases due to Actinomycetes respond to streptomycin therapy.

CHROMOBLASTOMYCOSIS (see Fig. 36–5 and Plate 102). Chromoblastomycosis is fre-quently seen in Panama, in Costa Rica, and, less frequently, in other Central and South American countries. It is characterized by warty nodules or ulcers, primarily of the lower extremities, that can coalesce to form large, cauliflower-like masses. Internal in-volvement has not been reported. The caus-ative organisms are *Hormodendrum* (*Fonse-caea*) *pedrosoi*, *H. compactum*, and *Phialophora verrucosa*. Therapy with oral po-tassium iodide is effective in some cases. Flu-cytosine orally has been effective. For early cases, curettage and electrodesiccation are successful.

COCCIDIOIDOMYCOSIS. Coccidioidomy-cosis, caused by *Coccidioides immitis*, is

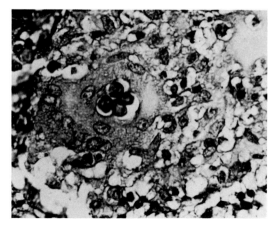

Figure 36–5. **Chromoblastomycosis.** Copper penny–like yeast cells with four buds inside giant cell. (*Drs. W. Schorr and F. Kerdel-Vegas*)

as common in the arid and desert areas of northern Mexico as it is in the southwestern part of the United States. Primary and secondary lesions can involve the skin. Systemic involvement is usually mild, but the disease can be fatal in rare instances.

SOUTH AMERICAN BLASTOMYCOSIS. South American blastomycosis, or *paracoccidioidomycosis* (Fig. 36–6) is a rare fungal disease, mainly of Brazilian farmers, caused by *Paracoccidioides brasiliensis*. Primary granulomatous lesions appear in or around the mouth, with secondary ulcers and nodules occurring around the face and the neck, along with a massive lymphadenopathy of the neck. This serious disease is responsive to oral ketoconazole. *Any patient must be monitored closely while on ketoconazole therapy, especially for hepatotoxicity.*

Arthropod Diseases

SCABIES. Scabies is a very common skin disease in Latin America, according to Dr. Failmezgar. Infants readily catch the disease from their mothers and siblings. The highest incidence is found among the lower economic groups, where there are crowded housing conditions.

Protozoal Diseases

LEISHMANIASIS (Fig. 36–7). Leishmaniasis is a protozoal infection of the reticuloendothelial cells of the viscera and the skin. The vec-

tors are sandflies of the genus *Phlebotomus;* humans and dogs serve as the reservoir. The disease occurs in three forms, caused by three species of *Leishmania,* which produce overlapping clinical pictures.

The visceral form, *kala-azar,* occurs in Paraguay, Argentina, and Brazil. A post–kala-azar dermal leishmaniasis characterized by depigmentation and nodules in the skin can occur some 2 years after the onset of the disease.

The cutaneous form is known as *oriental sore* and occurs in the tropical areas of Central and South America.

The mucutaneous form is very common in Central and South America. The causative protozoa is *Leishmania brasiliensis.* At least three clinical forms of this disease exist:

1. *Espundia* is characterized by deep and destructive lesions of the nose and the mouth and is found mainly in Brazil and other South American countries.
2. *Uta* is a form that affects the skin and only rarely the mucous membranes. Discrete ulcerating lesions, which heal with angular scars, occur usually on the face but can

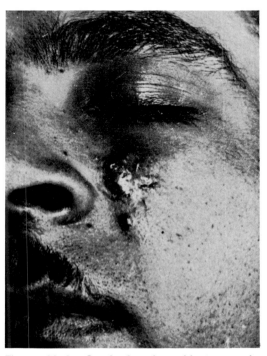

Figure 36–6. **South American blastomycosis.** Granulomatous nodule on the cheek. (*Dr. D. Grinspan, Argentina*)

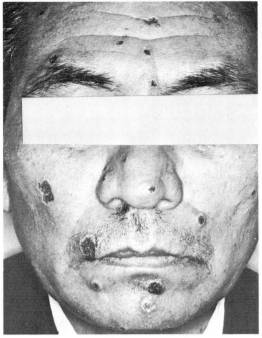

(A) Cutaneous leishmaniasis (oriental sore)

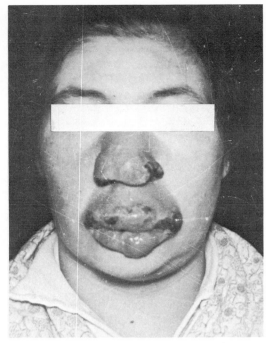

(B) Mucocutaneous form (espundia)

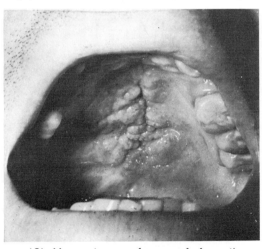

(C) Mucocutaneous form, roof of mouth

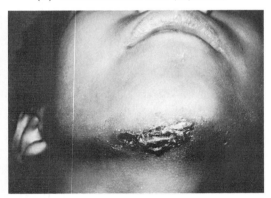

(D) Mucocutaneous lesion on chin

(E) Mucocutaneous chiclero ulcer of ear

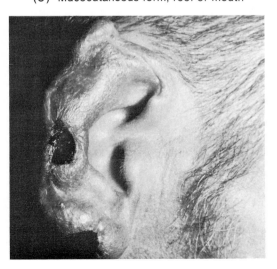

Figure 36–7. **Leishmaniasis.** (A, B, and C from Dr. D. Grinspan, Argentina; D and E from Dr. A. Gonza-lez-Ochoa, Mexico)

occur on any exposed area of the body. Verrucous lesions can develop. This form is endemic in the Andes.

3. *Chiclero ulcers* occur commonly in the chicle gatherers of Mexico and Central America. The lesion begins as a painful nodule of the ear, which can ulcerate and destroy all of the cartilage. There are no generalized symptoms.

Therapy for these mucocutaneous forms of leishmaniasis is disappointing. Amphotericin B has been used with some success, as has metronidazole.

TRYPANOSOMIASIS. Trypanosomiasis is a protozoal disease occurring in two forms: (1) the African form (sleeping sickness) and (2) the American form (Chagas' disease).

Chagas' disease is widely distributed in Argentina, Brazil, and other South American countries but is seen less frequently in Central America. It is caused by the protozoa *Trypanosoma cruzi* and is transmitted from human to human or animal to human by the reduviid, or "kissing" bugs.

Dermatologically, an early sign of the disease is a unilateral edema of an eyelid called Romaña's sign. Nonspecific eruptions of an urticarial or morbilliform nature can occur in the course of this severe systemic disease. There is no uniformly successful therapy.

CUTANEOUS AMEBIASIS (see Plate 102). Amebic dysentery caused by *Entamoeba histolytica* is a very common intestinal disease in Central and South America.

Skin lesions are less common, but, unless diagnosed early, the prognosis is very poor.

The ulcers or ulcerated granulomas, usually seen in a serpiginous configuration, are not characteristic. Examination of fresh tissue in saline reveals the ameba.

Lesions develop (1) from direct extension from the bowel, (2) from direct extension from an hepatic abscess, (3) after surgery in an infected person, or (4) from direct contact inoculation.

Treatment with injections of emetine is quite effective.

Helminthic Diseases

FILARIASIS BANCROFTI. This disease is caused by the presence of adult *Wuchereria bancrofti* in the lymphatic system or the connective tissues of humans. It is characterized clinically by several conditions related to the lymphatic system. The disease is present in Cuba and other West Indian islands, Colombia, Venezuela, Panama, and coastal areas of the Guianas and Brazil. Mosquitos of several species act as vectors and bite humans.

Clinically, a phase of inflammation of the lymphatic system is followed by an obstructive phase, which is marked by the eventual development of elephantiasis of the leg, the scrotum, the arm, or the breasts. Early treatment with diethylcarbamazine (Hetrazan) is quite successful.

ONCHOCERCIASIS. Onchocerciasis is another form of filarial infection, but it is confined to the southern states of Mexico and Guatemala. In these areas of coffee plantations, the disease is very common. The adult parasite, *Onchocerca volvulus*, is introduced into humans by the bite of species of *Simulium*, or black, or coffee flies. Clinically, one sees subcutaneous nodules on the scalp and the face caused by the migration or the disintegration of the microfilariae or the death of the adult worms. Other skin changes include facial redness and edema and severe pruritus of any of the body areas infected with the microfilariae. Involvement of the eye can lead to blindness. Early therapy with diethylcarbamazine kills the microfilaria, and intravenous administration of sodium suramin kills the adult worm.

Spirochetal Diseases

PINTA. Pinta, mal del Pinto, or carate (see Plate 102) is a nonvenereal treponemal infection caused by *Treponema carateum* that exists rather commonly in the West Indian islands and Mexico. Since the advent of penicillin therapy, the incidence of the disease has decreased considerably. Primary lesions are not observed clinically, but the secondary lesions, or pintids, begin as scaly papules on a red base. These areas progress to form bilateral and symmetrical areas of hyperpigmented and hypopigmented patches, usually on the palms, the soles, and the face. Hyperkeratotic lesions may also develop. Penicillin is curative, but the depigmented areas may not return to normal.

YAWS. Yaws, caused by *Treponema pertenue*, has been successfully treated with penicillin in the areas of the West Indies, Mexico, and Central America, where it was once prevalent. Some cases still exist in isolated areas of tropical South America. The primary lesion, or "mother yaw," is frequently found in children. Secondary skin lesions can appear in crops up to 5 years after the initial papule. These secondary skin lesions can be wartlike or papular, with ulceration, and appear in many configurations. The third-stage lesions are very destructive gummatous nodules or hyperkeratotic lesions of the palms and the soles. Bone lesions are common. Penicillin is curative, but the destructive changes are permanent.

Miscellaneous Conditions

VERRUGA PERUANA. This is the chronic dermatologic phase of *bartonellosis*. This disease is endemic along the steep valley slopes of Peru, Colombia, and Ecuador. The organism, *Bartonella bacilliformis,* is transmitted to humans by the bite of infected *Phlebotomus* sandflies.

The acute severe phase of the disease, Oroya fever, is characterized by high fever and a rapidly developing, often fatal, anemia. The cutaneous phase of bartonellosis, verruga peruana, can develop in the patient who survives Oroya fever, or it can develop as an initial manifestation of the disease. Verruga peruana is characterized by an eruption of hemangiomatous papules or nodules, varying in size from 1 to 2 cm. The larger nodules can ulcerate and hemorrhage severely and can last for several years before healing. There is no specific therapy for verruga peruana, but the mortality is very low.

PEMPHIGUS FOLIACEUS. Pemphigus foliaceus, or fogo selvagem, is an endemic form of pemphigus that occurs in the tropical regions of Brazil and Peru. Family groups can be affected with this disease. The initial lesions are flaccid bullae, which usually spread over the entire body, forming a generalized moist exfoliation. The course is chronic for several years, with death usually inevitable from intercurrent infection. Oral corticosteroids are beneficial. (For a general discussion of pemphigus, see Chapter 22.)

RHINOSCLEROMA. Rhinoscleroma is present in areas of higher altitude of Guatemala, El Salvador, and Venezuela, especially in persons with poor personal hygiene. The etiologic agent is believed to be *Klebsiella rhinoscleromatis,* but some believe it to be caused by a filtrable virus. Rhinoscleroma passes through three clinical stages, from a period of rhinitis, to a stage of plaques and masses on the septum, the lower part of the nostrils, and the larynx, to a final stage with large nodules and tumors. Treatment with chloromycetin is partially effective.

PIGMENTARY DISEASES. Pigmentary diseases such as melasma, vitiligo, postinflammatory changes, pityriasis alba, and tinea versicolor are of major cosmetic concern to dark-skinned Latin Americans.

"TROPICAL ECZEMA." This is an unclassified dermatitis that resembles generalized neurodermatitis or scabies in the young, according to Dr. Failmezgar. The condition is said to be precipitated by insect bites and consists of extensive, pruritic, lichenified patches that are often papular, symmetrically involving the extensor aspects of the extremities, fingers, face, and trunk.

ACNE. Acne is an important disease of the youth.

BIBLIOGRAPHY

Browne SC: Yaws. Int J Dermatol 21:220, 1982

Canizares O: A Manual of Dermatology for Developing Countries. New York, Oxford University Press, 1983

Elpern DJ: The dermatology of Kauai, Hawaii, 1981–1982. Int J Dermatol 24:647, 1985

Failmezgar TC: A clinical survey of skin diseases in selected Latin American countries. Int J Dermatol 17:583, 1978

Kerdel-Vegas F: American leishmaniasis. Int J Dermatol 21:291, 1982

Magana M: Mycetoma. Int J Dermatol 23:221, 1984

Nelson DA, Gustafson TL, Spielvogel RL: Clinical aspects of cutaneous leishmaniasis acquired in Texas. J Am Acad Dermatol 12:985, 1985

Radentz WH: Leishmaniasis. J Assoc Milit Dermatol 13(Fall):15, 1987

Talhari S, Souza Cunha MG, Mendes Schettin AP et

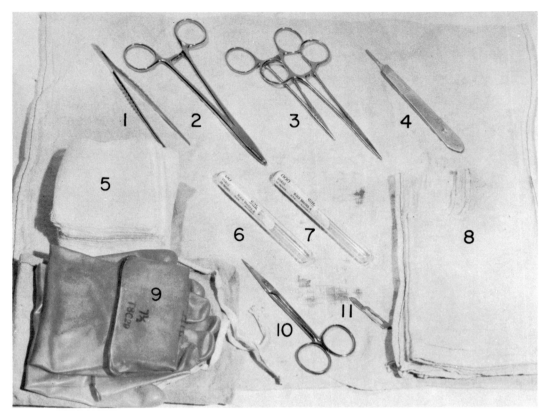

Figure 37–2. **Skin biopsy setup.**

Keyes, Miltex, #33-20, #33-24, #33-26, #33-28. Disposable biopsy punches are available.

OPTIONAL EQUIPMENT

Wood's light, Burton Fluorescing Ultra-Violet Light, #31501 (for diagnosing tinea of the scalp, tinea versicolor, and erythrasma)

Dry Ice Kit, Kidde Manufacturing Company, Bloomfield, NJ, #5605125 (for treating small hemangiomas, warts, seborrheic keratoses, and other superficial growths)

Liquid nitrogen and container. See p. 48.

Moto-Tool Hand Drill, Dremel Manufacturing Company, Racine, WI 53406, Model #2401, with steel cutters #9906 and #9908 (for debriding tinea of nails)

Magnifying visor, such as Optivisor, for close-up and fine work

Head lamp, such as the Lempert model, for adequate and directed illumination for examination and surgery

BIBLIOGRAPHY

Consult the surgical references and texts listed in Chapter 7.

Davis RS: New equipment and instruments for excisional surgery. Clin Dermatol 5:11, 1987

Grabski WJ, Salasche SJ, Lewis CW: Making the system work for you: Ordering surgical supplies and instruments. J Assoc Milit Dermatol 14(2):8, 1988

38

Where to Look For More Information About a Skin Disease

"Doctor, I saw a patient yesterday who was diagnosed as having epidermolysis bullosa. I understand this is quite a rare condition. Where can I find the latest information on this subject?"

This is a question frequently asked any teaching dermatologist. A computer will give you references, and some data bases will provide information about a dermatosis. But, assuming these are not readily available, there are other sources.

First, I would suggest that the inquiring physician or student check out the Dictionary-Index of this book. Even for rare conditions there will at least be a definition of the disease. The bibliographies at the end of each chapter can also point one in the right direction for books or papers on a given subject.

Second, there are several comprehensive general texts on dermatology that include rare diseases. The following are suggested:

Arnold HL Jr, Odum RB, James W: Andrew's Diseases of the Skin, 8th ed. Philadelphia, WB Saunders, 1989

Demis DJ, Dahl M, Smith EB, Thiers BH: Clinical Dermatology, 4 volumes, loose-leaf. Philadelphia, JB Lippincott. Yearly revisions.

Fitzpatrick TB, Eisen AZ, Wolff K, Freedberg IM, Austin KF: Dermatology in General Medicine, 3rd ed, 2 volumes. New York, McGraw-Hill Book Company, 1987

Moschella SL, Hurley HJ: Dermatology, 2nd ed, 2 volumes. Philadelphia, WB Saunders, 1985

Rook A, Wilkinson DS, Ebling FJG, Champion RH, Burton JL: Textbook of Dermatology, 4th ed, 3 volumes. Chicago, Year Book–Blackwell, 1986

These books fall into the category of color atlases:

Rassner G, Kahn G: Atlas of Dermatology. Baltimore, Urban & Schwarzenberg, 1983

Rosen T, Martin S: Atlas of Black Dermatology. Boston, Little, Brown & Co, 1981

Schaumburg-Lever G, Lever WF: Color Atlas of Histopathology of the Skin. Philadelphia, JB Lippincott, 1989

After these larger texts are consulted, then I would suggest that a computer search be done. A computer search on MEDLARS, or through other data bases, would direct one to pertinent references. MEDLARS (MEDical Literature Analysis and Retrieval System) provides computer-produced literature searches, using Index Medicus from 1966 to present. Available from the National Library of Medicine is a *Guide to MEDLARS Services* (Assistant to the Director, National Library of Medicine, 8600 Rockville Pike, Bethesda, MD 20014).

These journals are very pertinent:

Archives of Dermatology, a monthly journal published by the American Medical Association, Chicago. It is indexed in both the June and December issues.

Cutis, a monthly magazine for the general practitioner, published by Dun-Donnelley Publications, New York 10017.

Index Medicus, published monthly by the National Library of Medicine, and the *Cumulated Index Medicus,* published annually by the American Medical Association, Chicago. These contain current references to published papers and books, listed according to subject.

International Journal of Dermatology, a monthly journal, is the organ of the Society of Tropical Dermatology, published by JB Lippincott, Philadelphia.

Journal of the American Academy of Dermatology, a monthly journal, published by the American Academy of Dermatology, Evanston, IL 60201.

Journal of Investigative Dermatology, a monthly journal published by the Society of Investigative Dermatology, Baltimore, MD 21202.

Year Book of Dermatology is published annually by Year Book Medical Publishers, Chicago. The *Year Book* contains abstracts of the majority of important articles related to the field of dermatology.

There are also many excellent foreign journals. Those in English include *Acta Dermato-Venereologica,* Stockholm, and the *British Journal of Dermatology,* London.

Specialized journals include:

American Journal of Cosmetic Surgery, quarterly, American Board of Cosmetic Surgery, Los Angeles, California.

American Journal of Dermatopathology, quarterly, New York, Masson Publishing.

Clinics in Dermatology, quarterly, Philadelphia, JB Lippincott.

Pediatric Dermatology, quarterly, Boston, Blackwell.

Seminars in Dermatology, quarterly, New York, Thieme-Stratton.

Sexually Transmitted Diseases, quarterly, Philadelphia, JB Lippincott.

Reviews of dermatology include:

Callen JP et al (eds): Current Issues in Dermatology. Boston, GK Hall

Epstein E (ed): Controversies in Dermatology. Philadelphia, WB Saunders

Fleischmajer R (ed): Progress in Diseases of the Skin. New York, Grune & Stratton

Rook AJ, Maibach HI (eds): Recent Advances in Dermatology. New York, Churchill Livingstone, issued occasionally

For further specialized information on a subject the bibliography at the end of the appropriate chapters in this book should be helpful.

Here are a few additional books that cannot be readily classified:

Ackerman AB, Ragaz A: The Lives of Lesions. Chicago, Year Book Medical Publishers, 1983

Korting G: Practical Dermatology of the Genital Region. Philadelphia, WB Saunders, 1981

Krusinski PA, Flowers FP: Life-threatening Dermatoses. Boca Raton, FL, CRC Press, 1987

Shelley WB, Shelley ED: Advanced Dermatologic Therapy. Philadelphia, WB Saunders, 1987

Finally, a unique older publication is *A Dictionary of Dermatological Words, Terms and Phrases,* by Leider and Rosenblum. It was published by McGraw-Hill, New York, in 1968. Any interested student or physician will enjoy this dictionary and profit by perusing it.

For a list of dermatologic lay organizations and registries, consult volume 17 (1987), page 280 of the *Journal of the American Academy of Dermatology.*

Dictionary-Index

The purpose of the dictionary portion of this index is to define and classify some of the rarer dermatologic terms not covered in the text. Some very rare or unimportant terms have purposely been omitted, but undoubtedly some terms that are *not* rare and *are* important have also been omitted. Most of the histopathologic terms have been defined. Suggestions or corrections from the reader will be appreciated.

Abscess, 155

Acantholytic dermatosis, transient (Grover's disease). Characterized by intensely pruritic, small, firm, reddish-brown papules mainly on the upper torso, aggravated by sweating. Seen predominantly in white, older men. Histologically there is acantholysis of the epidermis.

Acanthoma, clear cell, 334

Acanthosis. An increase in thickness of the prickle cell layer.

Acanthosis nigricans, 263, 305

Achromia parasitica, 143, 352

Acid skin. An idiomatic term of black Americans for recurrent scaly eruptions, such as *tinea versicolor* or *seborrheic dermatitis*, thought to be caused by eating excess "acid" foods.

Acne, 123, 341
  conglobata, 158
  instruction sheet, 128
  necrotica miliaris, 154
  neonatal, 341
  rosacea, 131
  seborrhea complex, 7

Acne varioliformis. A chronic inflammatory disorder in adults on the scalp, the forehead, the nose and the cheeks, and rarely the trunk, characterized by the presence of papulopustular lesions that heal within a few days,

leaving a smallpox-like scar. Recurrent outbreaks can continue for months and years.

Acquired immunodeficiency syndrome (AIDS), 102, 197–203
  relevance to dermatology, 198
  and nails, 282
  in newborns, 342

Acrocyanosis. Characterized by constant coldness and bluish discoloration of the fingers and the toes, which is more intense in cold weather.

Acrodermatitis chronica atrophicans. This is a chronic, biphasic disease rather commonly seen in western Europe. The first phase begins with an erythematous patch on an extremity, which, in weeks or months, develops the second phase of skin atrophy. The cause is believed to be a mixed infection with group B arboviruses, transmitted by the wood tick *Ixodes ricinus*, and a penicillin-sensitive bacterium or spirochete.

Acrodermatitis enteropathica, 350

Acrodermatitis, papular, of childhood. *See* Gianotti-Crosti syndrome

Acrodermatitis perstans (Fig. DI–1). A chronic pustular dermatitis of hands and feet identical with or related to *pustular psoriasis, pustular bacterid,* and *dermatitis repens.*

Acrodynia, 350

Acrokeratosis, paraneoplastic (Bazex's syndrome). A specific sign of cancer of the upper respiratory and upper digestive tracts characterized by plum-colored acral skin lesions, paronychia, nail dysplasias, and keratoderma.

Acrokeratosis verruciformis. A rare disease affecting the dorsa of the hands and the feet characterized by flat warty papules. Probably hereditary. Differentiate from *flat warts* and from *epidermodysplasia verruciformis.*

Acromegaly, 259

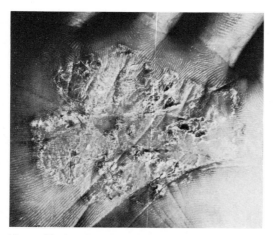

Figure DI–1. **Acrodermatitis perstans.**

riasis, scleroderma, prickly heat, vitamin A deficiency, and other diseases. Partial anhidrosis is produced by many antiperspirants.

Anhidrotic asthenia, tropical. Described in the South Pacific and in the desert in World War II. Soldiers showed increased sweating of neck and face and anhidrosis (lack of sweating) below the neck. It was accompanied by weakness, headaches, and subjective warmth and was considered a chronic phase of prickly heat.

Anonychia, 282

Anthralin. A proprietary name for dihydroxyanthranol, which is a strong reducing agent useful in the treatment of chronic cases of psoriasis. Its action is similar to that of chrysarobin.

Anthrax. A primary chancre-type disease caused by *Bacillus anthracis*, occurring in persons who work with the hides and the hair of infected sheep, horses, or cattle. A pulmonary form is known.

Antibody-mediated immunity, 101

Antimalarial agents. Dermatologically active agents include quinacrine (Atabrine), chloroquine (Aralen), and hydroxychloroquine (Plaquenil). Their mode of action is unknown, but these agents are used in the treatment of chronic discoid lupus erythematosus and the polymorphic actinic dermatoses (see p. 254).

Aphthous stomatitis, 184, 284

Apocrine adenomas, 335

Apocrinitis, 156

Argyll Robertson pupils. Small irregular pupils that fail to react to light but react to accommodation. This is a late manifestation of neurosyphilis, particularly tabes.

Argyria, 248

Arnold, Dr. Harry, 371

Arsenic. Inorganic arsenic preparations include Fowler's solution and Asiatic pills and are used in the treatment of resistant cases of psoriasis but can cause arsenical pigmentation and keratoses. Organic arsenic agents include neoarsphenamine and Mapharsen, used formerly in the treatment of syphilis.

Arsenical keratosis, 317
    pigmentation, 248

Arthritis, rheumatoid, 257

Arthropod dermatoses, 232

Arthus phenomenon. Characterized by local anaphylaxis in a site that has been injected repeatedly with a foreign protein.

Ashy dermatosis. Also known as erythema dyschromicum perstans. An uncommon pigmentary disorder characterized by ash-colored macules that slowly increase in size and number. The border may be erythema-

tous. Could be a variant of *erythema perstans.*

Astringents, 66

Ataxia-telangiectasia syndrome (Louis-Bar). Clinically shows oculocutaneous telangiectasia, progressive cerebellar ataxia, recurrent sinopulmonary infections, increased incidence of malignancy, x-ray hypersensitivity, and autosomal recessive inheritance.

Athlete's foot, 205

Atopic eczema. *See* Eczema, atopic

Atrophie blanche, 116, 361. Also see Atrophies of the skin.

Atrophies of the skin
  A. Congenital atrophies. Associated with other congenital ectodermal defects.
  B. Acquired atrophies
    1. Noninflammatory
       a. *Senile atrophy.* Often associated with senile pruritus and winter itch.
       b. *Linear atrophy (striae albicantes or distensae).* On abdomen, thighs, and breasts associated with pregnancy and obesity.
       c. *Secondary atrophy* from sunlight, x-radiation, injury, and nerve diseases.
       d. *Macular atrophy (anetoderma of Schweninger-Buzzi).* Characterized by the presence of small, oval, whitish depressions or slightly elevated papules, which can be pressed back into the underlying tissue. This may be an early form of von Recklinghausen's disease.
    2. Inflammatory
       a. *Acrodermatitis chronica atrophicans.* A moderately rare idiopathic atrophy in older adults, particularly women, characterized by the presence of thickened skin at the onset, with ulnar bands on the forearm, changing into atrophy of the legs below the knee and of the forearms. In the early stages this is to be differentiated from scleroderma. High doses of penicillin may be effective.
       b. *Folliculitis ulerythematosa reticulata.* A very rare reticulated atrophic condition localized to the cheeks of the face; seen mainly in young adults.
       c. *Ulerythema ophryogenes.* A rare atrophic dermatitis that affects the outer part of the eyebrows, resulting in redness, scaling, and permanent loss of the involved hair.
       d. *Macular atrophy (anetoderma of Jadassohn).* A very rare condition characterized by the appearance of circumscribed reddish macules that develop an atrophic center that pro-

Atrophies of the skin (*continued*)

gresses toward the edge of the lesion, seen mainly on the extremities.

e. *Lichen sclerosus et atrophicus (kraurosis vulvae, kraurosis penis, and balanitis xerotica obliterans)*, 256, 288, 319. An uncommon atrophic process, mainly of women, which begins as a small whitish lesion that contains a central hyperkeratotic pinpoint-sized dell. These 0.5-cm size or less whitish macules commonly coalesce to form whitish atrophic plaques. The most common localizations are on the neck, shoulders, arms, axillae, vulva, and perineum. Many consider kraurosis vulvae, kraurosis penis, and balanitis xerotica obliterans to be variants of this condition.

f. *Poikiloderma atrophicans vasculare (Jacobi)*. This rare atrophic process of adults is characterized by the development of patches of telangiectasis, atrophy, and mottled pigmentation on any area of the body. This resembles chronic radiodermatitis clinically and may be associated with dermatomyositis or scleroderma. May precede the development of a lymphoma.

g. *Hemiatrophy*. May be localized to one side of the face or may cover the entire half of the body. Vascular and neurogenic etiologies have been propounded, but most cases appear to be a form of *localized scleroderma*.

h. *Atrophoderma, idiopathic, of Pasini and Pierini*. Similar to morphea (localized scleroderma) but without induration. The round or irregular depressed atrophic areas are asymptomatic and appear mainly on the trunk of young females.

i. *Atrophie blanche*. A form of cutaneous atrophy characterized by scarlike plaques with a border of telangiectasis and hyperpigmentation that cover large areas of the legs and the ankles, mainly of middle-aged or older women.

j. *Secondary atrophy*. From inflammatory diseases such as syphilis, chronic discoid lupus erythematosus, leprosy, tuberculosis, scleroderma, etc.

Autoeczematization. *See* Id reaction

Autohemotherapy. A form of nonspecific protein therapy, administered by removing 10 ml of venous blood from the arm and then immediately injecting that blood intramuscularly into the buttocks. It has been shown to pro-

duce a fall in circulating eosinophils, presumably due to a mild increase in the adrenal steroid hormones.

Ayres, Dr. Samuel, III, 368

B cells, 94

Babinski's reflex. Extension of the toes instead of flexion following stimulation of the sole of the foot, due to lesions of the pyramidal tract from syphilis infection or other causes.

Bacterial infection, 150
  in Latin America, 377
  scalp, 273

Bacterid, pustular, 208, 210

Bacteriologic dermatoses, 150, 377

Balanitis, fusospirochetal, 288

Balanitis xerotica obliterans (Fig. DI–2), 288

Bangor, Maine, 368

Barber's itch, 154

Bartonellosis, 384

Basal cell carcinoma, 290, 319

Basal cell nevoid syndrome (Fig. DI–3). This is a rare hereditary affliction characterized primarily by multiple genetically determined basal cell carcinomas, cysts of the jaws, peculiar pits of the hands and the feet, and developmental anomalies of the ribs, the spine, and the skull.

Baths, 37, 46

Bazex's syndrome. *See* Acrokeratosis, paraneoplastic

Bazin's disease. *See* Erythema induratum

Beau's lines, 281

Becker's melanosis. Large localized hypermelanotic and hypertrichotic patches associated with underlying structural abnormalities.

Bedbug bites, 372

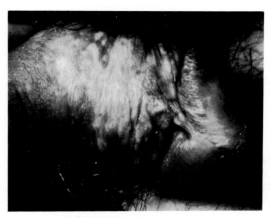

Figure DI–2. Balanitis xerotica obliterans of the penis. (*Dr. D. Morgan*)

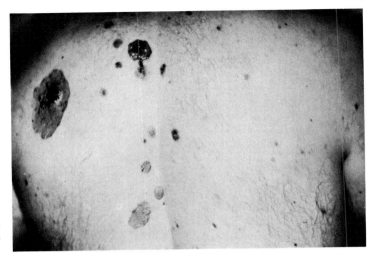

Figure DI–3. **Basal cell nevoid syndrome.** Back lesions. The patient also had radiographic evidence of bone cysts in the mandible.

Burn
    seaweed, 371
    sun, 289, 298
Burow's solution. A solution of aluminum acetate that in its original formula contained lead. A lead-free Burow's solution for wet dressings can be made by adding Domeboro tablets or powder to water to make a 1:20 or 1:10 solution.
Burton, Dr. Arthur, 368
Bypass syndrome. *See* Intestinal bypass syndrome

Cactus granuloma, 370
Café-au-lait spots, 266
Calcifying epithelioma (Malherbe), 335
Calcinosis. *Localized calcinosis* can occur in many tumors of the skin and following chronic inflammatory lesions, such as severe acne. *Metabolic calcinosis* may or may not be associated with an excess of blood calcium and is divided into universal calcinosis and circumscribed calcinosis.
Callus, 191. A hyperkeratotic plaque of the skin due to chronic pressure and friction.
    of mucous membranes, 319
Canada, 366
Cancer
    internal, 263
    skin. *See* Carcinoma
Candidiasis, 221
Canities. Gray or white hair.
Canker sores, 181, 284
Carbuncle, 156
Carcinoid syndrome, 335. A potentially malignant tumor of the argentaffin chromaffin cells of the appendix or the ileum. Some of these tumors or their metastases produce large amounts of serotonin (5-hydroxytryptamine), which causes transient flushing of the skin accompanied by weakness, nausea, abdominal pain, diarrhea, and sweating. The redness usually begins on the head and the neck and then extends down on the body. These episodes last from several minutes to a few hours. Repeated attacks of the erythema lead to the formation of permanent telangiectasias and a diffuse reddish-purple hue to the skin. The diagnosis can be made by the finding of over 25 mg of 5-hydroxyindoleacetic acid in a 24-hour urine.
Carcinoma
    basal cell, 290, 319
    metastatic, 336
    squamous cell, 290, 321
        with dermatomyositis, 257
    with skin lesions, 336

Carotinosis, 248
Caseation necrosis. Histologically, this is a form of tissue death with loss of structural detail leaving pale eosinophilic, amorphous, finely granular material. It is seen especially in tuberculosis, syphilis, granuloma annulare, and beryllium granuloma.
Cat-scratch disease, 342. Manifested by inflammation at the site of a cat scratch or bite obtained a few days previously. Malaise, headache, low-grade fever, chills, generalized lymphadenopathy, and splenomegaly occur. A maculopapular rash or erythema nodosum–like eruption occurs occasionally.
Caterpillar dermatitis. An irritating chemical is released when the hairs of some species of caterpillars penetrate the skin. The onset of irritation is quite immediate. Red macular lesions, then urticarial papules, and occasionally vesicles develop in areas exposed. Mild lesions can be gone in 12 hours, but more extensive cases can take several days to resolve. In these more severe cases occasionally there can be constitutional symptoms of restlessness and headache. Therapy is not very effective or necessary. Scotch tape over the affected skin might pull out some of the bristle-like hairs.
Causalgia. A condition characterized by burning pain aggravated by touching the neuralgic site.
Cell-mediated immunity, 102
Cellular elements, 1
Cellulitis, 158
    dissecting of the scalp, 158
    eosinophilic. *See* Eosinophilic cellulitis
Central American dermatoses, 374
Chagas' disease, 383
Chalazion. A small cyst of the meibomian glands of the eyelid.
Chamomile solution. A solution of whole chamomile flowers used in wet dressings for its mild anti-inflammatory action. The solution can be conveniently made by the addition of a Chamo-Powder (Dome) packet to 1 pint of tap water.
Chancre
    monorecidive. A relapsing form of syphilis characterized by the development of a lesion reduplicating the primary sore.
    primary, 167
Chancre-type, primary disease. *See* Primary chancre-type diseases
Chancroid, 163
Charcot joints. A type of joint destruction in patients with central nervous system syphilis of the paretic type.
Chédiak-Higashi syndrome. A fatal syndrome in children characterized by pigmentary dis-

Drill, 389
Drug eruptions, 85–92
    photosensitivity, 91, 293
Drugs
    internal, 44
    local, 36
    office, 42
Dry ice, 48
Dry ice kit, 389
Duhring's disease. *See* Dermatitis herpetiformis
Duke's disease, 350
Dyshidrosis (Fig. DI–4), 210. A syndrome charac-
    terized by blisters on the palms of hands
    and feet. If the cause is known, this term
    should not be used. The common causes of
    dyshidrosis, or *pompholyx*, are mycotic,
    contact dermatitis and drugs, and it is also
    associated as a manifestation of a general-
    ized skin disease.
Dyskeratoma, warty, 334
Dyskeratosis, benign. A histopathologic finding of
    faulty keratinization of individual epider-
    mal cells with formation of corps ronds and
    grains. Seen in Darier's disease and occa-
    sionally in familial benign chronic pemphi-
    gus.
Dykeratosis congenita. With pigmentation, dystro-
    phia unguis, and leukokeratosis oris, this is
    a rare syndrome characterized by a reticu-
    lated pigmentation, particularly of the neck,
    dystrophy of the nails, and a leukoplakia-
    like condition of the oral mucosa. Increased
    sweating and thickening of palms and soles
    may occur.
Dyskeratosis, malignant. A histopathologic finding
    in Bowen's disease and also in squamous
    cell carcinoma and senile keratosis in
    which premature and typical keratinization
    of individual cells is seen.

Ear fungus, 107
Ear piercing, 158
Ecchymoses. *See* Purpura
Eccrine tumors, 336
Echovirus infection, 196
Ecthyma, 153
Ectodermal defect, congenital, 303, 346
Ectodermosis erosiva pluriorificialis. A synonym for
    Stevens-Johnson form of erythema multi-
    forme.
Eczema
    in Arizona, 370
    atopic, 77, 266, 303
    craquelé. A French term for cracked-appearing
        skin, especially seen on the legs.
    infantile, 77
    nummular, 83
    pityriasis simplex variety, 350
    tropical, 384
Ehlers-Danlos syndrome, 305
Elastosis perforans serpiginosa. A rare asymptoma-
    tic disease in which keratotic papules occur
    in a circinate arrangement around a slightly
    atrophic patch, usually on the neck.
Electrocautery, 47
Electrocoagulation, 47
Electrodesiccation, 47
Electrolysis, 47
Electrosection, 47
Electrosurgery, 47
Elephantiasis, 383
    nostras (Fig. DI–5), 158
    from radiation, 292

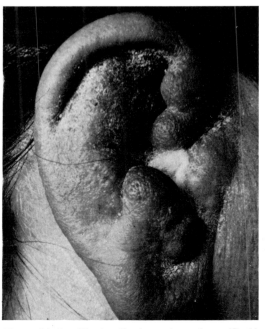

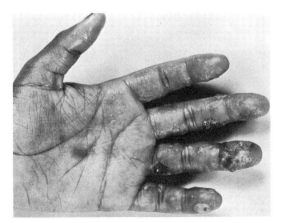

Figure DI–4. **Dyshidrosis with secondary infection in a black patient.**

Figure DI–5. **Elephantiasis nostras of ear.** (*Dr. M. Feldaker*)

Embolic nodules, 116. Emboli can come from a left atrial myxoma or from arteriosclerotic plaques.

Eosinophilic cellulitis (Well's syndrome). Characterized by sudden onset of pruritic, red, infiltrated, urticaria-like patches, which persist for 3 to 4 weeks and can recur.

Eosinophilic granuloma, 262

Ephelides, 338, 355

Epidermal tumors, 333

Epidermis, 3

Epidermodysplasia verruciformis. A rare, apparently hereditary disease manifested by papulosquamous and warty lesions present at birth with no site of predilection. The prognosis for life is poor because of the eventual development of squamous cell carcinomas from the lesions.

Epidermolysis bullosa, 236

Epidermophytid. A dermatophytid due to *Epidermophyton* infection. *See also* Id reaction

Epidermophytosis. A fungus infection due to *Epidermophyton.*

Epiloia. A triad of mental deficiency, epilepsy, and adenoma sebaceum. *See also* Adenoma sebaceum

Epithelioma
    apocrine, 335
    basal cell, 319
    calcifying, 335
    eccrine, 336
    sebaceous, 335
    squamous cell, 290, 321

Epulis. This term refers to any growth involving the gums.
    giant-cell. This is a solitary neoplasm or granuloma from the periosteum of the jaw bone in the gingival area.

Equipment, 386

Erosio interdigitale blastomycetica. A complex term signifying a candidal infection of the webs of the fingers.

Erysipelas, 158

Erysipeloid. A chancre-type infection on the hand occurring at the site of accidental inoculation with the organism *Erysipelothrix rhusiopathiae*, seen in butchers, veterinarians, and fishermen. A localized form runs its course in 2 to 4 weeks. A generalized form develops a diffuse eruption with occasional constitutional symptoms such as arthritis. A very rare systemic form exhibits an eruption, joint pains, and endocarditis.

Erythema ab igne (Fig. DI-6). A marmoraceous-appearing redness that follows the local application to the skin of radiant heat such as from a heating pad.

Erythema dyschromicum perstans. *See* Ashy dermatosis

Erythema elevatum diutinum. A persistent nodular,

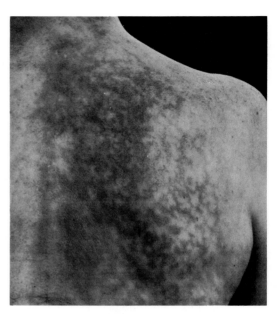

Figure DI-6. **Erythema ab igne from a hot water bottle.** (*K.U.M.C.*)

symmetrical eruption usually seen in middle-aged males with a rather characteristic histologic picture. This may be a deeper form of *granuloma annulare.*

Erythema induratum, 115

Erythema infectiosum, 195

Erythema Jacquet, 349

Erythema multiforme, 114
    in Arizona, 370
    bullosum, 241

Erythema of the ninth day. A morbilliform erythema of sudden onset appearing around the ninth day after the initiation of organic arsenic therapy for the treatment of syphilis. It may be accompanied by generalized lymphadenopathy and fever.

Erythema nodosum, 115

Erythema, palmar. Redness of the palms of the hands, which may be due to heredity, pulmonary disease, liver disease, rheumatoid arthritis, or pregnancy.

Erythema perstans (Fig. DI-7). Over a dozen entities have been described that fit into this persistent group of diseases that resemble erythema multiforme. The following entities are included in this group: *erythema annulare centrifugum (Darier)*; *erythema chronicum migrans (Lipschutz)*, which may be due to a tick bite, as in Lyme disease; *erythema gyratum perstans (Fox)*; *erythema figuratum perstans (Wende)*; and *erythema gyratum repens (Gammel).*

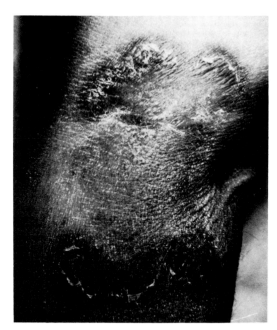

Figure DI–7. **Erythema perstans.** Chronic lesions on elbow. (*Drs. L. Grayson and H. Shair*)

Erythermalgia. *See* Erythromelalgia

Erythrasma, 158

Erythredema. *See* Acrodynia

Erythroderma(s), 242, 349

    T cell. *See* Sézary syndrome, 338

Erythrodermia desquamativa. Another term for Leiner's disease.

Erythromelalgia or erythermalgia. A rare disorder of hands and feet, most common in middle age; characterized by burning pain, which is activated by exertion or heat and is refractory to treatment.

Erythromelanosis follicularis faciei et colli. A very rare dermatosis of the cheeks and neck, seen usually in young males. Clinically one sees a slightly hyperpigmented scaly follicular eruption.

Erythroplasia of Queyrat, 334

Erythropoietic protoporphyria, 297

Erythrose pigmentaire peribuccale. A rare condition of middle-aged women, characterized by diffuse brownish red pigmentation about the mouth, the chin, and the neck with or without a slight burning sensation.

Espundia, 381

Exanthem subitum. Another term for roseola infantum or sixth disease.

Excisions, 57

Exclamation mark hairs, 272

Exfoliative dermatitis, 242, 349

External otitis, 107

Exudative discoid and lichenoid chronic dermatosis, 373–374

Fabry's disease, 305

Factitial dermatitis, 265

Failmezger, T. C., 376

Fall dermatoses, 28

Familial benign chronic pemphigus, 237

Fat necrosis

    of newborn, 349

    subcutaneous, with pancreatic disease, 115. Histologic picture is quite characteristic.

Fat tissue tumors, 336

Fatal granulomatous disease of childhood. A very rare, X-linked disease of males mainly characterized by eczematous lesions in infancy with progressive chronic granulomatous bacterial infections.

Favre-Racouchot syndrome. The term for multiple comedomes on the high cheek and temple areas in older persons.

Female-pattern hair loss, 270

Fever blisters, 181, 286

Fibroma, pedunculated, 311

Fibrosarcoma, 323, 336

Fifth disease, 195

Filariasis, 383

Fire ant stings, 371

Fixed drug eruption, 91

Flea bites, 372

Fluorinated corticosteroids, 43

Fluorouracil method, for actinic/senile keratoses, 317

Fogo selvagem, 384

Folliculitis, 153

    beard, 154

    decalvans, 154

    scalp, 154

    superficial, 154

Folliculitis, perforating, of the nose (Fig. DI–8). A folliculitis of the stiff hairs of the nasal mucocutaneous junction that penetrates deeply through to the external nasal skin. Unless the basic pathology is understood and corrected by plucking the involved stiff

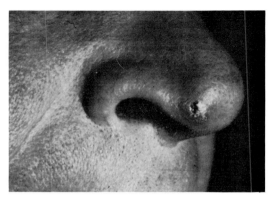

Figure DI–8. **Folliculitis, perforating, of the nose.** (*Dr. C. Lessenden*)

Folliculitis, perforating, of the nose (*continued*)
hair, the condition cannot be cured. The external papule can simulate a skin cancer.
Food testing, 11
Foot-and-mouth disease, 287
Fordyce's disease, 286
Foreign body granuloma, 228. *See also* Granuloma, foreign body
Formulary, 36
Foshay test. A 48-hour intradermal test that, if positive, indicates that the person has or has had *tularemia.*
Fourth disease. Another term for Duke's disease.
Fox-Fordyce disease (Fig. DI–9). A rare, intensely pruritic, chronic papular dermatosis of the axillae and the pubic area in women. The intense itching is due to the closure of the apocrine gland pore with rupture of the duct and escape of the apocrine sweat into the surrounding epidermis.
Fragrance products, 67
Frambesia. *See* Yaws
Freckles, 338, 355
Fröhlich's syndrome, 259
Frostbite. Exposure to cold can cause pathologic changes in the skin that are related to the severity of the exposure but vary with the susceptibility of the person. Other terms in use that refer to cold injuries under varying conditions include *trench foot, immersion foot, pernio,* and *chilblain. See also* Chilblain
Fulguration, 47
Fungus diseases, 204. *See also* Tinea
elements, 204
examination, 11

culture, 11
scraping, 11
infections, Latin America, 375
Furuncle, 155
Fusospirochetal balanitis, 288

Galveston, Texas, 370
Gangosa. A severe ulcerative and mutilating form of yaws affecting the palate, the pharynx, and nasal tissues.
Gangrene, symmetrical peripheral. A rare syndrome associated with a multitude of underlying medical problems. Disseminated intravascular coagulation occurs in many cases.
Gardner's syndrome. An autosomal dominant trait with osteomas, fibrous and fatty tumors, and epidermoid inclusion cysts of the skin, and multiple polyposes.
Gaucher's disease, 263
Gell and Coombs' classification, 97
General paresis. A psychosis due to syphilitic meningoencephalitis.
Genetic counseling, 299
Genodermatoses, 299
Gentian violet. A pararosaniline dye that destroys gram-positive bacteria and some fungi.
Geographic skin diseases
Central and South America, 311
North America, 366
Geographic tongue, 284
Geriatric dermatoses, 259, 355
Gianotti-Crosti syndrome (papular acrodermatitis of childhood). Characterized by acute onset of symmetrical, red or flesh-colored, flat-topped papules, usually 2 to 3 mm in diameter, mainly on the face and limbs. Nonpruritic, they last about 3 weeks. The cause is a virus, sometimes of the hepatitis type.
Glands
sebaceous, 7
sweat, 7
infections of, 156
Glandular appendages, 6
Glomus body, 5
tumor, 5, 337
Glossitis, 287
Glossitis rhomboidea mediana, 287
Glossodynia, 287
Glucagonoma syndrome. A glucagon-secreting islet cell neoplasm of the pancreas results in a polymorphous skin eruption characterized by superficial epidermal necrosis with fragile blister formation (necrolytic migratory erythema). The perioral area and intertriginous areas are frequently involved.
Gonorrhea, 167
Gonorrheal dermatosis, 167. *See also* Keratosis blenorrhagica

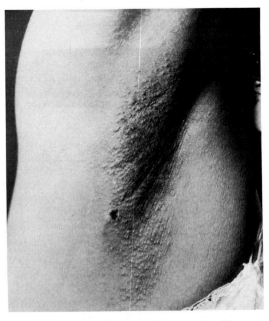

Figure DI–9. **Fox-Fordyce disease of axilla.**

Gottran papules. Flat reddish papules on the knuckles seen in 30% of the patients with advanced dermatomyositis.

Gougerot-Blum disease, 118

Graft-versus-host disease. Both the acute and chronic disease are accompanied by erythematous lesions that may develop into an erythroderma, with bullae and necrolysis. The chronic type can eventuate in sclerodermatous-like lesions with ulcerations. Nails and hair can be affected.

Grain itch. Due to a mite, *Pediculoides ventricosus*, that lives on insects that attack wheat and corn. This mite can attack humans working with the infested grain and cause a markedly pruritic papular and papulovesicular eruption.

Granular cell schwannoma, 336

Granuloma, 1, 228

    chronic cutaneous, 371

    foreign body, 228. A granulomatous reaction seen in the dermis due to the introduction, usually by trauma, of certain agents such as lipids, petrolatum, paraffin, indelible pencil, silica and silicates (talc), suture, hair, and zirconium from certain deodorants.

    swimming pool, 371. *See also* Swimming pool granuloma

Granuloma annulare, 230

Granuloma faciale. Typically occurs as brownish papules or plaques, multiple or single, usually on the face, in middle-aged or older persons (usually males).

Granuloma inguinale, 163

Granuloma pyogenicum, 163, 330, 336

Granuloma silica, 230

Granulomatosis

    allergic. *See* Allergic granulomatosis

    lymphomatoid. *See* Lymphomatoid granulomatosis

Granulomatous dermatoses, 228

Granulomatous disease of childhood, chronic. An inherited disorder of leukocyte function characterized by indolent infections of the skin, as well as lymph nodes, lungs, liver, spleen, bone, and bone marrow.

Granulosis rubra nasi, 350

Grenz ray therapy, 50

Griseofulvin therapy, 209

Ground substance, 3

Grover's disease. *See* Acantholytic dermatosis, transient

Gumma, 175

Habit-tic nail deformity, 283

Haeberlein, Dr. Robert W., Jr., 368

Hailey-Hailey disease, 237, 303

Hair

    diseases, 268

        rare, 274

    excess, 268

    facts, 6, 268

    fragility, 275

    follicles, 6

    gray, 268

    green, 275

    growth, 6

    ingrown, 275

    ingrown beard, 275

    kinking, 274

    lanugo, 6

    loss, 270

    spun-glass, 274

    twisted, 275

    vellus, 6

Hair casts, 235

Hair coloring, 64

Hair preparations, 63–64

Hair waving, 64

Halitosis, 287

Halo nevus, 328, 354

Hansen's disease, 166

Harlequin fetus, 300, 346

Hartnup disease, 298

Hapalonychia, 283

Helminthic dermatoses, 232, 383

Hemangioma, 323, 340

    capillary, 327

    cavernous, 325

    nuchal, 327

    port-wine, 327

    sclerosing, 323

    senile, 327

    spider, 326

    superficial, 325

Hematoma, subungual, 332

Hematomata. *See* Purpura

Hemochromatosis, 248. A rare hereditary metabolic disease characterized by a deposit of hemosiderin in the glandular tissues, and hemofuscin in the connective tissues, the spleen, and the smooth muscles.

Hemorrhagic telangiectasis, 305, 327

Hemorrhoids, 108

Hemostasis, 56

Henoch-Schönlein purpura, 118

Herald patch, 139

Hereditary skin diseases, 299

Herpangina, 196. A name applied to a primary form of virus infection of the herpes simplex type that occurs on the mucous membranes of the mouth in children. Fever and malaise accompany this acute infection, which lasts approximately 2 weeks. *See also* Herpes simplex

Herpes simplex, 181, 286

    in immunocompromised patients, 185

    recurrent genital, 184

Lymphogranulomatosis benigna. *See* Sarcoidosis

Lymphoma, 265, 332, 338

Lymphomatoid granulomatosis. This is a serious vasculitis, primarily of the lungs. Skin lesions occur in more than one third of patients, mainly erythematous papules, plaques, and subcutaneous nodules, which may ulcerate.

Lymphomatoid papulosis. Self-healing, erythematous, maculopapular lesions that occasionally ulcerate. Clinically these look benign, but histologically they appear malignant. The more chronic form may eventuate as a lymphoma, but most cases run a benign course.

Lynch, Dr. Peter J., 370

McAllen, Texas, 370

McGowan, Dr. Thomas, 366

Maculae cerulae, 235

Maddin, Dr. Stuart, 366

Majocchi's disease, 118

Majocchi's granuloma. A deep mycotic infection usually due to animal fungi.

Makeup products, 66

Male-pattern hair loss, 270

Malignant disease. *See* Cancer; Carcinoma

Malignant melanoma, 290, 331

Malherbe's tumor. Calcifying epithelioma. *See also* Tumors

Mange. A skin condition particularly of dogs caused by allergic eczema, seborrheic dermatitis, bacterial infection, or parasitic infestation of the skin.

Mask of pregnancy, 245

Mast cell disease, 98, 266

Mast cells, 3

Mastocytosis, 266

Measles, 194

Measles, German, 194

Mechanobulbous disorders, 303

Median canaliform dystrophy, 283

Mees' lines, 282

Melanocytes, 4

Melanocytic nevi, 328

Melanoma
    benign juvenile, 328, 354
    malignant, 290, 331

Melanonychia, 280

Melanosis of Riehl. A brownish pigmentation of the skin on the sun-exposed areas of the body that have come into contact with certain tars. *See* Poikiloderma of Civatte *and* Pigmentary disorders

Melasma, 245

Melioidosis. An infectious disease of rodents and humans with abscesses and pustules of the skin and other organs, similar to glanders.

Menopause state, 259

Menthol, 43

Mercury, ammoniated. This is an antiseptic chemical that, prior to the advent of the antibiotics, was useful in the treatment of impetigo and other pyodermas. It is valuable in the treatment of psoriasis. *See* p. 43.

Mesodermal tumors, 336

Miami, Florida, 371

Milia, 341

Miliara, 8
    rubra, 8, 156, 349, 378

Military dermatoses, 28

Milker's nodules, 368. A virus disease contracted from infected udders of cows. The lesions, usually on the hands, consist of brownish-red or purple firm nodules that subside in 4 to 6 weeks, conferring immunity.

Miller, Dr. Otis, 370

Millikan, Dr. Larry E., 371

Milwaukee, Wisconsin, 368

Moeller's glossitis, 287

Moisturizers, 66

Moles, *See* Nevus

Molluscum contagiosum, 192, 352

Mongolian spots, 340

Monilethrix, 275

Monilial intertrigo, 221, 346

Monilial paronychia, 221

Moniliasis, 221
    in South, 370

Monoclonal antibodies. These are specific antibodies produced from a hybrid cell. This hybrid cell results from the fusion of nuclear material from two cells.

Mononucleosis, infectious, 194

Morbilliform rash, 194

Morphea, 256, 350

Mosaic "fungus." This is not a fungus but an artifact commonly found in KOH slide preparations taken from the feet and the hands.

Mouth diseases, 284, 287

Mucinosis. When fibroblasts produce an excess amount of acid mucopolysaccharides (mucin), they may replace the connective tissue elements. This occurs in myxedema and localized pretibial myxedema. *See also* Myxedema, localized

follicular (alopecia mucinosa). This rare disease is characterized by one or more asymptomatic, well-circumscribed, indurated, slightly erythematous plaques with loss of hair. The most common site is the face. The plaques involute spontaneously after several months. Some cases are associated with a T-cell lymphoma.

papular. A rare cutaneous fibromucinous disease with a monoclonal serum protein of cathodal mobility. Clinically seen are localized or generalized papules, plaques, or nodules.

Papular mucinosis (*continued*) lesions are probably part of a systemic dysproteinemia. *See* Scleromyxedema

Papular urticaria, 349

Papulosis

lymphomatoid. *See* Lymphomatoid papulosis

malignant atrophying (Degos' disease). A predominantly fatal disease with spotty vascular lesions and subsequent atrophy of the overlying tissues, affecting the skin, intestines, and other organs including the brain, kidney and heart. It is differentiated from thromboangiitis obliterans and periarteritis nodosa.

Papulosquamous dermatoses, 133

Paracoccidioidomycosis, 381

Paraffinoma. A foreign body granuloma due to the injection of paraffin into the subcutaneous tissue for cosmetic purposes.

Parakeratosis. An example of imperfect keratinization of the epidermis resulting in the retention of nuclei in the horny layer. In areas of parakeratosis the granular layer is absent.

Parapsoriasis. A term for a group of persistent macular and maculopapular scaly erythrodermas. An acute form with the synonym *pityriasis lichenoides et varioliformis acuta (Mucha-Habermann)* (*see* entry) is now believed to be a distinct entity. One chronic form of parapsoriasis, *parapsoriasis guttata,* can resemble guttate psoriasis, pityriasis rosea, or seborrheic dermatitis. This condition does not itch and persists for years. A variant of this type of parapsoriasis is *pityriasis lichenoides chronica* (Juliusberg), which is a form of guttate psoriasis with slightly larger scaly areas. Another chronic form of parapsoriasis, *parapsoriasis en plaque,* is characterized by nonpruritic or slightly pruritic scaly brownish patches and plaques. A high percentage of patients that are given this diagnosis die with mycosis fungoides.

Parasitology, 232, 363

Parasitophobia, 233

Paronychia

bacterial, 221

candidal, 221

Pasini and Pierini atrophoderma. *See* Atrophies of the skin

Pediatric skin diseases, 340

Pediculosis, 234

Pedunculated fibromas, 311

Pellagra, 263, 298

Pemphigoid, 98

bullous, 98, 237

localized cicatricial (Brunsting-Perry), 237. In elderly patients recurrent blisters are seen, most commonly of the head and neck. Histology and immunofluorescence are similar to cicatricial mucosal pemphigoid but there is no mucous membrane involvement in this form. Heals with scarring.

Pemphigus

erythematosus, 238

familial benign chronic, 237

foliaceus, 238, 384

neonatorum, 151, 236

vegetans, 238

vulgaris, 99, 238

Perforating skin disorders. Several dermatoses exhibit epidermal perforation as a histologic feature. Many represent transepithelial elimination. Four diseases are essential perforating disorders: elastosis perforans serpiginosa, reactive perforating collagenosis, perforating folliculitis, and Kyrle's disease.

Perfumes, 67

Periadenitis mucosa necrotica recurrens, 287

Periateritis nodosa, 115

Perioral dermatitis, 69, 125

Perleche, 221

Pernio. *See* Chilblain *and* Frostbite

Petechiae, 18, 118

Peutz-Jeghers syndrome, 249

Phobias, 265

Photoallergic dermatitis, 100, 293

Photosensitivity dermatoses, 293

endogenous, 296

exogenous, 293

onycholysis, 283

reaction from drugs, 91, 293

Phrynoderma, 263

Phthiriasis. Infestation with the crab louse.

Physical agents, dermatoses of, 289

Piebaldism, 268, 304

Pigmentary dermatoses, 245, 304

classification, 248

Pigmented purpuric eruption, 118

Pili annulati, 275

Pili incarnati, 275

Pili torti, 275

Pilomatrixoma, 336

Pimples, 123

Pink disease. *See* Acrodynia

Pinta, 383

Pinworms, 108

Pitted keratolysis, 208

Pityriasis amiantacea. A distinct morphologic entity characterized by masses of sticky, silvery overlapping scales adherent to the hairs and scalp. When the thick patch of scales is removed, the underlying scalp is red and oozing and often has a foul odor. The underlying cause can be a pyoderma, neurodermatitis, or psoriasis.

Pityriasis lichenoides chronica (Juliusberg). A form of guttate parapsoriasis.

Pityriasis lichenoides et varioliformis acuta (Mucha-Habermann). This is an acute disease that appears as a reddish macular generalized eruption with mild constitutional signs including fever and malaise. Vesicles may develop and also papulonecrotic lesions. This disease gradually disappears in several months. Histologically this is characterized by a vasculitis that differentiates it from the parapsoriasis group of diseases.

Pityriasis rosea, 139

Pityriasis simplex faciei, 350, 353. A common disorder of children seen predominantly in the winter as a rather well-localized scaly oval patch on the cheeks. The end result is depigmentation of the area, but the normal pigment returns when the eruption clears up (usually in the summer). I believe this condition to be a mild form of atopic eczema.

Plantar warts, 191

"Planter's" warts, 191

Plasma cells, 3

Plummer-Vinson syndrome. A syndrome characterized by dysphagia, glossitis, hypochromic anemia, and spoon nails in middle-aged women. The associated dryness and atrophy of the mucous membranes of the throat may lead to leukoplakia and squamous cell carcinoma.

POEMS syndrome (*p*olyneuropathy, *o*rganomegaly, *e*ndocrinopathies, *M*-protein, and *s*kin changes). Cherry-type and subcutaneous hemangiomas are reported in this syndrome.

Poikiloderma atrophicans vasculare (Jacobi). *See* Atrophies of the skin

Poikiloderma of Civatte, 298, 335

Poikiloderma congenitale, 298. A rare syndrome characterized by telangiectasis, pigmentation, defective teeth, and bone cysts. This may be similar to dsykeratosis congenita.

Poison ivy dermatitis, 74

Poison oak dermatitis, 74

Polyarteritis nodosa, 259

Polymorphous light eruption, 297

Polysystemic disorders, 304

Pompholyx, 210. *See also* Dyshidrosis

Porokeratosis. A rare disorder that begins as a small, slightly elevated, wartlike papule that slowly enlarges, leaving an atrophic center with a keratotic ridgelike border. The small individual lesions may coalesce. A disseminated form (disseminated superficial actinic porokeratosis) develops in middle-aged persons on sun-exposed limbs.

Porphyria, 296
    cutanea tarda, 296
    familial variegate, 296

Port-wine hemangioma, 327

Potassium hydroxide preparation, 11

Potassium permanganate. An oxidizing antiseptic usually used as a wet dressing in the concentration of 1:10,000.

Potassium permanganate bath, 240

Powder bed, 240

Prausnitz-Küstner reaction. A demonstration of passive sensitization of the skin of a nonsensitive person. This is accomplished by the intradermal injection of serum from a sensitive patient into the skin of a nonsensitive person. After 24 to 48 hours the atopen to be tested is injected intracutaneously into the previously injected site on the nonsensitive person's skin. Passive transfer of the sensitivity is manifested by the formation of a wheal.

Precancerous tumors, 314

Pregnancy state, 258

Prickly heat, 8, 156, 349, 373

Primary chancre-type diseases. These include the following:
    Anthrax
    Blastomycosis, primary cutaneous type
    Chancroid
    Coccidioidomycosis, primary cutaneous type
    Cowpox
    Cutaneous diphtheria
    Erysipeloid
    Furuncle
    Milker's nodules
    Orf
    Sporotrichosis
    Syphilis (genital but also extragenital)
    Tuberculosis, primary inoculation type
    Tularemia (Fig. DI-10)
    Vaccinia

Progeria. Extremely rare autosomal dominant mutation condition. Noticed early in life with characteristics of the elderly but no mental changes. Most patients die between 10 and 15 years of age. A factor may be a defect of hyaluronic acid.

Protoporphyria, erythropoietic, 297

Protozoal dermatoses, 232, 381

Proud flesh, 336

Prurigo. This term is used more in Europe. It lacks a precise definition. *See* Jorizzo JL: J Am Acad Dermatol 4:723, 1981

    actinic. A chronic photodermatitis seen in native Americans.

Prurigo nodularis. A rare chronic dermatosis, usually of women, consisting of discrete nodular pruritic excoriated papules and tumors scattered over the arms and the legs.

Pruritic dermatoses, localized, 104

Pruritic hereditary localized patch on back (notalgia paresthetica). A rather common problem manifested by a single patch of approximately 4 × 4 cm, usually lichenified, on the back. Frequently the person rubs the area on the door jamb or similar scratching post.

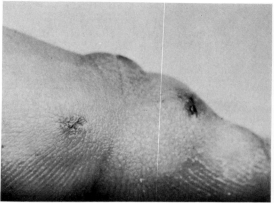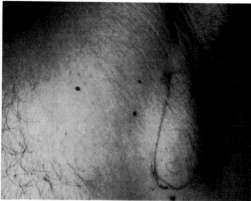

Figure DI–10.   **Primary chancre-type disease.** (*Left*) Tularemic chancre on finger. (*Right*) Axillary adenopathy in same patient. (*Dr. L. Calkins*)

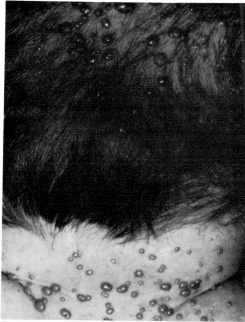
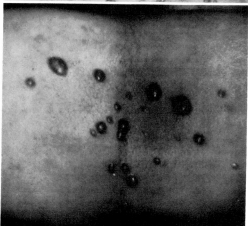

Figure DI–11. Xanthogranuloma. (*Top*) Back of head and neck of child. (*Bottom*) Arm of same child. (*Dr. D. Morgan*)

the stretched atrophic skin; endocrine disturbances, including diabetes mellitus, hypogonadism, and calcinosis; and faulty body growth. Believed to be related to *Rothmund's syndrome.*

Zits. Teenager's vernacular for "pimples" of acne.
Zoonoses. Animal-transmitted diseases due to fungi, bacteria, viruses, and rickettsiae.